nst
to Ch
Guidelines and
Protocols

Instant Access

to Chiropractic Guidelines and Protocols

Edited by:

Lew Huff, DC

Clinical Rotations Coordinator,
Assistant Professor,
Texas Chiropractic College,
Pasadena, Texas;
Private Practice,
Houston, Texas;
Fellow of the American Back Society

David M. Brady, DC, CCN, DACBN

Assistant Professor of Clinical Sciences,
University of Bridgeport College of Chiropractic,
Bridgeport, Connecticut;
Former Attending Clinician and Clinical Instructor,
Texas Chiropractic College,
Pasadena, Texas;
Private Practice,
The Center for the Healing Arts,
Orange, Connecticut

——————————— *with 13 contributors*

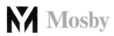 Mosby

A Harcourt Health Sciences Company

St. Louis   London   Philadelphia   Sydney   Toronto

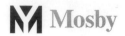

Mosby

A Harcourt Health Sciences Company

Publisher: John Schrefer
Executive Editor: Martha Sasser
Senior Developmental Editor: Amy Christopher
Project Manager: Carol Sullivan Weis
Senior Production Editor: Rick Dudley
Designer: Jen Marmarinos
Manufacturing Manager: Dave Graybill

Mosby, Inc.
11830 Westline Industrial Drive
St. Louis, Missouri 63146

Library of Congress Cataloging-in-Publication Data

Instant access to chiropractic guidelines and protocols / edited by
  Lew Huff, David Brady ; with 13 contributors.
      p.   cm.
   Includes bibliographical references and index.
   ISBN 0-323-00535-7
   1. Chiropractic–Handbooks, manuals, etc. 2. Pain–Treatment–
Handbooks, manuals, etc. I. Huff, Lew. II. Brady, David, D.C.
   [DNLM: 1. Chiropractic–methods handbooks. 2. Pain–therapy
handbooks. 3. Musculoskeletal Diseases–therapy handbooks. WB
39I59 1999]
RZ242.9.I57 1999
615.5'34–dc21
DNLM/DLC   98-33726

01   02   /   9   8   7   6   5   4   3

Contributors

Liza O. Banaag-Huff, MD

Physician, Private Practice,
Houston, Texas;
Graduated Baylor College of Medicine

Brian Batenchuk, DC, DACBR

Associate Professor,
Texas Chiropractic College,
Pasadena, Texas;
Private Practice,
Houston, Texas;
Graduated Palmer College of Chiropractic, Davenport, Iowa;
BS, Colorado State University

David M. Brady, DC, CCN, DACBN

Assistant Professor of Clinical Sciences,
University of Bridgeport College of Chiropractic,
Bridgeport, Connecticut;
Former Attending Clinician and Clinical Instructor,
Texas Chiropractic College,
Pasadena, Texas;
Private Practice,
The Center for the Healing Arts,
Orange, Connecticut;
Graduated Texas Chiropractic College, Pasadena, Texas

Darryl D. Curl, DDS, DC

Attending Clinician/Lecturer,
University of California at Los Angeles,
Los Angeles, California;
Professor,
Los Angeles College of Chiropractic,
Private Practice,
Whittier, California;
Graduated Los Angeles College of Chiropractic, Whittier, California

Brian Dannenfelser, DC

Former Attending Clinician,
Texas Chiropractic College,
Pasadena, Texas;
Private Practice,
Houston, Texas;
Graduated Parker College of Chiropractic, Dallas, Texas

Douglas Davison, DC

Dean of Clinical Sciences and Clinics,
Texas Chiropractic College,
Private Practice,
Houston, Texas;
Graduated Texas Chiropractic College, Pasadena, Texas

Jason Flanagan, DC

Attending Clinician,
Clinical Instructor,
Texas Chiropractic College,
Pasadena, Texas;
Graduated Texas Chiropractic College, Pasadena, Texas

Steven Foster, DC

Director of Clinics,
Texas Chiropractic College,
Pasadena, Texas;
Graduated Texas Chiropractic College, Pasadena, Texas

Ursula Funderburk, DC

Attending Clinician,
Texas Chiropractic College,
Pasadena, Texas;
Graduated Los Angeles College of Chiropractic, Whittier, California

Lew Huff, DC

Clinical Rotations Coordinator,
Assistant Professor,
Texas Chiropractic College,
Pasadena, Texas;
Private Practice,
Houston, Texas;
Fellow of the American Back Society
Graduated Cleveland Chiropractic College, Los Angeles

Mikell Suzanne Parsons, DC, CCN, DACBN

Assistant Professor of Clinical Sciences,
University of Bridgeport College of Chiropractic,
Bridgeport, Connecticut;
Former Attending Clinician and Clinical Instructor,
Texas Chiropractic College,
Pasadena, Texas;
Graduated Los Angeles College of Chiropractic, Whittier, California

Kevin Pringle, DC*

Former Clinical Instructor,
Attending Clinician,
Texas Chiropractic College,
Pasadena, Texas;
Graduated Los Angeles College of Chiropractic, Whittier, California

Donald C. Stran, DPM

Fellow of the American College of Foot and Ankle Surgeons,
Former Director of the Harris County, Texas Surgical Residency
    Foundation,
Private Practice,
Houston, Texas;
Graduated Pennsylvania College of Podiatric Medicine

Jeffrey Weiss, DC

Attending Clinician,
Texas Chiropractic College,
Pasadena, Texas;
Private Practice,
Houston, Texas;
Graduated Los Angeles College of Chiropractic, Whittier, California

Karlene Wise, DC, CCSP

Assistant Professor,
Director of Student Clinic,
Texas Chiropractic College,
Pasadena, Texas;
Graduated Texas Chiropractic College, Pasadena, Texas

---

*Special thanks to Dr. Pringle for his assistance in editorial review.

*This book is dedicated to my
daughter Jamaica and my wife Liza.*

Lew Huff

*A special acknowledgment and note of thanks is in order
to my wife Mikell for her unconditional support and love, and
for her sacrifice of time with her husband during this project and
many others. I promise, someday I will learn how to say no.*

David M. Brady

How to Use This Book

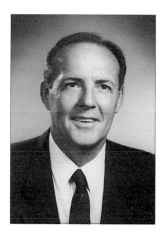

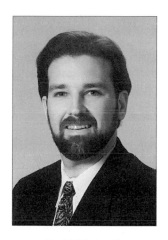

Lew Huff

David M. Brady

As Chiropractic approaches the mainstream of health care in the United States and throughout the world, there is a growing need to establish standards of care specific for those conditions within our scope of practice.

Instant Access to Chiropractic Guidelines and Protocols provides an accurate representation of scientifically valid procedures and modalities generally used and accepted throughout our profession.

Each topic has been formatted in a manner that allows "at-a-glance" accessibility. The format was designed to ensure easy retrieval of pertinent information. Examination and diagnostic criteria closely follow history and examination protocols currently used throughout chiropractic. Differential diagnosis, orthopedic, neurological, and radiographic sections briefly outline what you might expect to find with any given disorder, in a

Photo at right, © Mike Scalf Photography Inc.

quick-reference, telegraphic manner. The emphasis of the book, however, is on treatment protocol.

The management protocols are derived from many notable sources and we believe represent a solid outline of accepted modalities and procedures useful for each disorder. Home care protocols have been emphasized with a belief that patient participation is essential for rapid recovery. The authors have purposely stayed clear of questionable procedures or those that may lack firm scientific validity.

Regarding the management protocols, it should be noted that they are simply a list of treatment options or alternatives. They are not intended to be followed in a "cookbook fashion," nor are all the listed modalities or procedures intended to be used at one time on a patient. Rather, they represent a "menu" of accepted treatment choices according to the latest literature. Treatment should only continue if objective improvement is being made by the patient within an acceptable time frame. If improvement is not being made, a reassessment should be performed to determine if the diagnosis should be altered. Lack of improvement should also prompt the clinician to consider a change in treatment protocol, referral to another provider, or release of the patient with maximal medical improvement. Good clinical judgment should always take precedent in decision making with regard to any particular patient.

Outcome assessment questionnaires are included in Appendix C and are referenced throughout the book. Outcome assessment questionnaires are a valuable guide to assess levels of disability, patient progress, and/or a need to alter a patient's treatment plan.

At times in this book, nutritional and laboratory companies are mentioned. Lists of contact numbers for these companies are provided in Appendixes A and B. This is done solely as a convenience for the reader and is not meant as an attempt to provide advertisement or endorsement. Specific company identification was limited to those circumstances in which a specific formula or test was only available through a specific supplier or provider, or in cases in which the product or service was considered superior.

Only commonly encountered related systemic disorders are included in this text, primarily due to their likelihood of co-management and general good response to both chiropractic and nutritional care.

The authors understand that no set of standards can dictate a complete treatment protocol for any given case, given the variables of age, gender, complicating factors, and response to treatment. However, sound clinical judgment combined with established modes of treatment can pave the way to successful management of chiropractically treatable disorders.

Lew Huff, DC
David M. Brady, DC, CCN, DACBN

Disclaimer

The authors and publisher would like to acknowledge that this book is a *guide* to assist in the establishment of clinical chiropractic protocols. As you will note, in the management protocols section the word (Options) appears. Each set of management protocols represents a *menu* of accepted treatment alternatives that, according to the latest literature and scientific journals, are available to select from to treat such conditions.

It should be noted that the chiropractic community has a wide variety of techniques ranging from osseous manipulation to reflex-oriented techniques. The authors make no judgment as to the effectiveness of one technique over the other; however, emphasis is placed on techniques with literature support. In some circumstances a specific technique is described. This is done to clarify the use of that particular technique in relationship to the condition mentioned.

The authors and publisher further note that no set of standards can dictate a complete treatment protocol for any given case, given the variables of age, gender, complicating factors, individual response to treatment, psychosocial factors, work conditions, and other variables that may be present with any given case.

Treatment should only continue if objective improvement on the part of the patient is being made within an acceptable time frame. If improvement is not being made, a reassessment should be performed to determine if the diagnosis should be altered. Lack of improvement should also prompt the clinician to consider a change in the treatment protocol, referral to another provider, or release of the patient with maximal medical improvement. Good clinical judgment should always take precedent in decision making with regard to any particular patient.

Foreword

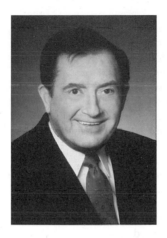

S.M. Elliott, DC

In recent years the chiropractic profession has been growing in many ways. Studies from around the world are illustrating the efficacy of our treatment methods and the importance of chiropractic care. Growing public awareness and a demand for conservative "nature-based" medicine has pushed chiropractic into the limelight of the health care arena. As we rapidly approach the "mainstream" in health care, the need for standardization of our health care delivery system grows.

Confronted with the enormous task of establishing standard-ized treatment protocols, we at Texas Chiropractic College dis-covered certain things about ourselves and chiropractic as a whole. We came to the realization that chiropractors share more in common than we once thought possible. We soon began to realize that it was not impossible to reach a consensus regarding what is considered appropriate and acceptable as opposed to those things considered "questionable." With the help of various sources, such as the Mercy Guidelines and numerous studies and texts, we were able to clarify those management protocols generally accepted and widely used within our profession. In so doing we were able to generate the first all-encompassing text establishing protocol guidelines for chiropractic care.

I am very proud of Dr. Huff and Dr. Brady for the hard work and diligence regarding this protocol project. Dr. Huff and Dr. Brady are outstanding members of the TCC family. Dr. Huff has been doing an exceptional job as liaison between the chiropractic and medical communities in our hospital rotations program.

It is our hope that this book will lead to a greater understanding of those things that we as chiropractors share in common. Historically we have been a profession divided; today we can be a profession united by the common thread that runs through us all.

S.M. Elliott, DC
President,
Texas Chiropractic College,
Pasadena, Texas

Foreword

This textbook provides a basis for comprehensive referral for chiropractic treatment. The information here is consistent with orthopedic practice for conservative management of musculoskeletal disorders, particularly pain of spinal origin. Chiropractic practice, as it has evolved, contributes to understanding of the mechanical aspects of lumbar and cervical pain. Mechanical assessment of the lumbar spine remains the foundation of musculoskeletal diagnosis and has become the standard for clinical evaluation of pain. As neurological assessment becomes an indispensable component of the evaluation of radicular pain, so chiropractic assessment of back pain similarly is becoming an integral adjunct to musculoskeletal evaluation.

This book is written in a concise manner with information tightly summarized and referenced. It is designed to supplement the knowledge of the mechanical component of low back pain that many practitioners possess. The information in the sections on cervical and lumbar treatment should be enlightening for orthopedic surgeons and practitioners of other disciplines dealing with pain originating from spinal disorders. The reader is encouraged to read this book from beginning to end. However, each maxim is designed to stand alone, as is each figure. This text provides an adequate working knowledge of the chiropractic approach to musculoskeletal disorders. I find this book to be a welcome and much-needed addition to the effort to standardize clinical diagnosis from the chiropractic point of view, as well as a reference for the conservative management of musculoskeletal injuries by other health care providers.

Alexander G. Hadjipavlou, MD, MSc, FACS, FRCS(C)
Professor of Orthopaedic Surgery and Neurosurgery,
Chief, Division of Spine Surgery,
The University of Texas Medical Branch at Galveston,
Galveston, Texas

Acknowledgments

Establishing protocols for a diverse profession is clearly no easy task. Without the help of the contributing authors and editors this book would not have been possible. I am grateful to those contributing authors and editors who spent hours pouring over textbooks and journal articles and computer files while inundated with interns, patients, and other obligations.

I would especially like to thank Drs. Brady, Pringle, and Batenchuk, whose knowledge and understanding of nutrition, case studies, radiology, and the Mercy Guidelines, along with their dedication to excellence, changed the character and outcome of this text. I cannot express enough special thanks to Dr. Brady. His persistence in editing and reediting this book cannot be overlooked. Without Dr. Brady's contributions in the realm of nutrition, established guidelines, and overall consistency, this book would not be what it is today. Anyone at TCC can affirm that nothing gets past Dr. Brady, and if we all could incorporate these principles and dedication to our profession, the whole world would have to take another look.

Drs. Davison, Foster, and Wise, in the midst of all their daily administrative tasks, problems, and students, took the time to add valuable insight and consistency in the development of this text, and to them I am grateful.

I would like to thank fellow attending clinicians, Drs. Parsons, Dannenfelser, Flanagan, Weiss, and Funderburk, who, although pressed for time and occupied with imparting excellent guidance to our interns, took the time to contribute to and edit this text.

Dr. Mandy Ngo and Dr. Agnus Nguyen helped tremendously by graciously researching and referencing topics during their busy internship.

A special thanks goes to Dr. Robert Taylor for his contribution of the excellent algorithms throughout this text.

In addition, I would like to thank my wife Liza and my daughter Jamaica, who spent years waiting for daddy while he was riding the computer on his never-ending book. It was they who inspired me to believe that such a book could be written (and finished!) and that perhaps such a book could help unify a profession.

Lew Huff, DC

Contents

SECTION I

Headaches

Cluster Headaches

Hypertensive Headaches

Migraine Headaches

Sinus Headaches

Cervicogenic Cephalgia

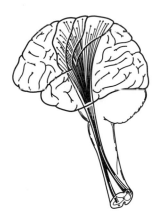

(Modified from Cramer GD, Darby SA: *Basic and clinical anatomy of the spine, spinal cord, and ANS,* St Louis, 1995, Mosby.)

Cluster Headaches

LEW HUFF AND DAVID M. BRADY

DEFINITION

An abrupt, severe unilateral headache characterized by one to three short-lived attacks of periorbital pain per day over a 4- to 8-week period. This is followed by a pain-free period that may last 3 to 18 months. Increased incidence among middle-aged men. No family history of headaches or evidence of organic disease.

ETIOLOGY

Attacks may be triggered by stress, glare, allergies, nitroglycerin use, or the ingestion of specific foods. These agents may be related to a vascular component or serotonergic mechanism. Blood flow increases and cerebral blood vessels dilate during an attack.

SIGNS AND SYMPTOMS

Location

Sudden unilateral periorbital pain often associated with ipsilateral nasal congestion. May affect orbital, supraorbital, and temporal regions.

Quality

Steady burning pain around the eye, deep and nonfluctuating pain, rarely pulsatile. Often described as stabbing, agonizing, steady ache, or deep burning.

Timing

May awaken the patient and typically begins at the same time each day or night. Pain usually starts abruptly and reaches maximum intensity quickly.

Systemic Manifestations

Horner's syndrome may occur transiently during attack or remain as a residual deficit between attacks. If suspected, an evaluation for Pancoast's tumor may be indicated. Other symptoms may include rhinorrhea and lacrimation, as well as nasal discharge or congestion, eyelid edema, and facial flushing.

Examination Findings

May include bloodshot eye, occluded nostril, ptosis, photophobia, facial flushing, tearing, or running nostril.

EXAMINATION

Check tension of masticatory and submandibular muscles. Rule out temporomandibular joint (TMJ) involvement. Check for hyperalgesia of skin zones in the cervical regions; trigger points of the neck and thorax; joint dysfunction of the cervicothoracic spine, acromioclavicular (AC) joint, and sternoclavicular joint; and inspect for anterior weight bearing, all of which would support a diagnosis of cervicogenic cephalgia as actual primary trigger or cause of these headaches (Table 1). Evaluate lung fields for apical tumor with Horner's syndrome.

DIFFERENTIAL DIAGNOSIS

Temporal arteritis
Cervicogenic cephalgia
Tooth disorder
Ocular disorder
Brain tumor

TABLE 1
Comparison of Cervicogenic Headache and Migraine Headache

Factor	Cervicogenic headache	Migraine headache
Anatomical area	From occiput to frontal	From frontal to occiput
Side (usually)	Unilateral	Bilateral
Relieved by rest	Yes	No
Photophobia	Yes	Yes (severe)
Phonophobia	Yes	Yes (severe)
Nausea	Mild	Severe
Frequency	Up to daily	Less than one per month
Intensity	Variable	Severe and constant
Response to analgesic medications	Yes (early)	No
Response to spinal manipulative therapy	Good	Minimal to none

LABORATORY WORK

Complete blood count (CBC), blood chemistry panel (SMAC), urinalysis (UA)

Findings may be coincidental

Clinical Note

Chronic recurring headache beginning for the first time in a patient over 50 years old may indicate a serious problem and requires thorough examination. Unrelenting headache of acute onset usually signals significant disease. The most common cause of severe recurrent headache in middle-aged men is the syndrome of cluster headache. The physician must consider temporal arteritis in any elderly patient with unilateral headache.[6]

TREATMENT GOALS

1. Identification of all related etiological or contributing agents, such as diet, food allergens, and medications
2. Acute headache relief

3. Modification of diet or activities directed toward prevention of recurrence and restoration of daily activities

MANAGEMENT PROTOCOL (OPTIONS)

- Moist heat applications to increase circulation, and for their antispasmodic and mild analgesic effects.
- Trigger point therapy (acupressure points): Apply moderate pressure to hypertonic nodules present in the muscle belly, hold for 5 to 7 seconds to force relaxation of the painful nodule. Repeat three times.
- Ultrasound (pulsed), at 0.5 to 1.0 W/cm^2 for 5 to 8 minutes. Ultrasound stimulates heat production, performs a micro-massage of tendon and ligamentous insertions, and pushes away inflammatory fluids.
- Spray-and-stretch techniques to reduce muscle spasms and myofascial trigger points.
- Adjust cervical and upper thoracic spine.
- Avoid stress and known allergic agents. Avoid glare associated with prolonged computer use.
- Identify and avoid known food allergens; monitor intake of salt and alcohol; monitor smoking; and monitor drinking of coffee, teas, and colas. Avoid monosodium glutamate (MSG), nitrates, aspartame (NutraSweet), metabisulfates, smoked meats, and dairy products.

NUTRITIONAL MANAGEMENT PROTOCOL (OPTIONS)

- Choline (500 mg twice daily)
- Lithium aspartate (150 mg 3 times daily) (supplying approximately 0.5 mg elemental lithium per dose) Non-prescription natural forms of lithium are available in the form of lithium aspartate, such as the product Lithate (Bio-Tech, Fayetteville, Ark), which will supply the above recommended dosage.
- Capsaicin (*Capsicum frutescens*/cayenne pepper) (0.025% or 0.075% ointments intranasally)
- Calcium/magnesium (800-1000 mg of each per day in divided dosages)
- Valerian root *(Valeriana officinalis)* (100 mg q4h while symptomatic)

- Passion flower *(Passiflora incarnata)* (100-200 mg q4h while symptomatic)

Many vendors offer formulary products with the above three elements, including Valerian Daytime/Calmicin Plus (Murdock Madaus Schwabe, Springville, Utah) and Myoplex/Myoplex PM (Metagenics, Inc., San Clemente, Calif).

Identifying any contributory food allergies and eliminating them from the diet can be helpful in many cases of migraine, as well as cluster headaches. Cheese, milk, chocolate, nitrates, nitrites, tyramine, tryptophan, MSG, and artificial sweeteners are the most common offenders. Screening for possible liver toxicity and treating it is also essential.

REFERENCES

1. Balch JF, Balch PA: *Prescription for natural healing,* Wayne, NJ, 1990, Avery Publishing.
2. Cohen JH, Schneider MJ: Receptor-tonus technique: an overview, *Chiropr Techn* vol 2, Feb 1990.
3. De Belleroche J, et al: Erythrocyte choline concentrations and cluster headache, *Br Med J* 288:268-270, 1984.
4. Diamond S: Cluster headaches, how to distinguish from migraines, *Consultant,* July 1996.
5. Dyken P: Headaches in children, *Am Fam Physician* 11(5):105-111, 1975.
6. Freemon F: Evaluation and treatment of headache, *Geriatrics* 33:82-85, 1978.
7. Gatterman M: *Chiropractic management of spine related disorders,* Baltimore, 1990, Williams & Wilkins.
8. Grabowski RJ: *Current nutritional therapy,* San Antonio, Tex, 1993, Image Press.
9. Hubka M, et al: A new look at the classification of headaches, *Chiropr Techn* (6)2, May 1994.
10. Kudrow L, Kudrow D: Inheritance of cluster headache and its possible link to migraine, *Headache* 34:400-407, 1994.
11. Lawrence D: *Fundamentals of chiropractic diagnosis and management,* Baltimore, 1991, Williams & Wilkins.
12. Liebenson C: *Rehabilitation of the spine,* Baltimore, 1996, Williams & Wilkins.
13. Lindahl O, Lindwall L: Double blind study of a valerian preparation, *Pharmacol Biochem Behav* 28(4):10065-10066, 1989.
14. *Manual of medical therapeutics (the Washington manual),* ed 27, Boston, 1992, Little, Brown.

15. Marks DR, et al: A double blind placebo-controlled trial of intranasal capsaicin for cluster headache, *Cephalgia* 13(2):114-116, 1993.

16. Nelson C: The reliability of an instrument used to evaluate primary headaches, *Proceedings of the International Conference on Spinal Manipulation,* Montreal, April 30-May 1, 1993.

17. Nimmo R: Receptor, effecters and tonus: a new approach, *J Natl Chiropr Assoc,* November 1957.

18. Rakel RE: *Textbook of family practice,* ed 5, Philadelphia, 1995, WB Saunders.

19. Schneider MJ: Chiropractic management of myofascial and muscular disorders. In Lawrence D, ed: *Advances in chiropractic,* vol 3, 1996, St Louis, Mosby.

20. Solomon SS, Lipton RB, Newman LC: Prophylactic therapy of cluster headaches, *Clin Neuropharmacol* 1492:116-130, 1991.

21. Speroni E, Minghetti A: Neuropharmacological activity of extracts from *Passiflora incarnata, Planta Med* 54(6):488-491, 1988.

22. Tierney LM, McPhee SJ, Papadakis MA: *Current medical diagnosis and treatment,* ed 35, Appleton & Lange, 1996, Norwalk, Conn.

23. Travell JG, Simons DG: *Myofascial pain and dysfunction: the trigger point manual,* vol 2, Baltimore, 1992, Williams & Wilkins.

24. Vernon H: The effectiveness of chiropractic manipulation in the treatment of headache: an exploration of the literature, *J Manipulative Physiol Ther* 18(9):611-617, 1995.

25. Vick D: The safety of manipulative treatment: a review of the literature from 1925 to 1993, *J Am Osteopath Assoc* 96:(2), 1996.

26. Weaver K: Magnesium and its role in vascular reactivity and coagulation, *Contemp Nutr* 12(3), 1987.

27. Werbach MR: *Nutritional influences on illness,* ed 2, Tarzana, Calif, 1996, Third Line Press.

28. Werbach MR, Murray MT: *Botanical influences on illness,* Tarzana, Calif, 1994, Third Line Press.

29. Yung CY: A review of clinical trials of lithium in neurology, *Pharmacol Biochem Behav* 21(suppl 1):57-64, 1984.

Hypertensive Headaches

MIKELL SUZANNE PARSONS AND LEW HUFF

DEFINITION

A pulsating suboccipital headache often occurring in the early mornings and subsiding during the day. Associated with hypertension, obesity, stress, lack of exercise, a high-salt diet, drug sensitivity, and renal or cardiovascular disease.

ETIOLOGY

Headache pain is secondary to an elevated systemic blood pressure of 200/120 mm Hg or greater. A sustained blood pressure of this magnitude is dangerous and warrants immediate referral.

SIGNS AND SYMPTOMS

Location

Usually throbbing pain at vertex, occiput, or frontal regions; pain may be generalized or unilateral. 'Hat band' distribution.

Quality

Dull, diffuse, throbbing or aching.

Intensity

Most often mild to moderate, but may be excruciating.

Timing

Worse in morning hours, may awaken the patient (4 to 6 AM), improves as day goes on. Pain is intermittent, lasting 15 minutes to 3 hours.

Eye Changes

Retinal changes, blurred vision, arteriovenous (A-V) nicking, papilledema, flame-shaped hemorrhage of eye reported. Copper wiring or cotton wool exudates may be seen.

Position

Headaches worsen when reclining. Pain is less severe when seated. Pain may be minimized by elevating head off the bed.

Systemic Manifestations

Elevated blood pressure, edema, anxiety, fatigue, nausea, and tinnitus reported.

EXAMINATION

Check tension of masticatory and submandibular muscles. Rule out TMJ involvement. Check for hyperalgesia of skin zones in the cervical regions and trigger points of the neck and thorax. Check joint dysfunction of the cervical and thoracic spine, AC joint, and sternoclavicular joint, and inspect for anterior weight bearing. Include a diet analysis to determine contributing agents, if any.

DIAGNOSIS

History
Family history
Examination findings

DIFFERENTIAL DIAGNOSIS

Migraine headaches
Cervicogenic headaches

Temporal arteritis
Myofascial pain syndrome

LABORATORY TESTS

Directed toward hypertensive workup
CBC, SMAC, UA
Thyroxine (T_4) ($\uparrow$)
Urinary free cortisol ($\uparrow$)

TREATMENT GOALS

1. Identification of all related etiological or contributing agents, such as diet, food allergens, and medications
2. Acute headache relief
3. Modification of diet or activities directed toward prevention of recurrence and restoration of daily activities

MANAGEMENT PROTOCOL (OPTIONS)

- Dietary modifications:
  1. High-fiber, low-salt diet.
  2. Avoid alcohol, high fat, sugar, caffeine, cheeses, wine, and MSG. Rule out food sensitivities.
- Manipulation of occiput, cervicals, and thoracics.[11]
- Advise regarding moderate exercise program.

NUTRITIONAL MANAGEMENT PROTOCOL (OPTIONS)

Treatment is directed toward hypertension:
- Calcium (1500 mg daily)
- Magnesium (1000 mg daily)
- Selenium (200 μmg daily)
- Garlic (500 mg tid)
- Coenzyme Q10 (100 mg)
- Taurine (3 g daily)
- Vitamin C (3000 mg daily)
- Potassium may need to be supplemented if patient is on hypertensive medications. Monitor blood work to make final decision.

REFERENCES

1. Balch JF, Balch PA: *Prescription for natural healing,* Wayne, NJ, 1990, Avery Publishing.
2. Dyken P: Headaches in children, *Am Fam Physician* 11(5):105-111, 1975.
3. Fauci A, et al: *Harrison's principles of internal medicine,* ed 13, New York, 1994, McGraw-Hill.
4. Freemon F: Evaluation and treatment of headache, *Geriatrics* 33:82-85, 1978.
5. Gatterman M: *Chiropractic management of spine related disorders,* Baltimore, 1990, Williams & Wilkins.
6. Grabowski RJ: *Current nutritional therapy,* San Antonio, Tex, 1993, Image Press.
7. Lawrence D: *Fundamentals of chiropractic diagnosis and management,* Baltimore, 1996, Williams & Wilkins.
8. Nelson C: The reliability of an instrument used to evaluate primary headaches, *Proceedings of the International Conference on Spinal Manipulation,* Montreal, April 30-May 1, 1993.
9. Paton D, Hyman B, Justice J: *Introduction to ophthalmoscopy,* Kalamazoo, Mich, 1985, Upjohn.
10. Tierney LM, McPhee SJ, Papadakis MA: *Current medical diagnosis and treatment,* ed 35, Norwalk, Conn, 1996, Appleton & Lange.
11. Vernon HT: The effectiveness of chiropractic manipulation in the treatment of headaches: an exploration in the literature, *J Manipulative Physiol Ther* 18(9), 1995.
12. Vick D: The safety of manipulative treatment: a review of the literature from 1925 to 1993, *J Am Osteopath Assoc* 96(2) 1996.
13. Weaver K: Magnesium and its role in vascular reactivity and coagulation, *Contemp Nutr* 12(3), 1987.
14. Werbach MR: *Nutritional influences on illness,* ed 2, Tarzana, Calif, 1996, Third Line Press.
15. Werbach MR, Murray MT: *Botanical influences on illness,* Tarzana, Calif, 1994, Third Line Press.

Migraine Headaches

LEW HUFF AND DAVID M. BRADY

DEFINITION

A unilateral or bilateral benign recurring headache. Often the patient can predict the occurrences before they begin. Usually characterized by an aura, with or without associated visual and gastrointestinal (GI) disturbances. Although any age may be affected, there is an increased incidence among females aged 10 to 30 years.

ETIOLOGY

Migraines may be caused by stress; excessive sleep; menstruation; pregnancy; use of oral contraceptives; and consumption of red wines, chocolates, nuts, or aged cheeses. Other factors may include hunger, fatigue, sleep disturbance, bright lights, and alcohol consumption.

MECHANISM

May be related to dilation and excessive pulsation of branches of the external carotid arteries. Focal disturbances of neurological function are attributed to the constriction of the internal carotid arteries.

SIGNS AND SYMPTOMS

Migraine Without Aura (80%)

Lasts 4 to 72 hours; unilateral or bilateral; pulsating; moderate to severe; and associated with nausea, vomiting, photophobia and phonophobia. Aggravated by physical activity.

Migraine With Aura (20%)

Preceded by one of the following:

  Visual: scotoma, photophobia, fortification spectra

  Sensory: paresthesia, numbness, unilateral weakness, speech disturbance

Systemic Manifestations

Cyanotic extremities, light-headedness, vertigo, chills, sweating, diarrhea, and sensitivity to odors.

Examination Findings

Prominent scalp arteries with an increased amplitude of pulse, scalp tenderness, pain increases with activities.

EXAMINATION

Check tension of masticatory and submandibular muscles. Rule out TMJ involvement. Check for hyperalgesia of skin zones in the cervical regions and trigger points of the neck and thorax. Check joint dysfunction of the cervical and thoracic spine, AC joint, and sternoclavicular joint, and inspect for anterior weight bearing. (See Table 1, pg. 4)

DIAGNOSIS

History
Clinical findings

DIFFERENTIAL DIAGNOSIS

Cervicogenic cephalgia
Cluster headaches
Sinus or ocular headaches
Temporal arteritis
Transient ischemic attack (TIA) or stroke

Clinical Note

Most chronic headaches exhibit clinical qualities of both tension and migraine headaches.[16]

TREATMENT GOALS

1. Identification of all related etiological or contributing agents, such as diet, food allergens, and medications
2. Acute headache relief
3. Modification of diet or activities directed toward prevention of recurrence and restoration of daily activities

MANAGEMENT PROTOCOL (OPTIONS)

- Avoid cheeses, wine, chocolate, coffee, teas, colas, sugar, MSG, smoked meats, dairy products, aspartame (NutraSweet), metabisulfates, and nitrates. Avoid any known food allergens, bright lights, and excessive fatigue.
- Trigger point therapy: Apply moderate pressure to hypertonic nodules present in the muscle belly, hold for 5 to 7 seconds to force relaxation of the painful nodule. Repeat 3 times.
- Deep tissue massage of suboccipitals.
- Ice packs for 15 minutes over suboccipital region to induce vasoconstriction.
- Adjust upper thoracic and cervical spine.

NUTRITIONAL MANAGEMENT PROTOCOL (OPTIONS)

- Feverfew *(Tanacetum parthenium)* (50 mg tid prophylactically, 1-2 g/day during acute attack)
- Ginger *(Zingiber officinale)* (500 mg of dried ginger q4h to alleviate visual aura and nausea)
- Ginko *(Gingko biloba)* (40 mg tid)
- EPA-DHA (omega-3 fatty acids) (1500 mg tid)
- Calcium/magnesium (800-1000 mg of each per day in divided dosages)

- Valerian root *(Valeriana officinalis)* (100 mg q4h while symptomatic)
- Passion flower *(Passiflora incarnata)* (100-200 mg q4h while symptomatic)
- A low dietary intake of foods high in tryptophan, tyramine, phenylalanine, and copper may be helpful. In patients with reactive hypoglycemia, avoidance of foods high in sucrose and simple carbohydrates in general has been shown to reduce migraine frequency.
- Identifying any contributing food allergies and eliminating them from the diet can be helpful in many cases of migraine headache. Cheese, milk, chocolate, nitrates, nitrites, tyramine, tryptophan, MSG, and artificial sweeteners are the most common offenders. Screening for possible liver toxicity and treating it is also helpful in difficult cases.

REFERENCES

1. Balch JF, Balch PA: *Prescription for natural healing,* Wayne, NJ, 1990, Avery Publishing.
2. Crook M: Migraine: a biochemical headache? *Biochem Soc Trans* 9(4):351-357, 1981.
3. DeFeudis FV: *Ginko biloba extract (ECb761): pharmacological activities and clinical applications,* New York, 1991, Reed Elsevier.
4. Dexter JD, et al: The five hour glucose tolerance test and effects of low sucrose diet in migraine, *Headache* 18:91-94, 1978.
5. Egger J, et al: Is migraine food allergy? A double-blind controlled trial of oligoantigenic diet treatment, *Lancet* 865-869, Oct 15, 1983.
6. Fauci A, et al: *Harrison's principles of internal medicine,* ed 13, New York, 1994, McGraw-Hill.
7. Freemon F: Evaluation and treatment of headache, *Geriatrics* 33:82-85, 1978.
8. Funfgeld EW, ed: *Rokan (Ginko biloba) recent results in pharmacology and clinic,* New York, 1988, Springer-Verlag.
9. Gatterman M: *Chiropractic management of spine related disorders,* Baltimore, 1990, Williams & Wilkins.
10. Grabowski RJ: *Current nutritional therapy,* San Antonio, Tex, 1993, Image Press.
11. Harrison DP: Copper as a factor in dietary precipitation of migraine, *Headache* 25(5):248-250, 1986.
12. Hasselmark L, et al: Effect of carbohydrate-rich diet, low in protein-tryptophane, in classic and common migraine, *Cephalgia* 7:87-92, 1987.

13. Hayes NA, Foreman JC: The activity of compounds extracted from feverfew on histamine release from rat mast cells, *J Pharm Pharmacol* 39:466-467, 1987.

14. Heptinstall S, et al: Extracts of feverfew inhibit granule secretion in blood platelets and polymorphonuclear leukocytes, *Lancet* i:1071-1074, 1985.

15. Heptinstall S, et al: Parthenolide content and bioactivity of feverfew *(Tanacetum parthenium)* (L.) (Schultz-Bip). Estimation of commercial and authenticated feverfew products, *J Pharm Pharmacol* 35:391-395, 1992.

16. Hubka M, et al: A new look at the classifications of headaches, *Chiropr Techn* 6(2), 1995.

17. Hughes EC, et al: Migraine: a diagnostic test for etiology of food sensitivity by nutritionally supported fast and confirmed by long-term report, *Ann Allergy* 55:28-32, 1985.

18. Kleijen J, Kipschild P: Ginko biloba, *Lancet* 340:1136-1139, 1992.

19. Lawrence D: *Fundamentals of chiropractic diagnosis and management,* Baltimore, 1991, Williams & Wilkins.

20. Lindahl O, Lindwall L: Double blind study of a valerian preparation, *Pharmacol Biochem Behav* 32(4):10065-10066, 1989.

21. Makheda AM, Baily JM: A platelet phospholipase inhibitor from the medicinal herb feverfew *(Tanacetum parthenium), Prostaglandins Leukot Med* 653-660, 1982.

22. *Manual of medical therapeutics (the Washington manual),* ed 27, Boston, 1992, Little, Brown.

23. *The Merck manual,* ed 16, Rahway, NJ, 1992, Merck.

24. Monroe J, et al: Migraine is a food allergic disease, *Lancet* 340:1136-1139, 1992.

25. Murphy JJ, et al: Randomized double-blind placebo-controlled trial of feverfew in migraine prevention, *Lancet* ii:189-192, 1988.

26. Nelson C: The reliability of an instrument used to evaluate primary headaches, *Proceedings of the International Conference on Spinal Manipulation,* Montreal, April 30-May 1, 1993.

27. Nimmo R: Receptor, effecters and tonus: a new approach, *J Natl Chiropr Assoc,* November 1957.

28. Perkins J, Hartje J: Diet and migraine: a review of the literature, *J Am Diet Assoc* 83:459, 1983.

29. Rakel RE: *Textbook of family practice,* ed 5, Philadelphia, 1995, WB Saunders.

30. Schneider MJ: Chiropractic management of myofascial and muscular disorders. In Lawrence D, ed: *Advances in chiropractic,* vol 3, St Louis, 1996, Mosby.

31. Seltzer S: Foods, and food and drug combinations, responsible for head and neck pain, *Cephalgia* 2(2):111-124, 1982.

32. Speroni E, Minghetti A: Neuropharmacological activity of extracts from *Passiflora incarnata, Planta Med* 54(6):488-491, 1988.
33. Tierney LM, McPhee SJ, Papadakis MA: *Current medical diagnosis and treatment,* ed 35, Norwalk, Conn, 1996, Appleton & Lange.
34. Travell JG, Simons DG: *Myofascial pain and dysfunction: the trigger point manual,* vol 2, Baltimore, 1992, Williams & Wilkins.
35. Unge G, et al: Effects of dietary protein-tryptophan restriction upon 5-HT uptake by platelets and clinical symptoms of migraine-like headache, *Cephalgia* 3(4):213-218, 1983.
36. Vernon H: The effectiveness of chiropractic manipulation in the treatment of headache: an exploration of the literature, *J Manipulative Physiol Ther* 18(9):611-617, 1995.
37. Vick D: The safety of manipulative treatment: a review of the literature from 1925 to 1993, *J Am Osteopath Assoc* 96(2), 1996.
38. Weaver K: Magnesium and its role in vascular reactivity and coagulation, *Contemp Nutr* 12(3), 1987.
39. Werbach MR: *Nutritional influences on illness,* ed 2, Tarzana, Calif, 1996, Third Line Press.
40. Werbach MR, Murray MT: *Botanical influences on illness,* Tarzana, Calif, 1994, Third Line Press.
41. Wilkinson CF: Return of migrinoid headaches associated with spontaneous hypoglycemia, *Am J Med Sci* 218:209-212, 1949.
42. Young K, Dhami M: The efficacy of cervical manipulation as opposed to pharmacological therapeutic treatment of migraine patients, *Transactions of the Consortium for Chiropractic Research,* June 1987.

Sinus Headaches

LEW HUFF, JASON FLANAGAN, AND DAVID M. BRADY

DEFINITION

Headache characterized by swollen sinuses, pain, and pressure over the cheeks, with possible radiation to the oral cavity.

ETIOLOGY

Inflammation of the mucosa of the sinuses resulting from allergies or bacterial or viral infections, such as the common cold. Precipitating factors are infection, nasal polyps, or deviated septum.

SIGNS AND SYMPTOMS

Location

Generally felt over the forehead and cheeks. Pain and pressure may refer to the upper incisor and canines. Occasionally the mastoid area is affected. Vague discomfort over nasal, frontal, and periorbital regions.

Quality

Dull ache and vague symptoms to severe pain reported. Gnawing or pressure pain.

Timing

Often worse in morning hours, aggravated by position. Pain may affect any age-group. Headache may be intermittent and daily. Sinus headache may be associated with cold or flu, especially poorly treated cold or flu.

Position

May be aggravated or relieved by head position that hinders or helps nasal drainage. Leaning forward usually exacerbates pain.

Aggravating Factors

Mastication, straining at stool, coughing or bending.

Other Manifestations

Nasal stuffiness and discharge. No nausea, vomiting, or prodrome. May affect any age-group.

EXAMINATION

Check tension of masticatory and submandibular muscles to rule out other causes of headaches. Rule out TMJ involvement. Check for hyperalgesia of skin zones in the cervical regions and trigger points of the neck and thorax. Check joint dysfunction of the cervical and thoracic spine, AC joint, and sternoclavicular joint, and inspect for anterior weight bearing. (See differential diagnosis of cervicogenic headache in Table 1, pg. 4). Inspect for diminished transillumination over affected sinus. Rhinorrhea may be clear, yellow, or green.

DIFFERENTIAL DIAGNOSIS

1. *Maxillary:* spreads to occiput, aggravated by position.
2. *Frontal:* spreads to parietal or temporal, aggravated by position.
3. *Sphenoidal:* uncommon, deep, dead center pain, position irrelevant.
4. *Ethmoidal:* rare, pain between eyes and into orbit, aggravated by cervical extension.
5. If *sphenoidal* or *ethmoidal* sinuses are affected, inquire as to previous injury or trauma to the head.

TREATMENT GOALS

1. Identification of all related etiological or contributing agents, such as diet, food allergens, and medications

2. Acute headache relief
3. Modification of diet or activities directed toward prevention of recurrence and restoration of daily activities

MANAGEMENT PROTOCOL (OPTIONS)

- Avoid known allergens; correct nasal polyps if contributing factor.
- Correct areas of cervical dysfunction.
- Vaporizer may be used to clear sinus congestion.
- Hot compresses over sinuses for 15 minutes using dry towels between the compress and the face. Use to induce sinus drainage.
- Short wave diathermy with butterfly electrode (only when draining).

NUTRITIONAL MANAGEMENT PROTOCOL (OPTIONS)

Treatment is directed at identifying and avoiding any environmental allergen if possible. Screening for possible contributory food allergies and eliminating them from the diet can be also helpful in many cases.

Symptomatic Nutritional Treatment:
Herbals:

- *Ephedra* leaf (ma huang) (200 mg tid)
- Ginger *(Zingiber officinale)* (100 mg tid)
- Licorice *(Glycyrrhiza glabra)* (100 mg tid)
- Turmeric rhizome *(Curcuma longa)* (100 mg tid)
- Feverfew *(Tanacetum parthenium)* (100 mg tid)

The above combination of herbals can be found in the product Sinuplex (Metagenics, Inc.). Significant symptomatic relief can be obtained by using this combination without the common side effects of the popular over-the-counter (OTC) medications.

CAUTION: If the patient is pregnant, nursing, or has hypertension, heart or thyroid disease, diabetes, or difficulty urinating because of prostate enlargement, or if taking monoamine oxidase (MAO) inhibitor medications: avoid usage of the above listed herbals. Reduce or discontinue use if the patient experiences nervousness, tremor, sleeplessness, loss of appetite, or nausea.

Prophylactic Nutrients:

- B complex (100 mg bid)
- Vitamin C (1000 mg tid)
- Mixed bioflavonoids (250 mg tid)
- Vitamin E (400 IU per day)
- Multidigestive enzymes (2 capsules with each meal)

Those with ulcers should avoid multienzyme supplements containing hydrochloric acid.

Homeopathic Remedies:

Various homeopathic remedies are available to help desensitize the patient's allergy response. A trial of homeopathic therapy may be attempted and long-term symptomatic improvement monitored.

REFERENCES

1. Amella M, et al: Inhibition of mast cell histamine release by flavonoids and bioflavonoids, *Planta Med* 51:16-20, 1985.
2. Balch JF, Balch PA: *Prescription for natural healing,* Wayne, NJ, 1990, Avery Publishing.
3. Butkus S, Mahan L: Food allergies: immunological reactions to food, *J Am Diet Assoc* 86:601, 1986.
4. Folkers K, et al: Biochemical evidence for a deficiency of vitamin B_6 in subjects reacting to monosodium-L-glutamate by the Chinese restaurant syndrome, *Biochem Biophys Res Commun* 100:972-977, 1981.
5. Freemon F: Evaluation and treatment of headache, *Geriatrics* 33:82-85, 1978.
6. Gatterman M: *Chiropractic management of spine related disorders,* Baltimore, 1990, Williams & Wilkins.
7. Grabowski RJ: *Current nutritional therapy,* San Antonio, Tex, 1993, Image Press.
8. Hayes NA, Foreman JC: The activity of compounds extracted from feverfew on histamine release from rat mast cells, *J Pharm Pharmacol* 39:466-467, 1987.
9. Heptinstall S, et al: Extracts of feverfew inhibit granule secretion in blood platelets and polymorphonuclear leukocytes, *Lancet* i:1071-1074, 1985.

10. Heptinstall S, et al: Parthenolide content and bioactivity of feverfew *(Tanacetum parthenium)* (L.) (Schultz-Bip). Estimation of commercial and authenticated feverfew products, *J Pharm Pharmacol* 44:391-395, 1992.

11. Hikrino H, et al: Anti-inflammatory principle of Ephedra herbs, *Chem Pharm Bull (Tokyo)* 28:2900-2904, 1980.

12. Hubka M, et al: A new look at the classifications of headaches, *Chiropr Techn* 6(2), 1995.

13. Kamimura M: Anti-inflammatory activity of vitamin E, *J Vitaminol* 18(4):204-209, 1972.

14. Lawrence D: *Fundamentals of chiropractic diagnosis and management,* Baltimore, 1991, Williams & Wilkins.

15. Makheda AM, Baily JM: A platelet phospholipase inhibitor from the medicinal herb feverfew *(Tanacetum parthenium), Prostaglandins Leukot Med* 8:653-656, 1982.

16. Middleton E Jr, Drzewiecki G: Flavonoid inhibition of human basophil histamine release stimulated by various agents, *Biochem Pharmacol* 33(21):333, 1984.

17. Nelson C: The reliability of an instrument used to evaluate primary headaches, Montreal, April 30-May 1, *Proceedings of the International Conference on Spinal Manipulation,* 1993.

18. Rakel RE: *Textbook of family practice,* ed 5, Philadelphia, 1995, WB Saunders.

19. Tierney LM, McPhee SJ, Papadakis MA: *Current medical diagnosis and treatment,* ed 35, Norwalk, Conn, 1996, Appleton & Lange.

20. Vernon HT: The effectiveness of chiropractic manipulation in the treatment of headaches: an exploration in the literature, *J Manipulative Physiol Ther* 18(9), 1995.

21. Werbach MR: *Nutritional influences on illness,* ed 2, Tarzana, Calif, 1996, Third Line Press.

22. Werbach MR, Murray MT: *Botanical influences on illness,* Tarzana, Calif, 1994, Third Line Press.

Cervicogenic Cephalgia

David M. Brady

DEFINITION

A cervicogenic headache characterized by a suboccipital and a temporal dull ache. Frequently characterized by a 'band,' or 'vise-like,' compressing around the scalp. Cervicogenic headache is often produced by sustained contraction of the muscles of the head and neck or segmental dysfunction of the neck articulations.

ETIOLOGY

May be due to upper cervical subluxations, trauma, postural strain, myofascial trigger points, TMJ syndrome, or tension. May be exacerbated by emotional stress, fatigue, noise, or glare.

SIGNS AND SYMPTOMS

Location

Often bilateral, including the occipitonuchal or bifrontal regions. May encircle the entire head. Often starts in occipital region and travels up and over the head into the frontal region.

Quality

Dull, nonpulsating pain, mild or moderate in intensity. Often described as steady and aching. Headache may be relieved by stress reduction or rest. Exercise to reduce stress is helpful prophylactically.

Timing

Typically begins in late afternoons and waxes and wanes in intensity. Onset is gradual or anxiety related. Headache may last from 4 hours to 2 days. Headaches can occur several times per week (much more frequent than migraine headaches).

Position

Pain may be increased with forward flexion. Not aggravated by physical activities.

Other Manifestations

No prodrome or vomiting. Mild nausea is sometimes reported but generally much less severe than with migraine headaches. Not associated with focal neurological symptoms. No evidence of organic disease. Phonophobia and photophobia may be present but less severe than in migraine headaches.

EXAMINATION

Check tension of masticatory and submandibular muscles. Rule out TMJ involvement. Check for hyperalgesia of skin zones in the cervical regions and trigger points of the neck and thorax. Check joint dysfunction of the cervical and thoracic spine, AC joint, and sternoclavicular joint, and inspect for anterior weight bearing. (See Table 1, pg. 4.)

DIFFERENTIAL DIAGNOSIS

1. Vascular headache (migraine)
2. Hypertensive headache
3. Brain tumor
4. Cluster headaches
5. Gum or tooth disease

Clinical Notes

In a 1977-1978 Ambulatory Care Survey, muscle tension headaches made up 90% of all headache diagnoses. Muscle tension headaches do not cause the amount of incapacitating pain as do migraine headaches, but they are far more frequent and result in a decreased level of productivity over time and a large consumption of OTC and prescribed medication, resulting in a subsequent diminished quality of life. Therefore patients seek out a variety of treatment approaches, including chiropractic, medical, and psychological therapies.[7]

In 1989, Stodolny and Chmielewski reported on 31 subjects with 'cervical migraine,' demonstrating that 100% had spinal segment blockage at C0-C1, 75% at C7-T1, and 25% between C1-C2 and C3. When manual manipulative techniques were used, the results were complete relief of headache in 75% of subjects, average increase in cervical range of motion of 9 degrees, fixations reduced in 28 of 31 subjects, and reports of dizziness in subjects greatly reduced.[7]

In the 1992 report by Vernon et al, it was reported that 84% of the control groups had fixation of at least two of the three upper cervical segments.[22]

A 1996 Rand Study concluded that cervical spine manipulation and/or mobilization may provide short-term relief for some patients with muscle tension (and other nonmigraine) headaches.[3]

When one compiles this data with those of previous studies, it can still be concluded that spinal manipulation appears to provide clinically significant levels of relief for benign headache types.[13]

TREATMENT GOALS

1. Identification of all related etiological or contributing agents, such as diet, food allergens, and medications
2. Acute headache relief
3. Modification of diet or activities directed toward prevention of recurrence and restoration of daily activities

MANAGEMENT PROTOCOL (OPTIONS)

- Deep massage of occipital and cervical paraspinal muscles.
- Ischemic compression, trigger point therapy of suboccipitals, sternocleidomastoid (SCM), and upper trapezius muscles.
- Ultrasound (pulsed): at 0.5 to 1.0 W/cm^2 for 5 to 8 minutes over upper trapezius and lower cervical paraspinal muscles, followed by moist heat applications for 15 minutes.
- Use ice over posterior neck in severe cervicogenic headaches.
- Adjust cervical and upper thoracic subluxations.
- Administration and utilization of an "outcome assessment" questionnaire, such as the Neck Disability Index and the Pain Disability Index, is strongly recommended to gauge patient progress, suggest alterations in treatment protocol, and determine the level of disability, if any.[19,22] (See Appendix C.)

NUTRITIONAL MANAGEMENT PROTOCOL (OPTIONS)

- Nutritional management of cervicogenic headache is directed mainly at the accompanying myospasm. Screening for food allergies and eliminating them from the diet can also be helpful.
  1. Valerian root *(Valeriana officinalis)* (100 mg q4h)
  2. Passion flower *(Passiflora incarnata)* (100-200 mg q4h)
  3. Magnesium (citrate) (100 mg q4h)
  4. Calcium (lactate) (50 mg q4h) Note: Use alternate calcium form if lactose intolerant.

Many vendors offer formulary products with the above elements, including Valerian Daytime/Calmicin Plus (Murdock Madaus Schwabe) and Myoplex/Myoplex PM (Metagenics, Inc.).

REFERENCES

1. Balch JF, Balch PA: *Prescription for natural healing,* Wayne, NJ, 1990, Avery Publishing.
2. Boline P: Chiropractic and pharmaceutical treatment for chronic muscle tension headaches: a randomized clinical trial, *Transactions of the Consortium for Chiropractic Research,* June, 1992.

3. Coulter ID, et al: The appropriateness of manipulation and mobilization of the cervical spine, *Rand Study,* 1996.
4. Fauci A, et al: *Harrison's principles of internal medicine,* ed 13, New York, 1994, McGraw-Hill.
5. Freemon F: Evaluation and treatment of headache, *Geriatrics* 33:82-85, 1978.
6. Gatterman M: *Chiropractic management of spine related disorders,* Baltimore, 1990, Williams & Wilkins.
7. Gatterman M: *Foundations of chiropractic: subluxation,* St Louis, 1995, Mosby.
8. Grabowski RJ: *Current nutritional therapy,* San Antonio, Tex, 1993, Image Press.
9. Hubka M, et al: A new look at the classifications of headaches, *Chiropr Techn* 6(2), 1995.
10. Lawrence D: *Fundamentals of chiropractic diagnosis and management,* Baltimore, 1991, Williams & Wilkins.
11. Lindahl O, Lindwall L: Double blind study of a valerian preparation, *Pharmacol Biochem Behav* 32(4):10065-10066, 1989.
12. *Manual of medical therapeutics (the Washington Manual),* ed 27, Boston, 1992, Little, Brown.
13. Nelson C: The reliability of an instrument used to evaluate primary headaches, Montreal, April 30-May 1, *Proceedings of the International Conference on Spinal Manipulation,* 1993.
14. Nimmo R: Receptor, effecters and tonus: a new approach, *J Natl Chiropr Assoc,* November 1957.
15. Rakel RE: *Conn's current therapy,* Philadelphia, 1996, WB Saunders.
16. Rakel RE: *Textbook of family practice,* ed 5, Philadelphia, 1995, WB Saunders.
17. Schneider MJ: Chiropractic management of myofascial and muscular disorders. In Lawrence D, ed: *Advances in chiropractic,* vol 3, St Louis, 1996, Mosby.
18. Speroni E, Minghetti A: Neuropharmacological activity of extracts from *Passiflora incarnata, Planta Med* 54(6):488-491, 1988.
19. Tait RC, et al: The Pain Disability Index: psychometric and validity data, *Arch Phys Med Rehabil* 68(7):438-441, 1987.
20. Tierney LM, McPhee SJ, Papadakis MA: *Current medical diagnosis and treatment,* ed 35, Norwalk, Conn, 1996, Appleton & Lange.
21. Travell JG, Simons DG: *Myofascial pain and dysfunction: the trigger point manual,* vol 2, Baltimore, 1992, Williams & Wilkins.
22. Vernon H, Mior S: The Neck Disability Index: a study of reliability and validity, *J Manipulative Physiol Ther* 15(1), 1992.
23. Vernon HT: The effectiveness of chiropractic manipulation in the treatment of headaches: an exploration in the literature, *J Manipulative Physiol Ther* 18(9), 1995.

24. Vernon HT, et al: Cervicogenic dysfunction in muscle contraction headache and migraine: a descriptive study, *J Manipulative Physiol Ther* 15:418-429, 1992.

25. Werbach MR: *Nutritional influences on illness,* ed 2, San Antonio, Tex, 1996, Third Line Press.

26. Werbach MR, Murray MT: *Botanical influences on illness,* San Antonio, Tex, 1994, Third Line Press.

SECTION II

Thoracic Outlet Syndromes

Anterior Scalene Syndrome

Cervical Rib Syndrome

Costoclavicular Syndrome

Pectoralis Minor Syndrome

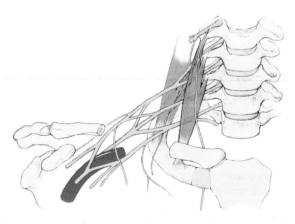

(Modified from Mathers LH, et al: *Clinical Anatomy Principles (CLASS)*, St Louis, 1996, Mosby.)

Anterior Scalene Syndrome

LEW HUFF AND DAVID M. BRADY

DEFINITION

A compression of the neurovascular bundle associated with spasm or hypertrophy of the scaleni anticus and medius muscles. A thoracic outlet syndrome (TOS).

ETIOLOGY

Spasm of the scalene muscles resulting from trauma or unusual or prolonged exercise, or may be secondary to hyperextension whiplash injury. Other causes include first or second rib subluxation, nerve root irritation, and postural changes.

SIGNS AND SYMPTOMS

Inspection

Anterior head carriage and hypertrophy of scalenes and SCM may be visualized.

Sensory

Numbness, tingling, and paresthesia of upper limbs. Pain may extend down the medial aspect of the arm and forearm into the little finger; typical of ulnar nerve.

Motor

Decreased grip strength may be a long-term effect.

Quality

A constant achiness with paresthesias.

Vascular

Diminished, irregular, or absent pulse with Adson's test. Late changes may include glossy skin, atrophy, nail bed changes. Edema, coldness, cyanosis, Raynaud's sign, and dry or excessive sweating are common.

Neurological

Muscle weakness may be present over the thenar, hypothenar, and interosseous muscles. Reflexes are generally unaffected. Hyperesthesia or hypesthesia over C8 and T1 dermatomes. The C5-C7 areas may be affected depending on nerve roots involved.

DIFFERENTIAL DIAGNOSIS

Vertebral subluxations
Disk herniation
Facet trophism
TMJ, carpal, or tunnel of Guyon syndromes
Trauma, fracture
Intervertebral foramen (IVF) encroachment

ORTHOPEDIC TESTS

Adson's, modified Adson's
Wright's hyperabduction
Allen's, EAST test
Flexion arm test, Phalen's maneuver
Costoclavicular, Eden's
Abduction and external rotation (AER) test/Roo's test is the most reliable provocative test for TOS
Caution: Pulsus obliterans is fairly common in asymptomatic population during Adson's test.

X-RAY FINDINGS

Biomechanical variations

TREATMENT GOALS

1. Promotion of soft tissue healing
2. Pain relief and prevention of recurrence

MANAGEMENT PROTOCOL (OPTIONS)

- Transcutaneous electrical stimulation (TENS) for pain syndrome: frequency 50 to 100 Hz, pulse width 20 to 60 ms, time 1 hour, set below motoric threshold to block pain.
- Ice applications for the first 24 hours to reduce swelling followed by moist hot pack applications to reduce scalene muscle spasms.
- Trigger point therapy: Apply moderate pressure over the painful nodule within the muscle belly for 5 to 7 seconds (repeat three times), inducing relaxation of the muscle.
- Ultrasound (pulsed) over related muscle tissues. Pulsed at 0.5 W/cm^2 at 5 to 8 minutes followed by stretching exercises and moist heat applications.
- Electrical muscle stimulation: Select setting that will induce muscle contraction to the point of fatigue.
- Correct cervical and upper thoracic subluxations. Assess the need for rib adjustments and thoracic extension technique.

Clinical Note

There is insufficient evidence to support or refute the use of cervical spine manipulation or mobilization for patients with chronic TOS. The literature indicates that manipulation and mobilization may be more effective in patients with acute or subacute symptoms.[3]

- Active stretching of involved muscles.
- Range of motion and stretching under hot shower to relieve muscle tension.
- Administration and utilization of an "outcome assessment" questionnaire, such as the Pain Disability Index, is strongly

recommended to gauge patient progress, suggest alterations in treatment protocol, and determine the level of disability, if any.[22] (See Appendix C.)

NUTRITIONAL MANAGEMENT PROTOCOL (OPTIONS)

Directed at muscle spasm:
- Valerian root *(Valeriana officinalis)* (100 mg q4h)
- Passion flower *(Passiflora incarnata)* (100-200 mg q4h)
- Magnesium (citrate) (100 mg q4h)
- Calcium (lactate) (50 mg q4h)

Many vendors offer formulary products with the above elements, including Valerian Daytime/Calmicin Plus (Murdock Madaus Schwabe) and Myoplex/Myoplex PM (Metagenics, Inc.).

REFERENCES

1. Balch JF, Balch PA: *Prescription for natural healing*, Wayne, NJ, 1990, Avery Publishing.
2. Brukner P: *Clinical sports medicine*, New York, 1993, McGraw-Hill.
3. Coulter ID, et al: The appropriateness of manipulation and mobilization of the cervical spine, *Rand Study*, 1996.
4. Downer AH: *Physical therapy procedures*, ed 4, Springfield, Ill, 1988, Charles C Thomas.
5. Fauci A, et al: *Harrison's principles of internal medicine*, ed 13, New York, 1994, McGraw-Hill.
6. Gatterman M: *Chiropractic management of spine related disorders*, Baltimore, 1990, Williams & Wilkins.
7. Gatterman M: *Foundations of chiropractic: subluxation*, St Louis, 1995, Mosby.
8. Grabowski RJ: *Current nutritional therapy*, San Antonio, Tex, 1993, Image Press.
9. Hammer W: *Functional soft tissue examination and treatment by manual methods*, Gaithersburg, Md, 1991, Aspen Publishers.
10. Lawrence D: *Fundamentals of chiropractic diagnosis and management*, Baltimore, 1991, Williams & Wilkins.
11. Liebenson C: *Rehabilitation of the spine*, Baltimore, 1996, Williams & Wilkins.
12. Lindahl O, Lindwall L: Double blind study of a *Valerian* preparation, *Pharmacol Biochem Behav* 32(4):10065-10066, 1989.
13. *Manual of medical therapeutics (the Washington manual)*, ed 27, Boston, 1992, Little, Brown.

14. *The Merck manual,* ed 16, Rahway, NJ, 1992, Merck Co.

15. Nimmo R: Receptor, effecters and tonus: a new approach, *J Natl Chiropr Assoc,* November 1957.

16. Rakel RE: *Conn's current therapy,* Philadelphia, 1996, WB Saunders.

17. Rakel RE: *Textbook of family practice,* ed 5, Philadelphia, 1995, WB Saunders.

18. Schestack R: *Handbook of physical therapy,* ed 3, New York, 1977, Springer-Verlag.

19. Schneider MJ: Chiropractic management of myofascial and muscular disorders. In Lawrence D, ed: *Advances in chiropractic,* vol 3, St Louis, 1996, Mosby.

20. Scully RM, Barnes MR: *Physical therapy,* Philadelphia, 1989, JB Lippincott.

21. Speroni E, Minghetti A: Neuropharmacological activity of extracts from *Passiflora incarnata, Planta Med* 54(6):488-491, 1988.

22. Tait RC, et al: The Pain Disability Index: psychometric and validity data, *Arch Phys Med Rehabil* 68(7):438-441, 1987.

23. Taylor RB: *Manual of family practice,* Boston, 1996, Little, Brown.

24. Tierney LM, McPhee SJ, Papadakis MA: *Current medical diagnosis and treatment,* ed 35, Norwalk, Conn, 1996, Appleton & Lange.

25. Travell JG, Simons DG: *Myofascial pain and dysfunction: the trigger point manual,* vol 2, Baltimore, 1992, Williams & Wilkins.

26. Vear HJ: *Chiropractic standards of practice and quality of care,* Gaithersburg, Md, 1992, Aspen Publishers.

27. Werbach MR: *Nutritional influences on illness,* ed 2, Tarzana, Calif, 1996, Third Line Press.

28. Werbach MR, Murray MT: *Botanical influences on illness,* Tarzana, Calif, 1994, Third Line Press.

Cervical Rib Syndrome

LEW HUFF AND DAVID M. BRADY

DEFINITION

A rudimentary rib at the C7 vertebral level associated with a number of brachial plexus–subclavian artery compression syndromes. A thoracic outlet syndrome.

ETIOLOGY

The lowest brachial trunk or subclavian artery is caught between the rudimentary cervical rib and the clavicle. Compression of the brachial plexus or subclavian artery may cause neurological or vascular symptoms. Frequently this may be asymtomatic.

NOTE: Although up to 1% of the population has a cervical rib, only 10% of those have any related symptomatology.

See caution statement on p. 36.

SIGNS AND SYMPTOMS

Location

Motor, vascular, and sensory symptoms of the upper limbs. Ulnar distribution of pain or paresthesia. Impaired light touch to the hands.

Palpation

Digital palpation reveals rudimentary rib at the base of the neck. The cervical rib is frequently bilateral at the C7 level. A downward compression of the shoulder or traction of the arm causes compression. Tenderness over the sternocleidomastoids and scalenes.

Motor Strength

Decreased grip strength, clumsiness. Wasting and weakness of the intrinsic muscles of the hand, especially the thenar eminence.

Vascular and Systemic Manifestations

Decreased, irregular, or absent radial pulse. Trophic skin ulcerations, brittle nails, glossy skin, ischemia, cyanosis, vasospasm may be present.

Differential

Ulnar distribution denotes possible cervical rib. Median nerve distribution denotes possible rupture of intervertebral (IV) disk.

CAUTION: The simultaneous presence of a cervical rib and TOS signs or symptoms does not definitively implicate the cervical rib as the cause.

DIFFERENTIAL DIAGNOSIS

Herniated disk
Scalenus anticus syndrome
Hyperabduction syndrome
IVF encroachment
Peripheral entrapment syndrome

ORTHOPEDIC/NEUROLOGICAL RESULTS

Possible (+) Adson's
Possible (+) costoclavicular
Possible (+) AER/Roo's

X-RAY FINDINGS

Cervical rib visible

TREATMENT GOALS

1. Promote soft tissue healing.
2. Relieve pain and prevent recurrence.
3. Increase pain-free ranges of motion.

MANAGEMENT PROTOCOL (OPTIONS)

- Reduce all cervical and upper thoracic subluxations.

Clinical Note

There is insufficient evidence to support or refute the use of cervical spine manipulation and/or mobilization for patients with TOS. The literature indicates that manipulation and mobilization may be more effective in patients with acute or subacute symptoms.[3]

- Trigger point therapy: Apply moderate pressure over the painful nodule within the muscle belly for 5 to 7 seconds. This pressure induces ischemia followed by reactive vasodilation and forces muscle relaxation. Repeat three times.
- Cervical rib uplift technique: Patient seated, physician hooks thumb and index finger beneath the transverse process of the rudimentary rib, lifting superiorly six times while the patient inhales and exhales.
- Evaluate the need for manipulation of the first rib, sternoclavicular joint, and AC joint.
- Myofascial stripping techniques: Use a sticky massage cream, traction the skin and lock in, and very slowly apply moderate to strong pressure while moving slowly along the course of the involved muscle groups.
- Shoulder elevation exercises: Physician instructs patient to lift both shoulders up simultaneously, back (retraction) and then down; this stretches the muscles and improves posture.
- Ultrasound (pulsed) at 0.5 to 1.0 W/cm^2 over cervical paraspinal muscles followed by moist heat applications and range-of-motion exercises. Breaks up fibrotic adhesions, reduces muscle spasms, and increases range of motion.
- Active stretching of involved muscles.
- Taping and immobilization techniques: Taping to temporarily elevate the shoulder and relieve symptoms (use only if absolutely necessary).
- Administration and utilization of an "outcome assessment" questionnaire, such as the Pain Disability Index, is strongly

recommended to gauge patient progress, suggest alterations in treatment protocol, and determine the level of disability, if any.[20] (See Appendix C.)

NUTRITIONAL MANAGEMENT PROTOCOL (OPTIONS)

Directed at muscle spasms:
- Valerian root *(Valeriana officinalis)* (100 mg q4h)
- Passion flower *(Passiflora incarnata)* (100-200 mg q4h)
- Magnesium (citrate) (100 mg q4h)
- Calcium (lactate) (50 mg q4h)

Many vendors offer formulary products with the above elements, including Valerian Daytime/Calmicin Plus (Murdock Madaus Schwabe) and Myoplex/Myoplex PM (Metagenics, Inc.).

HOME CARE PROTOCOL (OPTIONS)

- Avoid hyperflexion and hyperextension of the neck.
- Posture exercises, including shoulder elevation exercises, should be advocated.

REFERENCES

1. Balch JF, Balch PA: *Prescription for natural healing,* Wayne, NJ, 1990, Avery Publishing.
2. Brukner P: *Clinical sports medicine,* New York, 1993, McGraw-Hill.
3. Coulter ID, et al: The appropriateness of manipulation and mobilization of the cervical spine, *Rand Study,* 1996.
4. Fauci A, et al: *Harrison's principles of internal medicine,* ed 13, New York, 1994, McGraw-Hill.
5. Gatterman M: *Chiropractic management of spine related disorders,* Baltimore, 1990, Williams & Wilkins.
6. Gatterman M: *Foundations of chiropractic: subluxation,* St Louis, 1995, Mosby.
7. Grabowski RJ: *Current nutritional therapy,* San Antonio, Tex, 1993, Image Press.
8. Halstead WS: An experimental study of circumscribed dilation of an artery immediately distal to partially occluding band and it's bearing on the dilation of the subclavian artery observed in certain cases of cervical rib, *J Exp Med* 24:271, 1916.
9. Hammer W: *Functional soft tissue examination and treatment by manual methods,* Gaithersburg, Md, 1991, Aspen Publishers.

10. Lawrence D: *Fundamentals of chiropractic diagnosis and management,* Baltimore, 1991, Williams & Wilkins.
11. Lindahl O, Lindwall L: Double blind study of a *Valerian* preparation, *Pharmacol Biochem Behav* 21(4):10065-10066, 1989.
12. *Manual of medical therapeutics (the Washington manual),* ed 27, Boston, 1992, Little, Brown.
13. *The Merck manual,* ed 16, Rahway, NJ, 1992, Merck Co.
14. Nimmo R: Receptor, effecters and tonus: a new approach, *J Natl Chiropr Assoc,* November 1957.
15. Rakel RE: *Conn's current therapy,* Philadelphia, 1996, WB Saunders.
16. Rakel RE: *Textbook of family practice,* ed 5, Philadelphia, 1995, WB Saunders.
17. Schneider MJ: Chiropractic management of myofascial and muscular disorders. In Lawrence D, ed: *Advances in chiropractic,* vol 3, St Louis, 1996, Mosby.
18. Shekelle PG, et al: The appropriateness of spinal manipulation for low back pain. Indications and ratings by an all-chiropractic expert panel, *Rand Study,* 1991.
19. Speroni E, Minghetti A: Neuropharmacological activity of extracts from *Passiflora incarnata, Planta Med* 54(6):488-491, 1988.
20. Tait RC, et al: The Pain Disability Index: psychometric and validity data, *Arch Phys Med Rehabil* 68(7):438-441, 1987.
21. Taylor RB: *Manual of family practice,* Boston, 1996, Little, Brown.
22. Tierney LM, McPhee SJ, Papadakis MA: *Current medical diagnosis and treatment,* ed 35, Norwalk, Conn, 1996, Appleton & Lange.
23. Travell JG, Simons DG: *Myofascial pain and dysfunction: the trigger point manual,* vol 2, Baltimore, 1992, Williams & Wilkins.
24. Werbach MR: *Nutritional influences on illness,* ed 2, Tarzana, Calif, 1996, Third Line Press.
25. Werbach MR, Murray MT: *Botanical influences on illness,* Tarzana, Calif, 1994, Third Line Press.
26. White AA, Panjabi MM: *Clinical biomechanics of the spine,* Philadelphia, 1990, JB Lippincott.
27. Zahid M, Jordan D: Bilateral cervical rib syndrome, *Am J Chiropr Med* 1(2):71-74, 1987.

Costoclavicular
Syndrome

LEW HUFF AND DAVID M. BRADY

DEFINITION

A neurovascular compression of the shoulder girdle characterized by pain, numbness, and paresthesias of the upper extremities. There is an increased incidence in 35- to 55-year-old women. Classified as a thoracic outlet syndrome.

ETIOLOGY

Caused by a narrowing of the space between the clavicle and the first rib, with compression of the brachial plexus and the subclavian artery. May relate to poor posture, trauma, fatigue, or emotional stress.

SIGNS AND SYMPTOMS

Inspection

May see cyanosis, edema, or distal gangrene of hands.

Palpation

Trigger points around the neck and clavicular regions. Palpate for diminished or absent pulse either unilaterally or bilaterally.

Pain Pattern

Pain and numbness radiates to neck and upper extremities or anterior chest wall. Abduction and retraction of shoulder increases pain and paresthesia.

Timing

Pain increases in severity during the night and early morning hours.

Neurological

Painful side shows various degrees of sensory impairment over the C8 to T1 dermatomes. No muscle weakness.

Vascular

Vascular and autonomic changes of the upper limbs, such as cyanosis, edema, Raynaud's phenomenon, and distal gangrene may be noted.

Other

Symptoms may be transient.

DIFFERENTIAL DIAGNOSIS

Anterior scalene syndrome
Vertebral subluxations
Cervical rib syndrome
Pancoast's tumor
IVF encroachment
Discopathy

ORTHOPEDIC/NEUROLOGICAL EXAMINATION

Adson's test
Soto-Hall sign
Foraminal compression
Costoclavicular sign
AER/Roo's
SPECIAL STUDY: photoelectric plethysmogram

ORTHOPEDIC/NEUROLOGICAL RESULTS

(+) Costoclavicular sign
(+) Adson's
(+) AER/Roo's

TREATMENT GOALS

1. Pain relief and prevention of recurrence
2. Restoration of normal strength and stability to joint

MANAGEMENT PROTOCOL (OPTIONS)

- Auscultate for bruit and rule out Pancoast's tumor.
- Moist heat and ultrasound followed by muscle stripping, stretching, and trigger point therapy to reduce muscle spasms.
- Check joint dysfunction of cervicothoracic spine, AC joint, and sternoclavicular joint, and inspect for anterior weight bearing.
- Reduce all occipital, cervical, and upper thoracic subluxations.

Clinical Note

There is insufficient evidence to support or refute the use of cervical spine manipulation and/or mobilization for patients with TOS. The literature indicates that manipulation and mobilization may be more effective in patients with acute or subacute symptoms.[3]

- Active stretching of involved muscles.
- Corrective posture exercises and shoulder elevation exercises.
- Reduction of myofascial trigger points in cervical, upper thoracic, and shoulder muscles with ischemic compression techniques applying pressure for 5 to 7 seconds. Repeat three times.
- Administration and utilization of an "outcome assessment" questionnaire, such as the Pain Disability Index, is strongly recommended to gauge patient progress, suggest alterations in treatment protocol, and determine the level of disability, if any.[19] (See Appendix C.)

NUTRITIONAL MANAGEMENT PROTOCOL (OPTIONS)

Directed at muscle spasms:
- Valerian root *(Valeriana officinalis)* (100 mg q4h)
- Passion flower *(Passiflora incarnata)* (100-200 mg q4h)
- Magnesium (citrate) (100 mg q4h)
- Calcium (lactate) (50 mg q4h)

Many vendors offer formulary products with the above elements, including Valerian Daytime/Calmicin Plus (Murdock Madaus Schwabe) and Myoplex/Myoplex PM (Metagenics, Inc.).

HOME CARE PROTOCOL (OPTIONS)

Avoid poor posture, heavy lifting, high heels, and shoulder straps on purses.

REFERENCES

1. Balch JF, Balch PA: *Prescription for natural healing,* Wayne, NJ, 1990, Avery Publishing.
2. Brukner P: *Clinical sports medicine,* New York, 1993, McGraw-Hill.
3. Coulter ID, et al: The appropriateness of manipulation and mobilization of the cervical spine, *Rand Study,* 1996.
4. Downer AH: *Physical therapy procedures,* ed 4, Springfield, Ill, 1988, Charles C Thomas.
5. Fauci A, et al: *Harrison's principles of internal medicine,* ed 13, New York, 1994, McGraw-Hill.
6. Gatterman M: *Chiropractic management of spine related disorders,* Baltimore, 1990, Williams & Wilkins.
7. Gatterman M: *Foundations of chiropractic: subluxation,* St Louis, 1995, Mosby.
8. Grabowski RJ: *Current nutritional therapy,* San Antonio, Tex, 1993, Image Press.
9. Hammer W: *Functional soft tissue examination and treatment by manual methods,* Gaithersburg, Md, 1991, Aspen Publishers.
10. Lawrence D: *Fundamentals of chiropractic diagnosis and management,* Baltimore, 1991, Williams & Wilkins.
11. Lindahl O, Lindwall L: Double blind study of a *Valerian* preparation, *Pharmacol Biochem Behav* 32(4):10065-10066, 1989.
12. *Manual of medical therapeutics (the Washington manual),* ed 27, Boston, 1992, Little, Brown.
13. *The Merck manual,* ed 16, Rahway, NJ, 1992, Merck Co.
14. Nimmo R: Receptor, effecters and tonus: a new approach, *J Natl Chiropr Assoc,* November 1957.

15. Rakel RE: *Textbook of family practice,* ed 5, Philadelphia, 1996, WB Saunders.

16. Schestack R: *Handbook of physical therapy,* ed 3, New York, 1977, Springer-Verlag.

17. Schneider MJ: Chiropractic management of myofascial and muscular disorders. In Lawrence D, ed: *Advances in chiropractic,* vol 3, St Louis, 1996, Mosby.

18. Speroni E, Minghetti A: Neuropharmacological activity of extracts from *Passiflora incarnata, Planta Med* 54(6):488-491, 1988.

19. Tait RC, et al: The Pain Disability Index: psychometric and validity data, *Arch Phys Med Rehabil* 68(7):438-441, 1987.

20. Taylor RB: *Manual of family practice,* Boston, 1996, Little, Brown.

21. Tierney LM, McPhee SJ, Papadakis MA: *Current medical diagnosis and treatment,* ed 35, Norwalk, Conn, 1996, Appleton & Lange.

22. Travell JG, Simons DG: *Myofascial pain and dysfunction: the trigger point manual,* vol 2, Baltimore, 1992, Williams & Wilkins.

23. Vernon H: The role of plethysmography in the chiropractic management of costoclavicular syndromes: review of principles and case report, *J Manipulative Physiol Ther* 5(1):17-20, 1982.

24. Werbach MR: *Nutritional influences on illness,* ed 2, Tarzana, Calif, 1996, Third Line Press.

25. Werbach MR, Murray MT: *Botanical influences on illness,* Tarzana, Calif, 1994, Third Line Press.

26. White AA, Panjabi MM: *Clinical biomechanics of the spine,* Philadelphia, 1990, JB Lippincott.

27. Wright I: The neuromuscular syndrome produced by hyperabduction of the arms, *Am Heart J* 29(1):1-19, 1945.

Pectoralis Minor Syndrome

LEW HUFF AND DAVID M. BRADY

DEFINITION

Also known as *hyperabduction syndrome,* a compression of the brachial plexus and/or axillary artery about the coracoid process. The pectoralis minor muscle lies beneath the pectoralis major muscle and lowers the scapula and depresses the shoulder girdle. A thoracic outlet syndrome.

ETIOLOGY

May be due to pectoralis minor spasm, first or second rib subluxation, or overexertion and overuse of the pectoralis muscle. A high incidence of TOSs are found in people working with cash registers, typists, computer operators, packers, and assembly line workers because of awkward work postures and repetitive motion that produces continuous muscle tension.

SIGNS AND SYMPTOMS

Inspection

Rubor, edema, and ulcerations of the hands may be present.

Palpation

Hypertrophy and tenderness of the pectoralis muscle.

Pain Pattern

Pain and paresthesia of the arms, hands, fingers, and forearms. Aching pain with weakness and fatigue is common.

Timing

Symptoms occur mostly at night and early morning hours.

Radiation

Paresthesia is common over the C8 to T1 dermatomes, distally to the fourth and fifth fingers.

Neurological Findings

Numbness most frequently involves the fingers and less frequently the forearms and arms. Deep tendon reflexes are not altered.

Vascular

Ischemic symptoms include discoloration, numbness, weakness, and coldness. Edema of the hand and base of fourth fingers.

Other manifestations

Symptoms are identical to anterior scalene or costoclavicular syndrome. Raynaud's may be present.

DIFFERENTIAL DIAGNOSIS

Anterior scalene syndrome
Costoclavicular syndrome
Cervical rib syndrome
Trauma, fracture
IVF encroachment
Disk herniation

ORTHOPEDIC/NEUROLOGICAL RESULTS

(+) Wright's test
(+) Allen's test

(+) AER/Roo's test
(+) Doppler vascular test

TREATMENT GOALS

Pain relief and prevention of recurrence

MANAGEMENT PROTOCOL (OPTIONS)

- Short wave diathermy: Remove metallic objects, treat involved areas; treatment time is 20 minutes.
- Short wave infrared: Place heat source 18 inches from the body part, use one towel between the heat source and the body part. Treatment time is 20 minutes.
- Identify painful trigger points often seen in pectoralis major and minor, anterior deltoid, sternalis, and sternocleidomastoids. Apply moderate pressure to the tender module for 5 to 7 seconds, inducing muscle relaxation. Repeat three times.
- Active stretching of involved muscles.
- Identify faulty posture, rounded shoulders, superior ribs, and anterior weight bearing. Correct all cervical and upper thoracic subluxations, and do shoulder mobilization techniques.

Clinical Note

There is insufficient evidence to support or refute the use of cervical spine manipulation and/or mobilization for patients with TOS. The literature indicates that manipulation and mobilization may be more effective in patients with acute or subacute symptoms.[3]

- Reduce any first and second rib subluxations.
- Posture and shoulder shrugging exercises.
- Ultrasound (pulsed) over related muscle tissues. Pulsed at 0.5 W/cm^2 at 5 to 8 minutes followed by stretching exercises and moist heat applications.
- Myofascial stripping techniques: Use a sticky massage

cream, traction the skin and lock in, and very slowly apply moderate to strong pressure while moving slowly along the course of the involved muscle groups.
- Administration and utilization of an "outcome assessment" questionnaire, such as the Pain Disability Index, is strongly recommended to gauge patient progress, suggest alterations in treatment protocol, and determine the level of disability, if any.[22] (See Appendix C.)

NUTRITIONAL MANAGEMENT PROTOCOL (OPTIONS)

Directed at muscle spasms:
- Valerian root *(Valeriana officinalis)* (100 mg q4h)
- Passion flower *(Passiflora incarnata)* (100-200 mg q4h)
- Magnesium (citrate) (100 mg q4h)
- Calcium (lactate) (50 mg q4h)

Many vendors offer formulary products with the above elements, including Valerian Daytime/Calmicin Plus (Murdock Madaus Schwabe) and Myoplex/Myoplex PM (Metagenics, Inc.).

REFERENCES

1. Balch JF, Balch PA: *Prescription for natural healing,* Wayne, NJ, 1990, Avery Publishing.
2. Brukner P: *Clinical sports medicine,* New York, 1993, McGraw-Hill.
3. Coulter ID, et al: The appropriateness of manipulation and mobilization of the cervical spine, *Rand Study,* 1996.
4. Downer AH: *Physical therapy procedures,* ed 4, Springfield, Ill, 1988, Charles C Thomas.
5. Fauci A, et al: *Harrison's principles of internal medicine,* ed 13, New York, 1994, McGraw-Hill.
6. Gatterman M: *Chiropractic management of spine related disorders,* Baltimore, 1990, Williams & Wilkins.
7. Gatterman M: *Foundations of chiropractic: subluxation,* St Louis, 1995, Mosby.
8. Grabowski RJ: *Current nutritional therapy,* San Antonio, Tex, 1993, Image Press.
9. Hammer W: *Functional soft tissue examination and treatment by manual methods,* Gaithersburg, Md, 1991, Aspen Publishers.
10. Lawrence D: *Fundamentals of chiropractic diagnosis and management,* Baltimore, 1991, Williams & Wilkins.
11. Liebenson C: *Rehabilitation of the spine,* Baltimore, 1996, Williams & Wilkins.

12. Lindahl O, Lindwall L: Double blind study of a *Valerian* preparation, *Pharmacol Biochem Behav* 32(4):10065-10066, 1989.
13. *Manual of medical therapeutics (the Washington manual)*, ed 27, Boston, 1992, Little, Brown.
14. *The Merck manual*, ed 16, Rahway, NJ, 1992, Merck Co.
15. Nimmo R: Receptor, effecters and tonus: a new approach, *J Natl Chiropr Assoc*, November 1957.
16. Rakel RE: *Conn's current therapy*, Philadelphia, 1996, WB Saunders.
17. Rakel RE: *Textbook of family practice*, ed 5, Philadelphia, 1995, WB Saunders.
18. Schestack R: *Handbook of physical therapy*, ed 3, New York, 1977, Springer-Verlag.
19. Schneider MJ: Chiropractic management of myofascial and muscular disorders. In Lawrence D, ed: *Advances in chiropractic*, vol 3, St Louis, 1996, Mosby.
20. Scully RM, Barnes MR: *Physical therapy*, Philadelphia, 1989, JB Lippincott.
21. Speroni E, Minghetti A: Neuropharmacological activity of extracts from *Passiflora incarnata*, *Planta Med* 54(6):488-491, 1988.
22. Tait RC, et al: The Pain Disability Index: psychometric and validity data, *Arch Phys Med Rehabil* 68(7):438-441, 1987.
23. Taylor RB: *Manual of family practice*, Boston, 1996, Little, Brown.
24. Tierney LM, McPhee SJ, Papadakis MA: *Current medical diagnosis and treatment*, ed 35, Norwalk, Conn, 1996, Appleton & Lange.
25. Travell JG, Simons DG: *Myofascial pain and dysfunction: the trigger point manual*, Baltimore, 1992, Williams & Wilkins.
26. Vear HJ: *Chiropractic standards of practice and quality of care*, Gaithersburg, Md, 1992, Aspen Publishers.
27. Werbach MR: *Nutritional influences on illness*, ed 2, Tarzana, Calif, 1996, Third Line Press.
28. Werbach MR, Murray MT: *Botanical influences on illness*, Tarzana, Calif, 1994, Third Line Press.
29. White AA, Panjabi MM: *Clinical biomechanics of the spine*, Philadelphia, 1990, JB Lippincott.

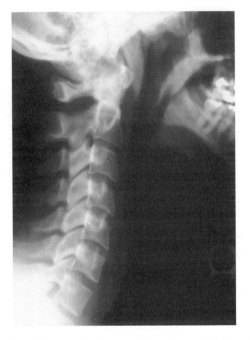

(Modified from Marchiori DM: *Clinical imaging: with skeletal, chest, and abdomen pain differentials,* St Louis, 1999, Mosby.)

SECTION III

Facial and Neck Pain Syndromes

Temporomandibular Joint Dysfunction

MIKELL SUZANNE PARSONS, DAVID M. BRADY, LEW HUFF, AND DARRYL D. CURL

DEFINITION

A dysfunction of the joint between the temporal bone and the mandible characterized by pain, popping or clicking of the TMJ, and/or an inability to fully open the mouth.

ETIOLOGY

May be associated with dental malocclusion, bruxism, faulty dentures, emotional strain, or hypertonicity and imbalance of the muscles of mastication. Affects approximately 40% of the U.S. population, with a female-to-male ratio of 4 to 1.

SIGNS AND SYMPTOMS

Inspection

Hypomobility of the TMJ evident by an inability to place less than 3 fingertips in the open mouth. Observe for mandibular protrusion, disturbed chewing pattern, and altered opening or closing patterns.

Palpation

Tenderness of muscles of mastication, spasm of internal and external pterygoid muscles. Crepitus indicates damaged disk.

Synovial swelling may be present. Facial tenderness may be present.

Joint Sounds

Loud audible clicking and popping. Possible crepitus on auscultation.

Neurological

Jaw reflex is often diminished.

Range of Motion

Patient should be able to insert 3 fingers between the upper and lower incisor teeth (3-finger test). Restricted or aberrant motion could be evaluated by placing tongue depressors between the upper and lower teeth and assessing the ranges of motion. Therapeutic progress can be monitored by the patient's ability to accommodate more tongue depressors between the teeth.

Pain Pattern

Facial pain and cervicogenic headaches caused by facilitation of the trigeminal nerve. Pain increases later in the day as a result of talking and chewing. Unilateral pain typically radiates to the head, neck, eye, or shoulders.

Systemic Manifestations

Tinnitis, ear pain, vertigo, dysphagia, sore throat, arm numbness, low back pain, sinus pain, and tooth pain may accompany this syndrome.

DIFFERENTIAL DIAGNOSIS

Myofascial pain syndrome
Osteoarthritis of TMJ
Ear or sinus infection
Dental malocclusion, bruxism

X-RAY FINDINGS

Usually negative
Biomechanical changes, sclerosis

Clinical Note

Check for *exceptional soleus pain,* a term coined by Janet Travell, MD, for an observed phenomenon in which a trigger point in the soleus muscle can produce referred pain to the TMJ.[19]

TREATMENT GOALS

1. Promote soft tissue healing.
2. Relieve pain and prevent recurrence.
3. Increase pain-free ranges of motion.
4. Restore normal motion and stability to joint.
5. Reduce contributing or secondary myofascial trigger points in facial and cervical musculature and restore functional balance to the TMJ musculature.

MANAGEMENT PROTOCOL (OPTIONS)

Acute Phase:

- Ice applications for the first 24 to 48 hours to reduce swelling. May be followed by moist hot pack applications and mobilization techniques.
- TENS for pain syndrome: frequency 50 to 100 Hz, pulse width 20 to 60 ms, time 1 hour, set below motoric threshold to block pain.
- Vapor coolant spray over external facial muscles.

Subacute Phase:

- Trigger point therapy (Nimmo/receptor tonus[13]): Apply moderate pressure to patient's tolerance, over the nodule located within the taut band of muscle for 5 to 7 seconds, then release. Treat each point up to 3 times per session and a maximum of every other day. This will induce muscle relaxation by resetting abnormal reflex. This procedure should be performed externally to the temporalis, digastric, masseter, and cervical musculature, as well as internally (wearing gloves) to the internal and external pterygoids.

- Ultrasound (pulsed) over related muscle tissues. Do not use directly over the TMJ because this may aggravate already inflamed tissues.
- Patient attempts to open jaw against resistance for 5 minutes, 6 times per day as instructed by doctor.
- TMJ adjustments (generalized approach):
1. A 20-second inferior distraction of the mandible with a rocking motion to reinsert joint into proper alignment
2. Nail point one (pisiform) contact driving superior to inferior with patient supine and head turned away from subluxated side
3. Short-amplitude, high-velocity thrust along the angle of the jaw
- Adjust cervical and upper thoracic subluxations.
- TMJ treatment may be necessary each time patient receives dental work.
- Administration and utilization of an "outcome assessment" questionnaire, such as the Pain Disability Index, is strongly recommended to gauge patient progress, suggest alterations in treatment protocol, and determine the level of disability, if any.[18] (See Appendix C.)

NUTRITIONAL MANAGEMENT PROTOCOL (OPTIONS)

Directed mainly at accompanying myospasm:
- Valerian root *(Valeriana officinalis)* (100 mg q4h)
- Passion flower *(Passiflora incarnata)* (100-200 mg q4h)
- Magnesium (citrate) (100 mg q4h)
- Calcium (lactate) (50 mg q4h)
- Many vendors offer formulary products with the above elements, including Valerian Daytime/Calmicin Plus (Murdock Madaus Schwabe) and Myoplex/Myoplex PM (Metagenics, Inc.).

REFERENCES

1. Balch JF, Balch PA: *Prescription for natural healing,* Wayne, NJ, 1990, Avery Publishing.
2. Cohen JH, Schneider MJ: Receptor-tonus technique: an overview, *Chiropr Techn* vol 2, February 1990.

3. Curl DD: Acute closed lock of the temporomandibular joint: manipulation paradigm and protocol, *Journal of Chiropractic Techniques* 3(1):13-18, 1991.

4. Curl DD: Advances in craniofacial disorders. In Lawrence D, ed: *Advances in chiropractic,* St Louis, 1995, Mosby.

5. Curl DD: *Chiropractic approach to temporomandibular disorders,* Philadelphia, 1990, Williams & Wilkins.

6. Curl DD: Discovery of a myofascial trigger point in the buccinator mechanism: a case report, *Craniology* 7(4):339-45, 1989.

7. Curl DD: The VROM scale: a method for analysis of mandibular gait in a chiropractic setting, *J Manipulative Physiol Ther* 15(2):115-122, 1992.

8. Curl DD, Saghafi D: Manual reduction of adhesion in the temporomandibular joint, *Journal of Chiropractic Techniques,* February 1995.

9. Curl DD, Shapiro CE: Literature searching by a field doctor: a comparison of manual versus computerized methods, *Journal of Chiropractic Techniques* 5(1):15-21, 1993.

10. Curl DD, Stanwood G: Management of capsulitis of the temporomandibular joint for relief of headaches and head pains: case report and review of the literature, *J Orofacial Pain,* June 1993.

11. Grabowski RJ: *Current nutritional therapy,* San Antonio, Tex, 1993, Image Press.

12. Lindahl O, Lindwall L: Double blind study of a *Valerian* preparation, *Pharmacol Biochem Behav* 32(4):10065-10066, 1989.

13. Nimmo R: Receptor, effecters and tonus: a new approach, *J Natl Chiropr Assoc,* November 1957.

14. Saghafi D, Curl DD: Chiropractic manipulation of anteriorly displaced disc with adhesion, *J Manipulative Physiol Ther* 18(2), 1995.

15. Schneider M: *Principles of manual trigger point therapy,* Pittsburgh, 1994, Michael Schneider.

16. Schneider MJ: Chiropractic management of myofascial and muscular disorders. In Lawrence D, ed: *Advances in chiropractic,* vol 3, St Louis, 1996, Mosby.

17. Speroni E, Minghetti A: Neuropharmacological activity of extracts from *Passiflora incarnata, Planta Med* 54(6):488-491, 1988.

18. Tait RC, et al: The Pain Disability Index: psychometric and validity data, *Arch Phys Med Rehabil* 68(7):438-441, 1987.

19. Travell JG, Simons DG: *Myofascial pain and dysfunction: the trigger point manual,* vol 2, Baltimore, 1992, Williams & Wilkins.

20. Werbach MR: *Nutritional influences on illness,* ed 2, Tarzana, Calif, 1996, Third Line Press.

21. Werbach MR, Murray MT: *Botanical influences on illness,* 1994, Tarzana, Calif, Third Line Press.

Injuries to the Cervical Spine: General Overview

Lew Huff

CERVICAL SPINE INJURIES

The cervical spine is vulnerable to a number of injuries and conditions, primarily because of a greater flexibility relative to the thoracic and lumbar regions. Poor posture and sports and occupational injuries may lead to degenerative changes visible on radiographic examination. Segmental dysfunction of the cervical spine has been implicated as a major causative factor in headaches.[6]

SITE OF PAIN

Pain may be localized to the lateral neck, suboccipital regions, shoulders, and midthoracic region. Pain may be intensified by active or passive ranges of motion.

EXAMINATION (FIG. 1)

On deep palpation, the following may be observed: edema, pinpoint tenderness, myospasms, nodules, adhesions, and trigger points.

Full passive ranges of motion with restricted active ranges of motion may indicate muscle weakness as a cause.

Pain on resistive ranges of motion may indicate a strain, whereas pain with passive ranges of motion may indicate ligamentous involvement.

With restriction of passive range of motion, look for bony or soft tissue blockage.

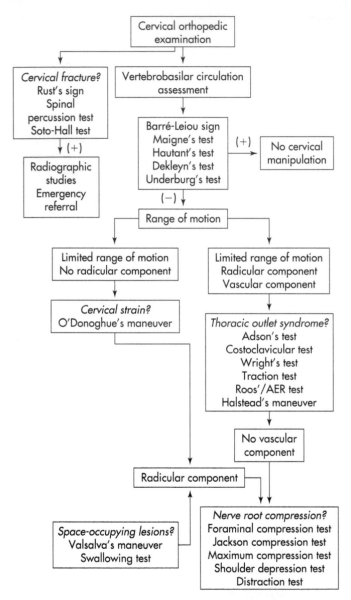

FIG. 1 Examination and diagnosis flow diagram.

RADIATION, REFERRED PAIN

Painful radiation from the neck to the C5-C8 nerve roots dermatomes seen in radiculopathy or whiplash. Numbness and tingling of distal dermatomal patterns may be seen. Pain may radiate to the occiput or anterior chest wall.

MUSCLES

The muscle groups involved in cervical spine injuries may include the suboccipitals, scalenes, levator scapulae, splenius capitis, longus capitis, and SCMs.

LIGAMENTS

Ligaments are often affected or weakened by capsular fibrosis, loss of extensibility, or capsular hypertrophy. Cervical injuries may cause macroscopic or microscopic tearing of the anterior and posterior longitudinal ligaments, interspinous ligaments, or intertransverse ligaments.

ACTIVITIES OF DAILY LIVING

Cervical spine injuries can lead to bizarre symptoms, such as dizziness, blurred vision, tinnitus, Horner's syndrome, head-aches, loss of balance, chest pain, dysphagia, nausea, or vomiting. This, coupled with difficulty sleeping and weakness, may adversely affect the activities of daily living.

TIME FRAMES

Note: The need for all phases of care, as well as the time frames suggested, is highly dependent on the severity of the initial injury and the level of dysfunction. Correctional care and rehabilitation are stages used only if clinical signs warrant the need for continued care.

1. *Acute Care:* Pain is felt at rest, often over a diffuse area, and aggravated by activity. Movements are restricted by pain and guarding. Goals are to promote anatomical rest, decrease myospasm, diminish inflammatory reactions, alleviate pain to a tolerable level, and improve overall function. Acute injuries may be superimposed on degen-

erative conditions, anomalies, or prior trauma, which may slow or complicate the healing process.

Clinical Note

In general, some evidence of measurable clinical improvement (objective or subjective) should be noted within eight visits or 2 to 4 weeks to justify continued care.[8]

---

2. *Active/Correctional Care:* Characterized by little or no pain at rest; pain increases with activity. Pain is generally localized at this stage. Goals are to further reduce symptoms, improve function, and return patient to preinjury status.
3. *Rehabilitation:* Goals are to restore strength and endurance, increase physical work capacity, and improve function to preinjury status. Continue rehabilitation to maximum medical improvement whether or not preinjury status has been achieved. Rehabilitation should include therapeutic exercises and activities of daily living training. Active range of motion (ROM) exercises help disperse edema and prevent the formation of adhesions. ROM exercises should not be performed in planes that stress the joint.
4. *Lifestyle Adaptations:* To modify social and recreational activities, to diminish work environmental risk factors, and to adapt to psychological factors related to the disorder.

Clinical Notes

Proceed to rehabilitation as quickly as possible to avoid or minimize dependency on passive forms of treatment.[4]

Singer et al describe a relationship between three descriptive factors in the episode history noted at the time of patient consultation and the duration of conservative care: pain intensity and duration before consultation, number of prior episodes, and, in general, more severe pain at onset were associated with longer treatment times.[4]

1990 Rand Consensus Panel unanimously agreed: recommend a

trial course of 2 weeks each using alternative manipulative procedures before considering treatment to have failed. Without evidence of improvement over this time frame, spinal manipulation is no longer indicated.[2]

1996 Rand Study revealed that cervical spine manipulation and/or mobilization may provide at least short-term pain relief and ROM enhancement in persons with subacute or chronic neck pain.[2]

DISCLAIMER: The following time frames are controversial. Note that each case must be evaluated separately by a clinician to establish an adequate treatment plan and duration.

Preconsultation duration of symptoms: Pain less than 8 days: no anticipated delay in recovery. Pain more than 8 days: recovery many take 1.5 times longer.[4]

Typical severity of symptoms: Mild pain: no anticipated delay in recovery. Severe pain: recovery may take up to 2 times longer.[4]

Number of previous episodes: 0-3: no anticipated delay in recovery. 4-7: recovery may take up to 2 times longer.[4]

Injury superimposed on preexisting condition: Skeletal anomaly: may increase recovery time by 1.5 to 2 times. Structural pathology: may increase recovery time by 1.5 to 2 times.[4]

REINJURY/FLARE-UP

Restrict aggravating activities, continue care, and start low-impact rehabilitative exercises.

HOME CARE

ROM exercises, passive stretching, stretching under the shower, and the use of a cervical pillow may be emphasized. Surgical tubing exercises, ice applications, or compresses may be appropriate.

WHEN TO DISCHARGE

When patient has reached maximum medical improvement or the need for referral is established.

Clinical Note

Return to work usually can be commenced at 80% to 90% level of preinjury status.[4]

REFERRAL

If fracture, dislocation, or neurological complications are present. Daily treatment exceeding 2 weeks may signal the need for a second opinion or referral.

Treatment exceeding 4 weeks or temporary disability for longer than 4 weeks with no objective signs of improvement, or worsening of the condition within the first 2 weeks, may signal the need for a second opinion or referral.

Suspected fracture, bone pathology, spinal motion instability, contraindication for spinal manipulation, systemic disease, infection, or closed head injury signals the need for referral.[5]

REFERENCES

1. Clemente C: *Anatomy: a regional atlas of the human body,* ed 3, Baltimore, 1987, Williams & Wilkins.
2. Coulter ID, et al: The appropriateness of manipulation and mobilization of the cervical spine, *Rand Study,* 1996.
3. Gatterman M: *Chiropractic management of spine related disorders,* Baltimore, 1990, Williams & Wilkins.
4. Haldeman S, et al: Guidelines for chiropractic quality assurance & practice parameters, *The Proceedings of the Mercy Center Consensus Conference,* Gaithersburg, Md, 1993, Aspen Publishers.
5. Hansen DT: *Chiropractic standards of practice and utilization guidelines in the care and treatment of injured workers,* 1988, Washington State Department of Labor & Industries.
6. Lawrence D: *Fundamentals of chiropractic diagnosis and management,* Baltimore, 1991, Williams & Wilkins.
7. Schestack R: *Handbook of physical therapy,* ed 3, New York, 1977, Springer-Verlag.
8. Vear HJ: *Chiropractic standards of practice and quality of care,* Gaithersburg, Md, 1992, Aspen Publishers.

Cervical Radiculopathy

MIKELL SUZANNE PARSONS, DAVID M. BRADY,
AND LEW HUFF

DEFINITION

An acute or chronic neuromusculoskeletal disorder caused by degeneration of the posterior cervical joints and discopathy in which the nerve roots are impinged.

ETIOLOGY

Causes include degenerative joint disease, osteophyte formation, discopathy, and trauma. Frequently affects the 30-year-old and above age-groups.

SIGNS AND SYMPTOMS

Location

Sites of pain are the lateral neck, suboccipital regions, shoulders, and midthoracic region. Pain increases with hyperextension or deviation of head to involved side. Pain intensified by active or passive range of motion.

Radiation

Painful radiation from the neck to the C5-C8 nerve roots dermatomes. Numbness and tingling of distal dermatomal patterns.

Palpation

Tenderness over spinous processes; nonspecific muscle spasms of suboccipital and lateral neck muscles.

Other Findings

Decreased ranges of motion in all planes. Possible muscle wasting and weakness of upper limbs. Thoracic outlet symptoms, such as paresthesia, pain along dermatomal patterns, and vascular changes.

Neurological Testing

Muscle testing, reflexes, and sensory testing.

NEUROLOGICAL FINDINGS

Motor weakness at encroached level. Sensory changes at encroached level; atrophy. Possible loss of associated deep tendon reflexes (DTRs).

DIFFERENTIAL DIAGNOSIS

Osteoarthritis of facets
Lateral disk herniation
Cervical trauma
Pancoast's tumor
Lateral canal stenosis
Myofascial trigger points

ORTHOPEDIC RESULTS

Adson's may be (+)
Cervical compression may be (+)
Distraction may be (+)
Other TOS tests may be (+)

X-RAY FINDINGS

Loss of lordosis
Narrowed disk space

Osteophytes (posterior and posterolateral are significant)
Foraminal encroachment seen on oblique views
(See Fig. 1.)

POSTERIORLY DIRECTED OSTEOPHYTES

SPECIAL NOTE: All cervical lateral films with spondylosis must be checked for posteriorly directed osteophytes. Although anterior osteophytes may be very apparent and striking in appearance, the posterior directed spurs are of major clinical significance. They are, however, often overlooked. The posterolaterally directed spur has the ability to occlude the intervertebral foramen and cause IVF encroachment, resulting in nerve root compression syndromes. It can also cause cervical canal stenosis and impinge the cord if it is directed posteriorly. The canal diameter must be measured (from the most posterior portion of the spur to the spinolaminar junction) and compared with minimum safe values for the segmental level involved.[31] If cervical canal stenosis is present, **manipulation should not be performed** at that level. Traction and myofascial modalities should be used. If clinical symptoms or signs of cord compression exist, magnetic resonance imaging (MRI) with axial images and a referral for a neurosurgical consultation are warranted.

TREATMENT GOALS

1. Promote soft tissue healing.
2. Relieve pain and prevent recurrence.
3. Increase pain-free ranges of motion.
4. Restore normal strength and stability to joint.
5. Quickly change to rehabilitation or restoration of function.

MANAGEMENT PROTOCOL (OPTIONS)

In the absence of severe neurological deficits, conservative treatment is effective.

- Cervical collar to reduce pain and provide rest periods.
- Ice in acute stage, moist heat in chronic stage.
- Myofascial stripping techniques: use a sticky massage cream, traction the skin and lock in, very slowly apply moderate to strong pressure while moving slowly along the course of the involved muscle groups.

- Trigger point therapy (Nimmo/receptor tonus): Apply moderate pressure to patient's tolerance, over the nodule located within the taut band of muscle for 5 to 7 seconds, then release. Treat each point up to 3 times per session and a maximum of every other day. This will induce muscle relaxation by resetting the abnormal reflex.
- Ultrasound (pulsed) at 0.5 to 1.0 W/cm^2 over cervical paraspinal muscles followed by moist heat applications and ROM exercises.
- Surgical tubing exercises to strengthen involved muscle groups. Graded levels and low speed through partial ranges of motion in the beginning. Later use high speed through-out the entire ranges of motion.
- Active (by the patient) and passive (by the doctor) ROM exercises.
- Postural exercises to regain lost strength.
- Correct spinal subluxations of the cervical, occiput, and upper thoracic spine.

Clinical Note

1996 Rand Study revealed that cervical spine manipulation and/or mobilization may provide at least short-term pain relief and ROM enhancement in persons with subacute or chronic neck pain.[5]

- Prompt referral in cases of severe pain, advancing motor or sensory deficits.
- Administration and utilization of an "outcome assessment" questionnaire, such as the Neck Disability Index, is strongly recommended to gauge patient progress, suggest alterations in treatment protocol, and determine the level of disability, if any.[28] (See Appendix C.)

NUTRITIONAL MANAGEMENT PROTOCOL (OPTIONS)

Inflammation:
- Proteolytic enzymes, such as trypsin, chymotrypsin, and bromelin (3 to 4 tablets qid between meals). CAUTION: Do not give to patients with ulcers.

- Bioflavonoids, such as quercetin, hesperidin, rutin (200 mg of mixed bioflavonoids q2h acute phase).
- Herbals, such as boswellia, ginger, turmeric, cayenne (400 mg, 300 mg, 200 mg, 50 mg, respectively, q2h acute phase).

The above proteolytic enzymes can be obtained in Biozyme (Metagenics, Inc., San Clemente, Calif.) or Lyso-Lyph Forte (Nutri-West, Inc., Douglas, Wyo.). Inflavonoid Intensive Care (Metagenics, Inc.) will provide the above bioflavonoids and herbals.

- Vitamin C (3000 mg daily)

Myospasms:
- Valerian root *(Valeriana officinalis)* (100 mg q4h)
- Passion flower *(Passiflora incarnata)* (100-200 mg q4h)
- Magnesium (citrate) (100 mg q4h)
- Calcium (lactate) (50 mg q4h)

Many vendors offer formulary products with the above elements, including Valerian Daytime/Calmicin Plus (Murdock Madaus Schwabe, Springville, Utah) and Myoplex/Myoplex PM (Metagenics, Inc.).

HOME CARE PROTOCOL (OPTIONS)

- Use a cervical pillow.
- Restrict movements of the cervical spine at first.
- Avoid hyperextension or hyperflexion of the spine.
- Moist heat or ice applications: always use dry towel between the ice or heat source and the patient. Use 20 minutes every 2 hours.
- Gradually work into isometric or surgical tubing exercises to strengthen the neck. Never exercise if it causes pain or leaves the patient with residual pain.

REFERENCES

1. Balch JF, Balch PA: *Prescription for natural healing,* Wayne, NJ, 1990, Avery Publishing.
2. Bracker M, Ralph L: Problem-oriented diagnosis: the numb arm and hand, *Am Fam Physician* 51(1):103-116, 1995.
3. Bucci LR: *Nutrition applied to injury rehabilitation and sports medicine,* Boca Raton, Fla, 1995, CRC Press.
4. Cichoke AJ, Marty L: The use of proteolytic enzymes with soft-tissue athletic injuries, *Am Chiropr,* October 1981, p 32.
5. Coulter ID, et al: The appropriateness of manipulation and mobilization of the cervical spine, *Rand Study,* 1996.

6. Downer AH: *Physical therapy procedures,* ed 4, Springfield, Ill, 1988, Charles C Thomas.

7. Gatterman M: *Chiropractic management of spine related disorders,* Baltimore, 1990, Williams & Wilkins.

8. Grabowski RJ: *Current nutritional therapy,* San Antonio, Tex, 1993, Image Press.

9. Hall T, Quintner J: Responses to mechanical stimulation of the upper limb in painful cervical radiculopathy, *Aust J Physiol* 42:277-286, 1996.

10. Hammer W: *Functional soft tissue examination and treatment by manual methods,* Gaithersburg, Md, 1991, Aspen Publishers.

11. Havsteen B: Flavinoids, a class of natural products of high pharmacological potency: *Biochem Pharmacol* 33(24):3933-3939, 1984.

12. Lawrence D: *Fundamentals of chiropractic diagnosis and management,* Baltimore, 1991, Williams & Wilkins.

13. Lindahl O, Lindwall L: Double blind study of a *Valerian* preparation, *Pharmacol Biochem Behav* 32(4):10065-10066, 1989.

14. Malanga G: The diagnosis and treatment of cervical radiculopathy, *Med Sci Sports Exerc* 29(7):S236-245, 1997.

15. *Manual of medical therapeutics (the Washington manual),* ed 27, Boston, 1992, Little, Brown.

16. Mariano K, et al: Double crush syndrome: chiropractic care of an entrapment neuropathy, *J Manipulative Physiol Ther* 14(4):262-265, 1991.

17. Nimmo R: Receptor, effecters and tonus: a new approach, *J Natl Chiropr Assoc,* November 1957.

18. Rakel RE: *Conn's current therapy,* Philadelphia, 1996, WB Saunders.

19. Rakel RE: *Textbook of family practice,* ed 5, Philadelphia, 1995, WB Saunders.

20. Schneider MJ: Chiropractic management of myofascial and muscular disorders. In Lawrence D, ed: *Advances in chiropractic,* vol 3, St Louis, 1996, Mosby.

21. Scully RM, Barnes MR: *Physical therapy,* Philadelphia, 1989, JB Lippincott.

22. Speroni E, Minghetti A: Neuropharmacological activity of extracts from *Passiflora incarnata, Planta Med* 54(6):488-491, 1988.

23. Taraye JP, Lauressergues H: Advantages of combination of proteolytic enzymes, flavonoids and ascorbic acid in comparison with non-steroid inflammatory drugs, *Arzneimittelforschung* 27(1):1144-1149, 1977.

24. Taylor RB: *Manual of family practice,* Boston, 1996, Little, Brown.

25. Tierney LM, McPhee SJ, Papadakis MA: *Current medical diagnosis and treatment,* ed 35, Norwalk, Conn, 1996, Appleton & Lange.

26. Travell JG, Simons DG: *Myofascial pain and dysfunction: the trigger point manual,* vol 2, Baltimore, 1992, Williams & Wilkins.

27. Vear HJ: *Chiropractic standards of practice and quality of care,* Gaithersburg, Md, 1992, Aspen Publishers.
28. Vernon H, Mior S: The Neck Disability Index: a study of reliability and validity, *J Manipulative Physiol Ther* 15(1), 1992.
29. Werbach MR: *Nutritional influences on illness,* ed 2, Tarzana, Calif, 1996, Third Line Press.
30. Werbach MR, Murray MT: *Botanical influences on illness,* Tarzana, Calif, 1994, Third Line Press.
31. Yochum TR, Rowe LJ: *Essentials of skeletal radiology,* ed 2, Baltimore, 1995, Williams & Wilkins.

Cervical Spondylosis

DAVID M. BRADY, KEVIN PRINGLE, AND LEW HUFF

DEFINITION

A chronic disorder characterized by osteoarthritic changes of the facet joints, IV disk space narrowing, and osteophyte formation, with or without neurological symptoms.

ETIOLOGY

Cervical strains/sprains and repetitive trauma can lead to disk injuries. Postsurgical changes and metabolic disorders of articular cartilage may also be causative factors.

SIGNS AND SYMPTOMS

Pain Patterns

Neck pain may be limited to the posterior neck muscles or may radiate to the occiput, anterior chest wall, shoulders, arms, or hands. Pain may be increased by passive or active movements of the neck. Pain and paresthesia may be distributed along dermatomal patterns over the arms.

Other Findings

Diminished ranges of motion of the neck. Associated cervicogenic headaches. Disk degeneration is more common after the age of 40 years but is a normal part of the aging process. Degenerative changes may lead to vertebrobasilar ischemia, ataxia, and vertigo.

RADIOGRAPHIC FINDINGS

Decreased cervical lordosis, decreased disk height, osteophytosis, sclerosis, and eburnation of the uncovertebral joints
Subchondral osteoporosis
IVF encroachment
Anterior/posterior osteophytes

POSTERIORLY DIRECTED OSTEOPHYTES

SPECIAL NOTE: All cervical lateral films with spondylosis must be checked for posteriorly directed osteophytes. Although anterior osteophytes may be very apparent and striking in appearance, the posteriorly directed spurs are of major clinical significance. They are, however, often overlooked. The posterolaterally directed spur has the ability to occlude the intervertebral foramena and cause IVF encroachment, resulting in nerve root compression syndromes. It can also cause cervical canal stenosis and impinge the cord if it is directed posteriorly. The canal diameter must be measured (from the most posterior portion of the spur to the spinolaminar junction) and compared with minimum safe values for the segmental level involved.[36] If cervical canal stenosis is present, manipulation should not be performed at that level. Traction and myofascial modalities should be used. If clinical symptoms or signs of cord compression exist, MRI with axial images and a referral for a neurosurgical consultation is warranted.

DIFFERENTIAL DIAGNOSIS

Strains/sprains
Herniated disk
Compression fracture
Diffuse idiopathic skeletal hyperostosis (DISH)
Ankylosing spondylitis
(See Fig. 1, pg. 58)

TREATMENT GOALS

1. Promote soft tissue healing.
2. Relieve pain and prevent recurrence.
3. Increase pain-free ranges of motion.

4. Restore normal strength and stability to joint structure.
5. Quickly change to rehabilitation or restoration of function.

MANAGEMENT PROTOCOL (OPTIONS)

- Wear cervical collar throughout majority of the day for 2 weeks to decrease pain and separate joint spaces in severe cases.
- Cervical traction: Start with 10 lb or 5% of body weight. Increase weight by 2 lb per session until reaching 40 lb maximum. Head held at 25 to 58 degrees of flexion, seated or supine.
- Myofascial stripping techniques: Use a sticky massage cream, traction the skin and lock in, very slowly apply moderate to strong pressure while moving slowly along the course of the involved muscle groups.
- Ultrasound (pulsed) at 0.5 to 1.0 W/cm^2 over cervical paraspinal muscles followed by moist heat applications and ROM exercises. Breaks up fibrotic adhesions, reduces muscle spasms, and increases range of motion.
- Adjust cervical and upper thoracic subluxations.

Clinical Note

1996 Rand Study revealed that cervical spine manipulation and/or mobilization may provide at least short-term pain relief and ROM enhancement in persons with subacute or chronic neck pain.[5]

- Active and passive ROM exercises with rest periods using a cervical pillow.
- Trigger point therapy: Apply moderate pressure over the painful nodule within the muscle belly for 5 to 7 seconds. Release and repeat 3 times. This pressure induces ischemia and forces muscle relaxation via resetting of the abnormal reflex arc.
- Administration and utilization of an "outcome assessment" questionnaire, such as the Neck Disability Index, is strongly recommended to gauge patient progress, suggest alterations

in treatment protocol, and determine the level of disability, if any.[31] (See Appendix C.)

NUTRITIONAL MANAGEMENT PROTOCOL (OPTIONS)

- Glucosamine sulfate (1500 mg per day in divided dosages)
- Vitamin C (3000-6000 mg per day in divided dosages)
- Iron (glycinate) (8-12 mg per day in divided dosages)
- Alpha-ketoglutaric acid (15 mg per day in divided dosages)

The above three nutrients are required for the hydroxylation of L-proline to L-hydroxyproline, which is needed for the production of quality collagen.

- Calcium (400 mg tid)
- Vitamin E (200 IU per day)
- Zinc (glycinate) (12-18 mg per day in divided dosages)
- Copper (glycinate) (600-900 µg per day in divided dosages)
- Manganese (glycinate) (4-6 mg per day in divided dosages)

The four above provide an antioxidant effect and serve as free radical scavengers to help remove cellular debris and promote healing. Zinc, copper, and manganese act as cofactors and catalysts for the potent antioxidant enzyme superoxide dismutase (SOD) and are therefore referred to as the *SOD induction complex.*

Most of the above nutrients can be obtained in the formulary product Collagenics Intensive Care (Metagenics, Inc.). Other manufactures make similar formulary products designed to aid in degenerative joint disease and usually contain glucosamine and/or chondroitin sulfate. Consult the catalog of the reputable venders you use for alternate products.

HOME CARE PROTOCOL (OPTIONS)

- Avoid rapid neck movements.
- Avoid cervical hyperextension and hyperflexion.
- Stretching and ROM exercises under a moderately hot shower.

REFERENCES

1. Balch JF, Balch PA: *Prescription for natural healing,* Wayne, NJ, 1990, Avery Publishing.
2. Bland JH, Cooper SM: Osteoarthritis: a review of the cell biology involved and evidence for reversibility, management rationally

related to known genesis and pathophysiology, *Semin Arthritis Rheum* 14(2):106, 1984.

3. Brukner P: *Clinical sports medicine,* New York, 1993, McGraw-Hill.

4. Bucci LR: *Nutrition applied to injury rehabilitation and sports medicine,* Boca Raton, Fla, 1995, CRC Press.

5. Coulter ID, et al: The appropriateness of manipulation and mobilization of the cervical spine, *Rand Study,* 1996.

6. D'Ambrosio E, et al: Glucosamine sulfate: a controlled clinical investigation in arthrosis: *Pharmatherapeutica* 2(8):504-508, 1981.

7. Davis CD, Greger JL: Longitudinal changes of manganese-dependent superoxide dismutase and other indexes of manganese and iron status in women, *Am J Clin Nutr* 55:747, 1992.

8. Downer AH: *Physical therapy procedures,* ed 4, Springfield, Ill, 1988, Charles C Thomas.

9. Drovanti A, et al: Oral glucosamine sulfate in osteoarthritis: a placebo controlled double-blind investigation, *Clin Ther* 3(4):260-272, 1980.

10. Fauci A, et al: *Harrison's principles of internal medicine*, ed 13, New York, 1994, McGraw-Hill.

11. Gatterman M: *Chiropractic management of spine related disorders,* Baltimore, 1990, Williams & Wilkins.

12. Grabowski RJ: *Current nutritional therapy,* San Antonio, Tex, 1993, Image Press.

13. Hammer W: *Functional soft tissue examination and treatment by manual methods,* Gaithersburg, Md, 1991, Aspen Publishers.

14. Kamimura M: Anti-inflammatory activity of vitamin E, *J Vitaminol* 18(4):204-209, 1972.

15. Lawrence D: *Fundamentals of chiropractic diagnosis and management,* Baltimore, 1991, Williams & Wilkins.

16. Liebenson C: *Rehabilitation of the spine,* Baltimore, 1996, Williams & Wilkins.

17. MacMillan D: Cervical spondylosis, *J Can Chiropr Assoc* 9(5), 1965.

18. *Manual of medical therapeutics (the Washington manual),* ed 27, Boston, 1992, Little, Brown.

19. Niki E: Interaction of ascorbate and alpha-tocopherol, *Third Conference on Vitamin C* 498:187-189, 1987.

20. Nimmo R: Receptor, effecters and tonus: a new approach, *J Natl Chiropr Assoc,* November 1957.

21. Rakel RE: *Textbook of family practice,* ed 5, Philadelphia, 1996, WB Saunders.

22. Resnick D: *Diagnosis of bone and joint disorders,* vol 3, ed 2, Philadelphia, 1987, WB Saunders.

23. The role of distraction in improving the space available for the cord in cervical spondylosis, *Spine* 20(7), 1995.

24. Schneider MJ: Chiropractic management of myofascial and muscular disorders. In Lawrence D, ed: *Advances in chiropractic,* vol 3, D. Lawrence, Mosby -Year Book, Inc. 1996

25. Schwartz RI, et al: Ascorbate can act as an inducer of collagen pathway because most steps are tightly coupled, *Third Conference on Vitamin C* 498:172-184, 1987.

26. Scully RM, Barnes MR: *Physical therapy,* Philadelphia, 1989, JB Lippincott.

27. Tenderness at motor points: an aid in the diagnosis of pain in the shoulder referred from the cervical spine, *J Am Osteopath Assoc* 77(30), 1977.

28. Tierney LM, McPhee SJ, Papadakis MA: *Current medical diagnosis and treatment,* ed 35, Norwalk, Conn, 1996, Appleton & Lange.

29. Travell JG, Simons DG: *Myofascial pain and dysfunction: the trigger point manual,* vol 2, Baltimore, 1992, Williams & Wilkins.

30. Vear HJ: *Chiropractic standards of practice and quality of care,* Gaithersburg, Md, 1992, Aspen Publishers.

31. Vernon H, Mior S: The Neck Disability Index: a study of reliability and validity, *J Manipulative Physiol Ther* 15(1), 1992.

32. Weaver K: Magnesium and its role in vascular reactivity and coagulation, *Contemp Nutr* 12(3), 1987.

33. Werbach MR: *Nutritional influences on illness,* ed 2, Tarzana, Calif, 1996, Third Line Press.

34. Werbach MR, Murray MT: *Botanical influences on illness,* Tarzana, Calif, 1994, Third Line Press.

35. White AA, Panjabi MM: *Clinical biomechanics of the spine,* Philadelphia, 1990, JB Lippincott.

36. Yochum TR, Rowe LJ: *Essentials of skeletal radiology,* ed 2, Baltimore, 1995, Williams & Wilkins.

37. Zhixiang S: Manipulative treatment of 12 cases of cervical spondylosis with trigeminal neuralgia, *J Tradit Chin Med* 2(2), 1982.

Herniated Cervical Disk

MIKELL SUZANNE PARSONS AND LEW HUFF

DEFINITION

A rupture of the anulus fibrosus, which may allow the nucleus to impinge on a cervical nerve root or the thecal sac, causing pain and paresthesia. Usually unilateral but may be central and involve both nerve roots. Most often the C5 or C6 nerve root is involved.

ETIOLOGY

Progressive degenerative processes set the stage for disk herniation. Trauma or whiplash may induce a sudden herniation. Most patients have no history of trauma.

SIGNS AND SYMPTOMS (WITHOUT CORD INVOLVEMENT)

Location

Lower neck pain, which may radiate to the extremities or chest. Pain over the trapezius, tip of shoulder, anterior upper arm, hands, and thumb.

Timing

Exacerbations and remissions are common, with increased pain and duration with each subsequent attack. Pain increases with forward flexion of the neck. Characterized by severe night pain. Pain may be relieved with upright posture and walking.

Observation

Head may be held in antalgic posture with neutral flexion and deviation away from side of pain. Decreased cervical range of motion with pain upon movements.

Palpation

Palpable tenderness over the neck muscles, cervical myospasms, hypoesthesia over the sixth and seventh cervical dermatomes. Local pain over the site of herniation.

Pain Pattern

Pain and paresthesia may radiate to arms and fingers, along the C6, C7, and C8 dermatome patterns. Aggravated by cough, sneeze, or strain. Pain and decreased ranges of motion with active and passive movements. Pain may be sudden and severe.

Neurological Manifestations

Weakness of affected muscles. Decreased deep tendon reflexes of the biceps, triceps, and/or brachioradialis. Weakness of forearms and hands associated with muscle atrophy.

COMPLICATIONS

There may be posterior ligamentous changes leading to a posterolateral herniation impinging on the spinal cord or nerve roots. A straight midline posterior herniation is an **acute surgical emergency** that can cause paraplegia or inhibit the breathing process. Cervical cord compression may lead to spastic paraparesis of the lower limbs.

ORTHOPEDIC FINDINGS

(+) Valsalva's maneuver
(+) Cervical compression
(+) Swallowing sign possible
(+) Bakody's sign
(See Fig. 1, pg. 58)

RADIOGRAPHIC FINDINGS

MRI is the study of choice, followed by computed tomography (CT) scan, electromyography (EMG), and nerve conduction velocity (NCV) study. Loss of cervical lordosis, scoliosis in the sagittal plane, narrowed IV disk spaces, disk material compressing a nerve root.

DIFFERENTIAL DIAGNOSIS

Subluxation complex
Trauma, fracture
Spinal stenosis, tumor
Facet trophism
TOS
Neoplasms
Myofascial pain syndrome
IVF encroachment

TREATMENT GOALS

1. Promote soft tissue healing.
2. Relieve pain and prevent recurrence.
3. Increase pain-free ranges of motion.
4. Restore normal strength and stability to joint structure.
5. Quickly change to rehabilitation or restoration of function.

MANAGEMENT PROTOCOL (OPTIONS)

- Bed rest: no longer than 3 days to decrease inflammation. Every additional day of bed rest may produce weeks of additional rehabilitation.[14]
- Soft or hard cervical collar: no longer than 10 to 14 days.
- Ice packs at 15 to 20 minutes over the cervical region when acute to reduce edema. During chronic stages, use moist hot packs followed by slow ROM exercises to increase ranges of motion and reduce scalene muscle spasms.
- Trigger point therapy (Nimmo/receptor tonus): Apply moderate pressure to patient's tolerance, over the nodule located within the taut band of muscle, for 5 to 7 seconds, then release. Treat each point up to 3 times per session and

a maximum of every other day. This will induce muscle relaxation by resetting the abnormal reflex.

- Ultrasound (pulsed) over related muscle tissues. Pulsed at 0.5 W/cm^2 at 5 to 8 minutes followed by stretching exercises and moist heat applications.
- Electrical muscle stimulation: select setting that will induce muscle contraction to the point of fatigue.
- In acute phase of cervical disk herniation with neurological deficits, manipulation and mobilization are **contraindicated** because of the high risk of spinal cord compression. Once a recovery of neurological deficits has occurred, manipulation may be attempted.
- Gentle adjusting of cervical and upper thoracic subluxations. Do not adjust with acute pain. When pain subsides, use gentle adjustments at first. Do not adjust in a position that reproduces pain.

Clinical Note

1996 Rand Study revealed that cervical spine manipulation and/or mobilization may provide at least short-term pain relief and ROM enhancement in persons with subacute or chronic neck pain.[7]

- A program of progressive exercises should be initiated after no longer than 2 to 3 days of bed rest.
- An objective functional assessment should occur if more than 2 weeks of treatment are required.
- Administration and utilization of an "outcome assessment" questionnaire, such as the Neck Disability Index, is strongly recommended to gauge patient progress, suggest alterations in treatment protocol, and determine the level of disability, if any.[34] (See Appendix C.)
- Check motor, sensory, and reflexes **each visit**. Consider a neurological consultation.
- If after 2 to 3 weeks of conservative care the patient shows no improvement or the condition worsens, an **MRI or referral** to a neurosurgeon may be appropriate.

NUTRITIONAL MANAGEMENT PROTOCOL (OPTIONS)

Muscle Spasms:
- Valerian root *(Valeriana officinalis)* (100 mg q4h)
- Passion flower *(Passiflora incarnata)* (100-200 mg q4h)
- Magnesium (citrate) (100 mg q4h)
- Calcium (lactate) (50 mg q4h)

Many vendors offer formulary products with the above elements, including Valerian Daytime/Calmicin Plus (Murdock Madaus Schwabe) and Myoplex/Myoplex PM (Metagenics, Inc.).

Inflammation:
- Proteolytic enzymes, such as trypsin, chymotrypsin, and bromelin (3-4 tablets qid between meals). **Caution**: do not give to patients with ulcers.
- Bioflavonoids, such as quercetin, hesperidin, and rutin (200 mg of mixed bioflavonoids q2h in acute phase).
- Herbals, such as boswellia, ginger, turmeric, cayenne (400 mg, 300 mg, 200 mg, 50 mg, respectively, q2h acute phase).

The above proteolytic enzymes can be obtained in Biozyme (Metagenics, Inc.) or Lyso-Lyph Forte (Nutri-West, Inc.). Inflavonoid Intensive Care (Metagenics, Inc.) will provide the above bioflavonoids and herbals.
- Vitamin C (3000 mg daily)

Tissue Healing:
- Glucosamine sulfate (1500 mg per day in divided dosages). Supplies the needed nutrients for the production of healthy ground substance.
- Vitamin C (3000-6000 mg per day in divided dosages).
- Iron (glycinate) (8-12 mg per day in divided dosages).
- Alpha-ketoglutaric acid (15 mg per day in divided dosages).

The above three nutrients are required for the hydroxylation of L-proline to L-hydroxyproline, which is needed for the production of quality collagen.
- Calcium (400 mg tid)
- Vitamin E (200 IU per day)
- Zinc (glycinate) (12-18 mg per day in divided dosages)
- Copper (glycinate) (600-900 µg per day in divided dosages)
- Manganese (glycinate) (4-6 mg per day in divided dosages)

The above provide antioxidant effect and serve as free radical scavengers to help remove cellular debris and promote healing.

The zinc, copper, and manganese act as cofactors and catalysts for the potent antioxidant enzyme SOD and are therefore referred to as the *SOD induction complex*. Oral supplementation with SOD can be attempted; however, it has been reported that it is often destroyed in the stomach and intestinal tract before assimilation. SOD can be obtained in Cell Guard (Biotec Foods).

All of the above tissue-healing nutrients can be obtained in the product Collagenics Intensive Care (Metagenics, Inc.).

HOME CARE PROTOCOL

- Bed rest with cervical halter traction: start with low weight (10 lb or 5% of body weight) and increase weight by 2 lb per session until you reach a maximum of 40 lb. Head at 25 to 58 degrees of flexion, seated or supine.
- Wear a light cervical collar for 23 hours per day for 2 weeks and reevaluate (severe cases only).
- Avoid activities that require hyperflexion or hyperflexion of the cervical spine.
- Use a cervical pillow.
- Get a lot of sleep (8 to 10 hours daily).
- Apply moist heat for muscle spasms.

REFERENCES

1. Balch JF, Balch PA: *Prescription for natural healing*, 1990, Avery Publishing.
2. Bland JH, Cooper SM: Osteoarthritis: a review of the cell biology involved and evidence for reversibility, management rationally related to know genesis and pathophysiology, *Semin Arthritis Rheum* 14(2):106, 1994.
3. Brouillette D, Gurske D: Treatment of cervical radiculopathy caused by a herniated cervical disc, *J Manipulative Physiol Ther* 17:119-123, 1994.
4. Brukner P: *Clinical sports medicine*, New York, 1993, McGraw-Hill.
5. Bucci LR: *Nutrition applied to injury rehabilitation and sports medicine*, Boca Raton, Fla, 1995, CRC Press.
6. Cichoke AJ, Marty L: The use of proteolytic enzymes with soft-tissue athletic injuries, *Am Chiropr*, October 1981, p 32.
7. Coulter ID, et al: The appropriateness of manipulation and mobilization of the cervical spine, *Rand Study*, 1996.

8. D'Ambrosio E, et al: Glucosamine sulfate: a controlled clinical investigation in arthrosis, *Pharmatherapeutica* 2(8):504-508, 1981.

9. Downer AH: *Physical therapy procedures*, ed 4, Springfield, Ill, 1988, Charles C Thomas.

10. Drovanti A, et al: Oral glucosamine sulfate in osteoarthritis: a placebo controlled double-blind investigation, *Clin Ther* 3(4):260-272, 1980.

11. Fauci A, et al: *Harrison's principles of internal medicine*, ed 13, New York, 1994, McGraw-Hill.

12. Gatterman M: *Chiropractic management of spine related disorders*, Baltimore, 1990, Williams & Wilkins.

13. Grabowski RJ: *Current nutritional therapy*, San Antonio, Tex, 1993, Image Press.

14. Hammer W: *Functional soft tissue examination and treatment by manual methods*, Gaithersburg, Md, 1991, Aspen Publishers.

15. Havsteen B: Flavinoids, a class of natural products of high pharmacological potency, *Biochem Pharmacol* 33(24):3933-3939, 1984.

16. Lawrence D: *Fundamentals of chiropractic diagnosis and management*, Baltimore, 1991, Williams & Wilkins.

17. Liebenson C: *Rehabilitation of the spine*, Baltimore, 1996, Williams & Wilkins.

18. Lindahl O, Lindwall L: Double blind study of a *Valerian* preparation, *Pharmacol Biochem Behav* 32(4):10065-10066, 1989.

19. *Manual of medical therapeutics (the Washington manual)*, ed 27, Boston, 1992, Little, Brown.

20. *The Merck manual*, ed 16, Rahway, NJ, 1992, Merck Co.

21. Nimmo R: Receptor, effecters and tonus: a new approach, *J Natl Chiropr Assoc*, November 1957.

22. Rakel RE: *Conn's current therapy*, Philadelphia, 1996, WB Saunders.

23. Rakel RE: *Textbook of family practice*, ed 5, Philadelphia, 1996, WB Saunders.

24. Schestack R: *Handbook of physical therapy*, ed 3, New York, 1977, Springer-Verlag.

25. Schneider M: *Principles of manual trigger point therapy*, 1994, Michael Schneider.

26. Schwartz RI, et al: Ascorbate can act as an inducer of collagen pathway because most steps are tightly coupled, *Third Conference on Vitamin C*, 498:172-184, 1987.

27. Scully RM, Barnes MR: *Physical therapy*, Philadelphia, 1989, JB Lippincott.

28. Speroni E, Minghetti A: Neuropharmacological activity of extracts from *Passiflora incarnata, Planta Med* 54(6):488-491, 1988.

29. Taraye JP, Lauressergues H: Advantages of combination of proteolytic enzymes, flavonoids and ascorbic acid in comparison with non-steroid inflammatory drugs, *Arzneimittelforschung* 27(1):144-149, 1977.

30. Taylor RB: *Manual of family practice,* Boston, 1996, Little, Brown.
31. Tierney LM, McPhee SJ, Papadakis MA: *Current medical diagnosis and treatment,* Norwalk, Conn, 1996, Appleton & Lange.
32. Travell J, Simons DG: *Myofascial pain and dysfunction: the trigger point manual,* vol 1, Baltimore, 1983, Williams & Wilkins.
33. Vear HJ: *Chiropractic standards of practice and quality of care,* Gaithersburg, Md, 1992, Aspen Publishers.
34. Vernon H, Mior S: The Neck Disability Index: a study of reliability and validity, *J Manipulative Physiol Ther* 15(1), 1992.
35. Werbach MR: *Nutritional influences on illness,* ed 2, Tarzana, Calif, 1996, Third Line Press.
36. Werbach MR, Murray MT: *Botanical influences on illness,* Tarzana, Calif, 1994, Third Line Press.
37. White AA, Panjabi MM: *Clinical biomechanics of the spine,* Philadelphia, 1990, JB Lippincott.

Whiplash Injury of the Cervical Spine: General Overview

DAVID M. BRADY

INITIAL EVALUATION

When confronted with a whiplash injury patient, a detailed explanation of the accident should be elicited along with the standard medical history information. The medical history can be collected by using a convenient mnemonic, such as OPPQRST, FAOMASH, and AMPLE. Patients who have suffered very minor trauma with minimal complaints, and those presenting with low-grade chronic symptomology from an accident that occurred a significant amount of time ago, can be examined in the normal fashion. If the history reveals that the patient has sustained a significant acute cervical spine trauma, it is most prudent to place the patient in a hard cervical collar. A brief physical examination should then be conducted, including vital signs and funduscopy and otoscopy. A brief assessment of the patient's neurological status should then be performed to include pupillary constriction, DTRs, motor and sensory of the upper and lower extremities, and cranial nerve examination. Any indication of concussion or closed head trauma should result in a **referral** for immediate neurological consultation. Radiographic assessment should then be conducted to include a neutral lateral view with the cervical collar on. If the patient was neurologically intact on initial examination and the neutral lateral scout film did not reveal any signs of unstable injury, the collar can be removed and a complete cervical trauma series (Davis series) completed to include AP, APOM, flexion, extension, oblique, and pillar views in addition to the initial neutral lateral film; and the rest of the physical examination, including ROM and orthopedic testing, can be performed. If the scout film is equivocal, the trauma series should be continued with the collar on until unstable injury is ruled out. If the patient is neurologically compromised, or if radiographs reveal an **unstable injury**, the patient should be transported to the hospital immediately.

TREATMENT

Several studies suggest that, even in cases involving considerable accident forces and significant cervical strain/sprain injuries, when no objective evidence of fracture, hematoma, or ligamentous damage is present, these conditions are self-limiting by nature. In a 4-year study on whiplash that was published in the April 1995 issue of *Spine*, a task force of 25 international experts, including a distinguished chiropractor, concluded that uncomplicated cases should follow a treatment protocol of (1) reassurance that the condition is benign and self-limiting; (2) nonnarcotic analgesics and nonsteroidal antiinflammatory agents for not more than three weeks (NOTE: I support and prefer the use of natural-based antiinflammatory agents, such as proteolytic enzymes [e.g., bromelin, trypsin], omega-3 and omega-6 fatty acids, and bioflavonoids. Natural muscle relaxants, such as valerian ropt, passiflora, magnesium, and hops can also be useful.); (3) instructions on ROM exercises; (4) a quick return to normal activities as tolerated; and (5) reassessment only if the patient is unable to resume his or her usual activities. However, **passive modalities,** such as ice, heat, electrical muscle stimulation, ultrasound, and massage, are considered optional during the first 3 weeks after injury only if objective evidence is present in the examination to warrant such care, such as swelling, muscle spasm, and loss of range of motion. An emphasis should be placed on return as soon as possible to normal activity. Spinal manipulation was also recognized in the study in *Spine* as beneficial in restoring proper joint biomechanics and aiding in complete recovery. This protocol is also fairly consistent with the *Mercy Guidelines for Uncomplicated Cases (Acute Episodes) (Chapter 8, pg. 125),* which recommends a 3- to 6-week trial of care. The study in *Spine* and the Mercy Guidelines are considered controversial within the chiropractic community because the recommended protocols propose much less lengthy passive care then has been customary in chiropractic. However, when these protocols are compared with the typical allopathic care, which consists of antiinflammatories, muscle relaxants, and, occasionally, analgesics, as well as no physical medicine, the above protocols are actually quite radical. I believe that typical allopathic and chiropractic treatment protocols for whiplash injuries are at opposite extremes and the most logical course of care lies somewhere in the middle.

The proposed treatment guidelines below are an attempt to find that middle ground. Hopefully, they will adequately take into account the need for comprehensive care for the patient, as well as the realities of cost-effective therapy as demanded in today's health care environment. In the proposed protocols, *daily treatments* are not considered as warranted for more than 1 week and should be reserved for only severe cases. A 3-times-per-week schedule is generally accepted as appropriate during the 3- to 6-week initial care period. Weekly to biweekly treatments, depending on the severity of the injury, are recommended during weeks 6 through 12. This frequency of treatment provides the best environment for tissue healing and yields the best therapeutic return for the cost. Further passive-based care should require documentation as to any complications in that particular case that would support continued long-term passive care with the clinician's reasoning for continued care. The condition is considered resolved when the patient is able to resume work or other activities, notwithstanding the presence of some residual pain or motion limitation. In cases of confirmed ligamentous laxity on flexion/extension radiographs, **manipulation is absolutely contraindicated** and immediate orthopedic and/or neurological referral would be indicated.

THERAPEUTIC GOALS

Therapeutic goals should be to improve the patient to pre-accident condition or as close to that as possible and not necessarily to achieve a pain-free status in a patient who has suffered chronic pain in the injured region before the accident. Once maximum improvement is attained, the patient should be released with documentation of residual pain or disability. *Passive therapy beyond 6 weeks in moderate whiplash and 12 weeks in severe whiplash is generally not appropriate,* although currently it is common in the chiropractic profession. The scientific literature strongly suggests that passive modalities lose their effectiveness after 3 to 4 weeks and also foster physician dependence and a feeling of helplessness in the patient. More than two modalities, in addition to manipulation, per visit have also been shown in the medical literature to be redundant and to offer diminishing clinical results that do not justify the expense of such treatment. Transition to more active-based rehabilitative care, a neurosurgical consult, or a referral to a pain management facility would be warranted if the patient does not respond favorably and return to preaccident status within 6 to 12 weeks, depending on the severity of the injury.

DOCUMENTATION

Quality documentation is critical in all patients in today's health care environment, but in few cases is it more critical than in whiplash injuries. Litigation is common in motor vehicle accidents, and the chiropractic clinician's notes are critical to this process. Third-party payers are also not willing to reimburse medical expenses, and rightly so, without proper documentation of injury and without clinical reasoning as to the efficacy of the care delivered.

The daily chart notes on these patients should clearly list subjective complaints by the patient and *visual-analog pain scale* ratings on each visit. Detailed objective findings, such as palpatory findings and any repeat examination results, should also be provided on each visit. There is also a requirement for periodic assessments on the patient's progress, including disability and pain questionnaires *(Oswestry, Neck Pain and Disability Index, VAS, etc.)* All procedures performed and treatments rendered must be listed. Exactly what area of the body on which these procedures were performed and the vertebral segmental levels involved in the manipulative procedures should be provided. Narrative reports provided commonly by chiropractic clinicians tend to only outline initial findings as of the first visit and do not reference any reevaluation findings. This is a mistake on the clinician's part because these reevaluation findings provide the data that acts as the actual documentation of patient improvement and tend to support efficacy of treatment and third-party reimbursement. If these guidelines are followed, the documentation will meet the standards as delineated in the *Mercy Guidelines for Chiropractic Quality Assurance and Practice Parameters* as minimal acceptable documentation standards for the chiropractic clinician.

Hyperflexion-Hyperextension Injury of the Cervical Spine (Whiplash Injury of the Cervical Spine)

David M. Brady and Lew Huff

DEFINITION

A hyperflexion-hyperextension injury (or vice versa) to the cervical spine involving a strain-sprain of the soft tissue structures of the cervical spine. Whiplash injuries may be complicated by fractures or dislocations.

ETIOLOGY

May be caused by automobile accident, sports injury, or work-related injury. Whiplash injuries can cause injuries to the muscle motor unit and decreased function resulting from muscle spasms, ischemia, and myositis. Chronic strain can lead to inflammatory reaction, congestion, oversecretion of fluids, increased fibrin production, and sticky adhesions between tendons and tissues.

SIGNS AND SYMPTOMS

Pain Pattern

Pain after an accident may be immediate or occur within 24 hours to weeks after trauma.[13,31] Pain may localize to shoulders and scapular regions. Pain may increase with lateral flexion, extension, or rotation of the spine. Pain is often relieved by recumbency and increased with weight bearing.

Radiation

Pain may radiate to the shoulders, midscapular region, arms to the hands.

Palpation

Moderate to severe paraspinal muscle spasms and localized myofascial trigger points. Pain and an increase in the interspinous space suggest possible interspinous ligament injury. Tenderness of the sternocleidomastoids, scalenes, and longus coli.

Systemic Manifestations

Tinnitis, Horner's syndrome, blurred vision, headaches, loss of balance, chest pain, dyspnea, nausea, vomiting, dysphagia. (See Fig. 1, pg. 58.)

Poor Recovery Signs

1. Numbness and pain in upper limbs
2. Sharp reversal of the cervical curve
3. Need for the use of a cervical collar over 12 weeks
4. Anterior head carriage

COMPLICATIONS

Retropharyngeal space should not exceed *4 mm* in an adult. Retrotracheal space should not exceed *22 mm*. (Increases may suggest inflammation or hematoma in the neck region. Significant hematoma is an indication for **immediate referral to an emergency facility**.) Atlantodental interspace (ADI) (between the odontoid and the posterior part of the anterior surface of C1) should not exceed *3 mm* in an adult or *5 mm* in a child. **Increased**

ADI is a contraindication to cervical manipulation! Degenerative joint disease (DJD) seen on x-rays of the uncovertebral joints may lead to vertebral basilar ischemia with ataxia and vertigo.

DIAGNOSIS

History
Clinical findings

ORTHOPEDIC EXAMINATION

Quadrant test
George's
Valsalva's
Foraminal compression

NEUROLOGICAL EXAMINATION

Cottonswab
Reflexes
Dermatomes
Motor challenge of the upper extremities

X-RAY FINDINGS

Loss of cervical curve, scoliosis in coronal plane
IVF encroachment, narrowed IV disk space, marked decreased flexion, rule out retropharyngeal hematoma

TREATMENT GOALS

1. Promote soft tissue healing.
2. Relieve pain and prevent recurrence.
3. Increase pain-free ranges of motion.
4. Restore normal strength and stability to joint structure.
5. Quickly change to rehabilitation and restoration of function.

DURATION

See Treatment and Therapeutic Goals sections of Whiplash Injury of the Cervical Spine: General Overview.

RECURRENCE

Rear-end collisions and having one or more dependents were associated with a higher rate of relapse or recurrence of symptoms of whiplash subjects.[35]

RETURN TO WORK

Immediate return to usual activities is recommended for grade I whiplash-associated disorders (WAD); work restrictions are not indicated. For grades II and III WAD, return to usual activity as soon as possible, typically in less than 1 week for grade II. Work alterations may be prescribed for grades II and III but should be temporary unless otherwise justified. The work alteration prescription should be reassessed within 3 weeks.[35]

Female gender, older age, married/cohabital status, and a greater number of dependents were the sociodemographic factors associated with a longer time of absence from work for whiplash. Being in a severe collision, in a vehicle other than a car or taxi, in a collision other than rear-end, and not using a seatbelt were the collision-related factors associated with a longer time of absence. Having multiple injuries was also an important prognostic factor.[35]

PHYSIOTHERAPY

Physiotherapy treatments should be given for relief of pain and to promote early mobility and are recommended primarily on the basis of consensus. Long-term physiotherapy without multidisciplinary evaluation is not justified.[35]

MANIPULATION

Manipulation by trained persons for the relief of pain and facilitating early mobility can be used in WAD. Long-term repeated manipulation without multidisciplinary evaluation is not justified.[35]

Cervical spine manipulation and/or mobilization may provide at least short-term pain relief and ROM enhancement in persons with subacute or chronic neck pain.[7]

SURGERY

Surgery for WAD patients is rarely indicated. Surgery is only indicated for WAD grade III patients with progressive neurologic deficit or persisting arm pain.[35]

MANAGEMENT PROTOCOL (OPTIONS)

Acute Phase:
- Pulsed ultrasound, electrical muscle stimulation (EMS), interferential, and ice may be used during acute inflammatory phase.

Clinical Note

Acute inflammatory phase is defined as 1 week or until patient has no pain at rest and can perform unstressed daily activities.[22]

- Apply ice packs for 15 to 20 minutes with a thin, dry towel between the patient and the ice packs. Use every 2 hours for pain reduction and reduction of edema. Ice massage: freeze ¾ cup water in Styrofoam cup, break off bottom of cup exposing about ¼ inch of frozen ice, slowly in a circular pattern massage the involved painful area for about 3 minutes.
- Instruct patient in stretching techniques under moderately hot shower at home, followed by ice applications and careful ROM exercises.
- During acute phase, use ice and gentle mobilization techniques and manipulation.[22]
- **For Severe Whiplash Cases:** Place patient in a hard cervical collar for the first 2 weeks and then reevaluate for need of continued use.

Subacute Phase:
- Subacute to chronic use moist hot packs, EMS, muscle stripping, trigger point therapy.
- In subacute phase: use pulsed ultrasound at 0.5 to 1.0 W/cm^2 at 6 to 8 minutes over affected musculature. Follow with moist hot packs heated to 270° F. With two towels between patient and hot packs, apply for 20 minutes.

- Isometric exercises and surgical tubing exercises may begin gradually. Do not begin rehabilitation until the inflammatory phase has subsided.[23] In rehabilitative phase, consider the use of short-wave diathermy and dynamic adjusting techniques.
- SPECIAL NOTE: Cervical Traction:
1. Do not use until 8th week.
2. Rule out dens (odontoid) fracture and increased apical dental interspace.
3. Start with 10 lb or 5% of body weight, increasing 2 lb per session to a maximum of 40 lb. Head held in 25 to 58 degrees of forward flexion, patient seated or supine.
4. First treatment: DJD 20 minutes, disk problem 10 minutes.
5. Discontinue if pain, dizziness, difficult breathing, increased paresthesia, or nausea develops.
- Rehabilitation:
1. Slow active stretching under the shower.
2. Slow easy ROM exercises.
3. Graduate to active range of motion with assistance, then to active range of motion with resistance.
- Timing: Subacute phase may last 4 to 6 weeks with minor to moderate injuries. Moderate to severe injuries may require 6 to 12 weeks. Added complications may prolong recovery time. A complicated case is defined as an injury with radiation of symptoms below the elbow that has lasted over 6 weeks. Soft tissue injuries are considered chronic if the patient is still experiencing pain at 16 weeks of treatment. Soft tissue healing is complete at this time except for the most severe cases.[23]
- Administration and utilization of an "outcome assessment" questionnaire, such as the Neck Disability Index, is strongly recommended to gauge patient progress, suggest alterations in treatment protocol, and determine the level of disability, if any.[39] (See Appendix C.)

Clinical Note

The early treatment of whiplash injuries helps prevent the development of facetal adhesions, dural sleeve adhesions, and osteophyte formation.

NUTRITIONAL MANAGEMENT PROTOCOL (OPTIONS)

Acute Pain and Inflammation:
- Proteolytic enzymes (trypsin, chymotrypsin, bromelin) (3-4 tablets qid in between meals). NOTE: Do not give to patients with ulcers!
- Bioflavonoids (quercetin, hesperidin, rutin, etc.) (200 mg mixed bioflavonoids q2h during acute phase)
- Herbals, such as boswellia, ginger, turmeric, cayenne (400 mg, 300 mg, 200 mg, 50 mg, respectively, q2h acute phase).

The above proteolytic enzymes can be obtained in Biozyme (Metagenics, Inc.) or Lyso-Lyph Forte (Nutri-West, Inc.). Inflavonoid Intensive Care (Metagenics, Inc.) will provide the above bioflavonoids and herbals.
- Vitamin C (3000 mg daily)

Acute Muscle Spasm:
- Valerian root *(Valeriana officinalis)* (100 mg q4h)
- Passion flower *(Passiflora incarnata)* (100-200 mg q4h)
- Magnesium (citrate) (100 mg q4h)
- Calcium (lactate) (50 mg q4h)

Many vendors offer formulary products with the above elements, including Valerian Daytime/Calmicin Plus (Murdock Madaus Schwabe) and Myoplex/Myoplex PM (Metagenics, Inc.).

Tissue Healing:
- Amino acids (glycine, L-cystine, L-proline, and L-lysine) (300-400 mg per day each in divided dosages). Supplies the amino acid pool necessary for the structural production of collagen.
- Glucosamine sulfate (1500 mg per day in divided dosages). Supplies the needed nutrients for the production of healthy ground substance.
- Vitamin C (3000-6000 mg per day in divided dosages).
- Iron (glycinate) (8-12 mg per day in divided dosages).
- Alpha-ketoglutaric acid (15 mg per day in divided dosages).

The above three nutrients are required for the hydroxylation of L-proline to L-hydroxyproline, which is needed for the production of quality collagen.
- Calcium (400 mg tid)
- Vitamin E (200 IU per day).
- Zinc (glycinate) (12-18 mg per day in divided dosages)
- Copper (glycinate) (600-900 µg per day in divided dosages)
- Manganese (glycinate) (4-6 mg per day in divided dosages)

The above provide antioxidant effects and serve as free radical scavengers to help remove cellular debris and promote healing. The zinc, copper, and manganese act as cofactors and catalysts for the potent antioxidant enzyme SOD and are therefore referred to as the *SOD induction complex.* Oral supplementation with SOD can be attempted; however, it has been reported that it is often destroyed in the stomach and intestinal tract before assimilation. SOD can be obtained in Cell Guard (Biotec Foods).

All the above tissue-healing nutrients can be obtained in the formulary product Collagenics (Metagenics, Inc.) with the exception of the glucosamine sulfate. For glucosamine sulfate, the sister product Collagenics Intensive Care (IC) must be used; however, this product does not contain the amino acid pool contained in Collagenics.

Other manufacturers make similar formulary products designed to aid in soft-tissue repair, such as Rehab Plus Complex (Professional Health Products). Consult the catalog of the reputable venders you use for alternate products.

HOME CARE PROTOCOL

- Daily gentle ROM exercises.
- Patient may swim backstroke only for first month.
- Sleep 8 to 12 hours per day.
- Do not lift over 10 lb.
- In severe cases, wear a cervical collar for the first 2 weeks, then reevaluate.
- Use a cervical pillow for sleeping.
- Gradually build to the use of surgical tubing exercises.

REFERENCES

1. Balch JF, Balch PA: *Prescription for natural healing,* 1990, Avery Publishing.
2. Bland JH, Cooper SM: Osteoarthritis: a review of the cell biology involved and evidence for reversibility, management rationally related to known genesis and pathophysiology, *Semin Arthritis Rheum* 14(2):106, 1984.
3. Brukner P: *Clinical sports medicine,* New York, 1993, McGraw-Hill.
4. Bucci LR: *Nutrition applied to injury rehabilitation and sports medicine,* Boca Raton, Fla, 1995, CRC Press.

5. Cichoke AJ, Marty L: The use of proteolytic enzymes with soft-tissue athletic injuries, *Am Chiropr,* October 1981, p 32.
6. *Common problems of the head and neck region,* Philadelphia, 1996, WB Saunders.
7. Coulter ID, et al: The appropriateness of manipulation and mobilization of the cervical spine, *Rand Study,* 1996.
8. Croft AC: Mild traumatic brain injuries after motor vehicular accidents, *Dynam Chiropr,* March 1994.
9. D'Ambrosio E, et al: Glucosamine sulfate: a controlled clinical investigation in arthrosis, *Pharmatherapeutica* 2(8):504-508, 1981.
10. Davis CD, Greger JL: Longitudinal changes of manganese-dependent superoxide dismutase and other indexes of manganese and iron status in women, *Am J Clin Nutr* 55:747, 1992.
11. Drovanti A, et al: Oral glucosamine sulfate in osteoarthritis: a placebo controlled double-blind investigation, *Clin Ther* 3(4):260-272, 1980.
12. Dvorak T, et al: Consensus and recommendations as to the side-effects and complications of manual therapy of the cervical spine, *J Man Med* (6)117-118, 1991.
13. Fauci A, et al: *Harrison's principles of internal medicine,* ed 13, New York, 1996, McGraw-Hill.
14. Gatterman M: *Chiropractic management of spine related disorders,* Baltimore, 1990, Williams & Wilkins.
15. Grabowski RJ: *Current nutritional therapy,* San Antonio, Tex, 1993, Image Press.
16. *Guidelines for chiropractic quality assurance and practice parameters, proceedings of the Mercy Center conference,* Gaithersburg, Md, 1993, Aspen Publishers.
17. Hammer W: *Functional soft tissue examination and treatment by manual methods,* Gaithersburg, Md, 1991, Aspen Publishers.
18. Hansen DT: *Chiropractic standards of practice and utilization guidelines in the care and treatment of injured workers,* 1988, Washington State Department of Labor & Industries.
19. Havsteen B: Flavinoids, a class of natural products of high pharmacological potency, *Biochem Pharmacol* 33(24):3933-3939, 1984.
20. Innes K: Double crush syndrome, *Dynam Chiropr,* April 1994.
21. Lawrence D: *Fundamentals of chiropractic diagnosis and management,* Baltimore, 1991, Williams & Wilkins.
22. Liebenson C: *Rehabilitation of the spine,* Baltimore, 1996, Williams & Wilkins.
23. Lindahl O, Lindwall L: Double blind study of a *Valerian* preparation, *Pharmacol Biochem Behav* 32(4):10065-10066, 1989.
24. *Manual of medical therapeutics (the Washington manual),* ed 27, Boston, 1992, Little, Brown.

25. *The Merck manual,* ed 16, Rahway, NJ, 1992, Merck Co.

26. Niki E: Interaction of ascorbate and alpha-tocopherol, *Third Conference on Vitamin C* 498:187-189, 1987.

27. Nimmo R: Receptor, effecters and tonus: a new approach, *J Natl Chiropr Assoc,* November 1957.

28. Rakel RE: *Conn's current therapy,* Philadelphia, 1996, WB Saunders.

29. Rakel RE: *Textbook of family practice,* ed 5, Philadelphia, 1996, WB Saunders.

30. Roland M, Morris R: Study of natural history of back pain. Part 1. Development of reliable and selective measure of disability in low back pain, *Spine* 8:141, 1983.

31. Schneider MJ: Chiropractic management of myofascial and muscular disorders. In Lawrence D, ed: *Advances in chiropractic,* vol 3, St Louis, 1996, Mosby.

32. Schwartz RI, et al: Ascorbate can act as an inducer of collagen pathway because most steps are tightly coupled, *Third Conference on Vitamin C,* 498:172-184, 1987.

33. Scully RM, Barnes MR: *Physical therapy,* Philadelphia, 1989, JB Lippincott.

34. Speroni E, Minghetti A: Neuropharmacological activity of extracts from *Passiflora incarnata, Planta Med* 54(6):488-491, 1988.

35. Spitzer O, et al: Scientific monograph of the Quebec task force on whiplash-associated disorders: redefining 'whiplash' and its management, *Spine* 20(85), 1995.

36. Taraye JP, Lauressergues H: Advantages of combination of proteolytic enzymes, flavonoids and ascorbic acid in comparison with non-steroid inflammatory drugs, *Arzneimittelforschung* 27(1):1144-1149, 1977.

37. Tierney LM, McPhee SJ, Papadakis MA: *Current medical diagnosis and treatment,* Norwalk, Conn, 1996, Appleton & Lange.

38. Travell JG, Simons DG: *Myofascial pain and dysfunction: the trigger point manual,* vol 2, Baltimore, 1992, Williams & Wilkins.

39. Vernon H, Mior S: The Neck Disability Index: a study of reliability and validity, *J Manipulative Physiol Ther* 7:409-415, 1991.

40. Watkinson A, et al: Prognostic factors in soft tissue injuries of the cervical spine, *Injury* 22(4):307-309, 1991.

41. Werbach MR: *Nutritional influences on illness,* ed 2, Tarzana, Calif, 1996, Third Line Press.

42. Werbach MR, Murray MT: *Botanical influences on illness,* Tarzana, Calif, 1994, Third Line Press.

43. White AA, Panjabi MM: *Clinical biomechanics of the spine,* Philadelphia, 1990, JB Lippincott.

Torticollis

LEW HUFF AND DAVID M. BRADY

DEFINITION

An acute spasm of the muscles of the cervical spine, resulting in a painful neck locked in a classic position of rotation with lateral flexion. Generally affects levels C2 to C7 and most commonly C2 to C3.

ETIOLOGY

May be due to a rotatory fixation of C1 and C2 secondary to vertebral subluxation, hyperextension, trauma, or recent dental work. 25% of cases have an insidious onset. Bruxism and recent sinus infection have been identified as causative factors. There are two mechanisms involved: synovial villi entrapment and the slow drift of the nucleus pulposus.

SIGNS AND SYMPTOMS

Pain Pattern

Type 1—synovial villi entrapment: sudden onset with movement, characterized by jabbing pillar pain.

Type 2—slow drift of nucleus pulposus: patient awakens with pain on one side of the neck.

Radiation

Normally there is a jabbing pain upon movement. Pain is localized to the pillar region but radiates to the gallbladder, stomach, or pericardium.

Position

Head is tilted to one side or rotated to the other side in a very antalgic position.

Palpation

Boggy end play of movements, shortened SCM muscles with intense spasms.

Ranges of Motion

Ranges of motion moderately restricted in lateral flexion and rotation.

DIFFERENTIAL DIAGNOSIS

Central nervous system (CNS) infection
Subluxation complex

ORTHOPEDIC/NEUROLOGICAL

Cervical ROM
Standard cervical ortho tests
(See Fig. 1, pg. 58)

X-RAY FINDINGS

Structural changes may be noted.

TREATMENT GOALS

1. Reduction of myospasms
2. Restoration of preinjury status
3. Restoration of full activities of daily living

MANAGEMENT PROTOCOL (OPTIONS)

- Myofascial stripping techniques: Use a sticky massage cream, traction the skin and lock in, very slowly apply moderate to strong pressure while moving slowly along the course of the involved muscle groups.
- Do not use traction.

- Short-wave diathermy: Remove metallic objects, treat involved areas; treatment time is 20 minutes. (Do not use if cause is infection.)
- Ultrasound (pulsed) at 0.5 to 1.0 W/cm^2 over cervical paraspinal muscles followed by moist heat applications and ROM exercises. Breaks up fibrotic adhesions, reduces muscle spasms, and increases range of motion. (Do not use if cause is infection.)
- Trigger point therapy: Apply moderate pressure over the painful nodule within the muscle belly for 5 to 7 seconds. This pressure induces ischemia and forces muscle relaxation. Repeat 3 times.
- Electrical muscle stimulation: Select setting that will induce muscle contraction to the point of fatigue.
- Transverse friction massage: A deep tissue massage at the site of involvement, stroking perpendicular to the fiber alignment to increase fiber mobility without longitudinal stress. This promotes orientation of fibers and induces hyperemia to hypovascular tissues.
- Adjust all subluxations, especially CO, C1, and C1, C2.

Clinical Note

Cervical spine manipulation and/or mobilization may provide at least short-term pain relief and ROM enhancement in persons with subacute or chronic neck pain.[3]

- Postcontraction stretch to SCM. Postisometric relaxation technique.
- Administration and utilization of an "outcome assessment" questionnaire, such as the Neck Pain Disability Index, is strongly recommended to gauge patient progress, suggest alterations in treatment protocol, and determine the level of disability, if any.[29] (See Appendix C.)

NUTRITIONAL MANAGEMENT PROTOCOL (OPTIONS)

Directed at muscle spasm:
- Valerian root *(Valeriana officinalis)* (100 mg q4h)
- Passion flower *(Passiflora incarnata)* (100-200 mg q4h)

- Magnesium (citrate) (100 mg q4h)
- Calcium (lactate) (50 mg q4h)

Many vendors offer formulary products with the above elements, including Valerian Daytime/Calmicin Plus (Murdock Madaus Schwabe) and Myoplex/Myoplex PM (Metagenics, Inc.).

REFERENCES

1. Balch JF, Balch PA: *Prescription for natural healing,* 1993, Avery Publishing.
2. Brukner P: *Clinical sports medicine,* New York, 1993, McGraw-Hill.
3. Coulter ID, et al: The appropriateness of manipulation and mobilization of the cervical spine, *Rand Study,* 1996.
4. Downer AH: *Physical therapy procedures,* ed 4, Springfield, Ill, 1988, Charles C Thomas.
5. Fauci A, et al: *Harrison's principles of internal medicine,* ed 13, New York, 1994, McGraw-Hill.
6. Gatterman M: *Chiropractic management of spine related disorders,* Baltimore, 1990, Williams & Wilkins.
7. Grabowski RJ: *Current nutritional therapy,* San Antonio, Tex, 1993, Image Press.
8. Hammer W: *Functional soft tissue examination and treatment by manual methods,* Gaithersburg, Md, 1991, Aspen Publishers.
9. Hammond B: Torticollis, *Eur J Chiropr* 31(3), 1983.
10. Hyman C: Chiropractic adjustments and congenital torticollis with facial asymmetry: a case study, *Int Rev Chiropr* 52(5), 1996.
11. Lawrence D: *Fundamentals of chiropractic diagnosis and management,* Baltimore, 1991, Williams & Wilkins.
12. Liebenson C: *Rehabilitation of the spine,* Baltimore, 1996, Williams & Wilkins.
13. Lindahl O, Lindwall L: Double blind study of a *Valerian* preparation, *Pharmacol Biochem Behav* 32(4):10065-10066, 1989.
14. *Manual of medical therapeutics (the Washington manual),* ed 27, Boston, 1992, Little, Brown.
15. *The Merck manual,* ed 16, Rahway, NJ, 1992, Merck Co.
16. Mootz R: Facilitating high-velocity manipulation in the cervical spine, *Chiropr Techn* 8(2), 1996.
17. Nimmo R: Receptor, effecters and tonus: a new approach, *J Natl Chiropr Assoc,* November 1957.
18. Rakel RE: *Conn's current therapy,* Philadelphia, 1996, WB Saunders.
19. Rakel RE: *Textbook of family practice,* ed 5, Philadelphia, 1995, WB Saunders.
20. Schestack R: *Handbook of physical therapy,* ed 3, New York, 1977, Springer-Verlag.

21. Schneider MJ: Chiropractic management of myofascial and muscular disorders. In Lawrence D, ed: *Advances in chiropractic,* vol 3, St Louis, 1996, Mosby.

22. Scully RM, Barnes MR: *Physical therapy,* Philadelphia, 1989, JB Lippincott.

23. Speroni E, Minghetti A: Neuropharmacological activity of extracts from *Passiflora incarnata, Planta Med* 54(6):488-491, 1988.

24. Taylor RB: *Manual of family practice,* Boston, 1996, Little, Brown.

25. Tierney LM, McPhee SJ, Papadakis MA: *Current medical diagnosis and treatment,* Norwalk, Conn, 1996, Appleton & Lange.

26. Toto B: Chiropractic correction of congenital muscular torticollis, *J Manipulative Physiol Ther* 16(8), 1993.

27. Travell JG, Simons DG: *Myofascial pain and dysfunction: the trigger point manual,* vol 2, Baltimore, 1992, Williams & Wilkins.

28. Vear HJ: *Chiropractic standards of practice and quality of care,* Gaithersburg, Md, 1992, Aspen Publishers.

29. Vernon H, Mior S: The Neck Disability Index: a study of reliability and validity, *J Manipulative Physiol Ther* 15(1), 1992.

30. Werbach MR: *Nutritional influences on illness,* ed 2, Tarzana, Calif, 1996, Third Line Press.

31. Werbach MR, Murray MT: *Botanical influences on illness,* Tarzana, Calif, 1994, Third Line Press.

32. White AA, Panjabi MM: *Clinical biomechanics of the spine,* Philadelphia, 1990, JB Lippincott.

SECTION IV

Injuries to the Shoulder Joint

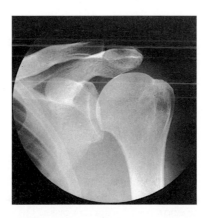

Injuries to the Shoulder Joint: General Overview

Lew Huff

DEFINITION

The glenohumeral joint relies exclusively on muscle control and tends to become dislocated with minimal injury to the ligaments. With complete tendon or ligament rupture, weakness without pain may be observed. Repair is compromised by hypovascularity. This leads to degeneration and failure of joint function.

SITE OF PAIN

The supraspinatus muscle is the most commonly ruptured of the shoulder girdle muscles.

The medial border of the scapula is a common site of referred pain from the cervical spine and shoulder muscle trigger points.

Initial pathology in shoulder injuries usually occurs in the tendons attached to the greater tuberosity, whereas the bursa is secondarily involved.

EXAMINATION

Upon deep palpation the following may be observed: edema, pinpoint tenderness, myospasms, nodules, adhesions, trigger points, and bursitis. A standing examination is preferred over a sitting one because gravity is in effect and it is easier to visualize a low shoulder and other anatomical signs. Passive extension of the elbow makes palpation easier. The nondominant shoulder is carried higher because of weaker muscles, whereas the dominant side is stronger, which pulls the shoulder girdle downward.

Full passive ranges of motion with restricted active ranges of motion may indicate muscle weakness as a cause.

With restriction of passive range of motion, look for bony or soft tissue blockage.

RADIATION, REFERRED PAIN

Pain at the glenohumeral joint is felt at the lateral brachial area and may radiate to the elbow. In shoulder tendinitis, pain may radiate to the arm and forearm. Pain may radiate from the elbow, TMJ, AC joint, cervical spine, gallbladder, liver, lungs, stomach, or spleen. Myocardial infarction (MI) may refer pain to the left shoulder. A herniated cervical disk may refer pain to the midline of the scapula.

MUSCLES

The muscle groups involved in shoulder injuries are commonly the rotator cuff muscles, or **SITS**: **s**upraspinatus, **i**nfraspinatus, **t**eres minor, and **s**ubscapularis.

SHOULDER LIGAMENTS

Shoulder ligaments are often affected or weakened by capsular fibrosis, loss of extensibility, or capsular hypertrophy.

ACTIVITIES OF DAILY LIVING

Shoulder tendinitis causes pain when putting on a jacket or reaching behind the back. Adhesive capsulitis may cause extreme difficulty when combing the hair, reaching into the hip pocket, or fastening bra or buttons.

UNINJURED AREA

Examination and, when necessary, radiographic assessment for bilateral comparison.

BURSITIS

With acute subdeltoid bursitis, intense, constant lateral brachial pain may be observed.

Most shoulder bursitis is associated with repeated microtrauma occurring in middle-age people, with degeneration of the tendon, muscle, or fibrous tissues.

Subacromial and subdeltoid bursa is easily palpated with the elbow in passive extension. Bursal thickening may be accompanied by crepitus.

Bursitis is often associated with demonstrable calcium deposition.

Predisposing factors of bursitis are bicipital tendinitis and acromioclavicular arthritis.

TENDINITIS

Commonly affects the supraspinatus in abduction, infraspinatus in external rotation, subscapularis in internal rotation, and biceps in elbow flexion.

Tendinitis is more common in short tendons without a sheath. Tenosynovitis (tendons with a sheath) is more common than tendinitis.

In shoulder tendinitis, a gradual onset of lateral brachial pain occurs.

Tendinitis is often due to aberrant biomechanics caused by a functionally weak shoulder muscle imbalancing the joint.

DURATION OF TREATMENT

Injury superimposed on preexisting condition, skeletal anomaly, and structural pathology may increase recovery time by 1.5 to 2 times.[3]

REINJURY/FLARE-UP

Restrict aggravating activities, continue care, and start low-impact rehabilitative exercises.

HOME CARE

ROM exercises, passive stretching, Codman's exercises, or wall walking may be emphasized. Surgical tubing exercises, ice applications, or compresses may be appropriate.

WHEN TO DISCHARGE

When patient has reached maximum medical improvement or the need for referral is established.

REFERRAL

If fracture, dislocation, or neurological complications are present. Daily treatment exceeding 2 weeks may signal the need for a second opinion or referral. Treatment exceeding 4 weeks or temporary disability for longer than 4 weeks with no objective signs of improvement, or worsening of the condition within the first 2 weeks, may signal the need for a second opinion or referral.

REFERENCES

1. Clemente C: *Anatomy: a regional atlas of the human body,* ed 3, Baltimore, 1987, Urban & Schwarzenberg.
2. Gatterman M: *Chiropractic management of spine related disorders,* Baltimore, 1990, Williams & Wilkins.
3. Haldeman S, et al: Guidelines for chiropractic quality assurance & practice parameters, *The Proceedings of the Mercy Center Consensus Conference,* Gaithersburg, Md, 1993, Aspen Publishers.
4. Lawrence D: *Fundamentals of chiropractic diagnosis and management,* Baltimore, 1991, Williams & Wilkins.
5. Schestack R: *Handbook of physical therapy,* ed 3, New York, 1977, Springer-Verlag.
6. Vear HJ: *Chiropractic standards of practice and quality of care,* Gaithersburg, Md, 1992, Aspen Publishers.

Acromioclavicular Joint Separation/Compression

Lew Huff and David M. Brady

DEFINITION

A traumatic separation or compression of the AC joint causing the capsule, fibers, and ligaments to be stretched beyond the plastic barrier.

ETIOLOGY

Injuries are commonly seen in sports such as volleyball, football, basketball, or skiing, or with heavy laborers and people in other occupational settings. AC joint dislocation implies a sprain of the AC and coracoclavicular ligaments.

SIGNS AND SYMPTOMS

Grade 1

Injuries without ligamentous instability, few fibers are torn, clavicle is not elevated.

Grade 2

Disruption of AC ligament, coracoclavicular ligaments remain intact. There is joint laxity, and the clavicle will subluxate less than the width of the clavicle.

Grade 3

Rupture of both the AC and coracoclavicular ligaments, clavicle will raise superior to the width of the clavicle.

Grade 4

Posterior displacement of clavicle is seen, complete ligamentous rupture.

Grade 5

Disruption of AC ligament, distal clavicle sits in a subcutaneous position toward base of neck.

Grade 6

Clavicle resides inferior to the coracoid process.

Inspection

The joint pops and clicks. Affected joint may protrude higher than the unaffected joint (Grade 3).

Pain Pattern

Local pain over the anterior shoulder (AC joint) especially with abduction or internal rotation. Pain increases with downward pressure or dangling of arm.

Differentiation

Pain upon approximation of the clavicle and acromion process indicates compression, whereas pain upon separation of the clavicle and acromion represents separation. Passive abduction and horizontal abduction produce pain. Contraction of shoulder cuff muscles or adduction is painless.

Other Manifestations

This can lead to degenerative arthritis of the joint.

DIFFERENTIAL DIAGNOSIS

Shoulder dislocation
Anterior humerus subluxation
Rotator cuff tear

ORTHOPEDIC EXAMINATION

Codman's arm drop
Apprehension
Dugas' test
Yergason's
ROM

X-RAY FINDINGS

Negative for fracture
Subluxation noted
Separation seen on x-ray

TREATMENT GOALS

1. Promote soft tissue healing.
2. Relieve pain and prevent recurrence.
3. Increase pain-free ranges of motion.
4. Restore normal strength and stability to joint structure.
5. Quickly change to rehabilitation or restoration of function.

MANAGEMENT PROTOCOLS (OPTIONS)

- Grades 1 and 2: Use conservative treatment.
- Grade 3: Try conservative treatments first, surgery possible, use Kenny-Howard brace (sling that cups elbow, causing a superior force to the AC joint while a pad applies caudal pressure to the lateral third of clavicle). Wear this brace 24 hours per day for 5 to 6 weeks.
- Adjust all cervical and thoracic subluxations.
- Adjust humerus and distal clavicle inferiorly.
- For AC separation: Approximate the clavicle and acromion 3 times per visit.
- For AC compression: Separate the clavicle from the acromion 3 times per visit.
- Ice applications for 20 minutes over AC joint.
- Gradually progress to passive and active ROM exercises.
- Isometric exercises, gradually progress to active shoulder stretching and strengthening exercises.
- Treat resulting myofascial trigger points, which may develop in rotator cuff and anterior chest musculature.

NUTRITIONAL MANAGEMENT PROTOCOL (OPTIONS)

Ligamentous Injury:
Acute Pain and Inflammation:

- Proteolytic enzymes (trypsin, chymotrypsin, bromelin) (3-4 tablets qid in between meals.) NOTE: Do not give to patients with ulcers!
- Bioflavonoids (quercetin, hesperidin, rutin, etc.) (200 mg mixed bioflavonoids q2h during acute phase)
- Herbals, such as boswellia, ginger, turmeric, cayenne (400 mg, 300 mg, 200 mg, 50 mg, respectively, q2h acute phase).

The above proteolytic enzymes can be obtained in Biozyme (Metagenics, Inc.) or Lyso-lymph Forte (Nutri-West, Inc.). Inflavonoid Intensive Care (Metagenics, Inc.) will provide the above bioflavonoids and herbals. Other manufacturers can provide quality proteolytic enzymes. Consult your product catalogs.

Tissue Healing:

- Amino acids (glycine, L-cystine, L-proline, and L-lysine) (300-400 mg per day each in divided dosages). Supplies the amino acid pool necessary for the structural production of collagen.
- Glucosamine sulfate (1500 mg per day in divided dosages). Supplies the needed nutrients for the production of healthy ground substance.
- Vitamin C (3000-6000 mg per day in divided dosages).
- Iron (glycinate) (8-12 mg per day in divided dosages).
- Alpha-ketoglutaric acid (15 mg per day in divided dosages).

The above three nutrients are required for the hydroxylation of L-proline to L-hydroxyproline, which is needed for the production of quality collagen.

- Calcium (400 mg tid)
- Vitamin E (200 IU per day)
- Zinc (glycinate) (12-18 mg per day in divided dosages)
- Copper (glycinate) (600-900 µg per day in divided dosages)
- Manganese (glycinate) (4-6 mg per day in divided dosages)

The above provide antioxidant effects and serve as free radical scavengers to help remove cellular debris and promote healing. The zinc, copper, and manganese act as cofactors and catalysts for the potent antioxidant enzyme SOD and are therefore referred to as the *SOD induction complex.* Oral supplementation with SOD can be attempted; however, it has been reported that it is often destroyed in the stomach and intestinal tract before assimilation. SOD can be obtained in Cell Guard (Biotec Foods).

All of the above tissue-healing nutrients can be obtained in the formulary product Collagenics (Metagenics, Inc.), with the exception of the glucosamine sulfate. For glucosamine sulfate, the sister product Collagenics Intensive Care (IC) must be used; however, this product does not contain the amino acid pool contained in the Collagenics. Other manufacturers make similar formulary products designed to aid in soft tissue repair, such as Rehab Plus (Professional Health Products). Consult the catalog of the reputable vendors you use for alternate products.

REFERENCES

1. Balch JF, Balch PA: *Prescription for natural healing,* Wayne, NJ, 1990, Avery Publishing.
2. Bland JH, Cooper SM: Osteoarthritis: a review of the cell biology involved and evidence for reversibility, management rationally related to known genesis and pathophysiology, *Semin Arthritis Rheum* 14(2):106, 1984.
3. Brukner P: *Clinical sports medicine,* New York, 1993, McGraw-Hill.
4. Bucci LR: *Nutrition applied to injury rehabilitation and sports medicine,* Boca Raton, Fla, 1995, CRC Press.
5. Cichoke AJ, Marty L: The use of proteolytic enzymes with soft-tissue athletic injuries, *Am Chiropr,* October 1981, p 32.
6. D'Ambrosio E, et al: Glucosamine sulfate: a controlled clinical investigation in arthrosis, *Pharmatherapeutica* 2(8):504-508, 1981.
7. Davis CD, Greger JL: Longitudinal changes of manganese-dependent superoxide dismutase and other indexes of manganese and iron status in women, *Am J Clin Nutr* 55:747, 1992.
8. Downer AH: *Physical therapy procedures,* ed 4, Springfield, Ill, 1988, Charles C Thomas.
9. Drovanti A, et al: Oral glucosamine sulfate in osteoarthritis: a placebo controlled double-blind investigation, *Clin Ther* 3(4):260-272, 1980.
10. Fauci A, et al: *Harrison's principles of internal medicine,* ed 13, New York, 1994, McGraw-Hill.
11. Grabowski RJ: *Current nutritional therapy,* San Antonio, Tex, 1993, Image Press.
12. Guidelines for chiropractic quality assurance and practice parameters, *Proceedings of the Mercy Center Conference,* Gaithersburg, Md, 1993, Aspen Publishers.

13. Hammer W: *Functional soft tissue examination and treatment by manual methods,* Gaithersburg, Md, 1991, Aspen Publishers.
14. Havsteen B: Flavinoids, a class of natural products of high pharmacological potency, *Biochem Pharmacol* 33(24):3933-3939, 1984.
15. Lawrence D: *Fundamentals of chiropractic diagnosis and management,* Baltimore, 1994, Williams & Wilkins.
16. Liebenson C: *Rehabilitation of the spine,* Baltimore, 1996, Williams & Wilkins.
17. Lindahl O, Lindwall L: Double blind study of a *Valerian* preparation, *Pharmacol Biochem Behav* 32(4):10065-10066, 1989.
18. *Manual of medical therapeutics (the Washington manual),* ed 27, Boston, 1992, Little, Brown.
19. *The Merck manual,* ed 16, Rahway, NJ, 1992, Merck Co.
20. Niki E: Interaction of ascorbate and alpha-tocopherol, *Third Conference on Vitamin C* 498:187-189, 1987.
21. Nimmo R: Receptor, effecters and tonus: a new approach, *J Natl Chiropr Assoc,* November 1957.
22. Rakel RE: *Conn's current therapy,* Philadelphia, 1996, WB Saunders.
23. Rakel RE: *Textbook of family practice,* ed 5, Philadelphia, 1995, WB Saunders.
24. Schestack R: Handbook of physical therapy, ed 3, New York, 1977, Springer-Verlag.
25. Schneider MJ: Chiropractic management of myofascial and muscular disorders. In Lawrence D, ed: *Advances in chiropractic,* vol 3, St Louis, 1996, Mosby.
26. Schwartz RI, et al: Ascorbate can act as an inducer of collagen pathway because most steps are tightly coupled, *Third Conference on Vitamin C* 498: 172-184, 1987.
27. Scully RM, Barnes MR: *Physical therapy,* Philadelphia, 1989, JB Lippincott.
28. Speroni E, Minghetti A: Neuropharmacological activity of extracts from *Passiflora incarnata, Planta Med* 54(6):488-491, 1988.
29. Taraye JP, Lauressergues H: Advantages of combination of proteolytic enzymes, flavonoids and ascorbic acid in comparison with non-steroid inflammatory drugs, *Arzneimittelforschung* 27(1):1144-1149, 1977.
30. Taylor RB: *Manual of family practice,* Boston, 1996, Little, Brown.
31. Tierney LM, McPhee SJ, Papadakis MA: *Current medical diagnosis and treatment,* Norwalk, Conn, 1996, Appleton & Lange.
32. Travell JG, Simons DG: *Myofascial pain and dysfunction: the trigger point manual,* vol 2, Baltimore, 1992, Williams & Wilkins.
33. Werbach MR: *Nutritional influences on illness,* ed 2, Tarzana, Calif, 1996, Third Line Press.

34. Werbach MR, Murray MT: *Botanical influences on illness,* Tarzana, Calif, 1994, Third Line Press.
35. White AA, Panjabi MM: *Clinical biomechanics of the spine,* Philadelphia, 1990, JB Lippincott.
36. Yochum TR, Rowe LJ: *Essentials of skeletal radiology,* ed 2, Baltimore, 1995, Williams & Wilkins.

Rotator Cuff Tear

DOUGLAS DAVISON, LEW HUFF, AND DAVID M. BRADY

DEFINITION

A common injury of the shoulder joint involving a tear or multiple tears of the rotator cuff muscles (SITS).

ETIOLOGY

May be due to a fall on an outstretched arm, overuse, impingement, abduction injury, or minor stresses in the elderly. Rotator cuff tears may be secondary to DJD or rheumatoid arthritis. These injuries are not usually due to a single event.

SIGNS AND SYMPTOMS

Grade 1

First-degree strain, minor pain, and weakness.

Grade 2

Second-degree strain, moderate impairment, and disability.

Grade 3

Third-degree strain, severe shoulder pain, 6 to 12 hours of no pain followed by gradual increase in pain and disability.

Pain Pattern

Painful or painless weakness is the chief complaint. Pain may be referred to the neck or deltoid insertion. Often pain is worse at night and localized to the region of the biceps tendon. Pain may radiate to neck.

Palpation

Palpable tenderness over the upper end of the humerus and over the individual muscles. Deltoid, supraspinatus, and infraspinatus atrophy may be present.

Ranges of Motion

Painful and diminished shoulder abduction. Large tears are characterized by inability to abduct and externally rotate the shoulder. Passive range of motion is essentially normal.

Neurological

Muscle atrophy of the supraspinatus and infraspinatus may occur within 2 to 3 weeks. Characterized by severe muscle weakness at the extreme range of shoulder abduction. The amount of weakness may help determine if it is a partial or complete tear. Muscle weakness is due to disuse atrophy. The initial weakness is due to loss of continuity of the tendon.

Other Manifestations

The healing process occurs only when torn edges are in contact; if not, fibrous tissue will fill in the spaces. Patients who have had cuff corticosteroid injections are more likely to develop tears.

Differentiation of Tendinitis and Tear

Evaluate by isometric muscle testing, which would indicate pain and relative strength with tendinitis or pain and weakness with rotator cuff tears.[23] Note that weakness may be due to pain-induced inhibition in tendinitis. Try icing to numbness before strength testing.

DIFFERENTIAL DIAGNOSIS

DJD
Cervical arthrosis

Radiculopathy
Osteophytosis
Disk herniation
Impingement syndrome
Myofascial pain syndrome

ORTHOPEDIC EXAMINATION

Codman's arm drop
Apprehension
Dugas'
Yergason's
Painful arc

X-RAY FINDINGS

Inferior malposition of humerus
Leakage of joint capsule with contrast dye
Arthrogram or MRI may be necessary
Chronic tear may reveal sclerosis and irregularity of the greater
  tuberosity
Narrowing of acromiohumeral interval to 5 mm or less

TREATMENT GOALS

1. Promote soft tissue healing.
2. Relieve pain and prevent recurrence.
3. Increase pain-free ranges of motion.
4. Restore normal strength and stability to joint structure.
5. Quickly change to rehabilitation or restoration of function.

MANAGEMENT PROTOCOL (OPTIONS)

Acute Phase:
- Apply ice packs for 15 to 20 minutes with dry towel between
  the patient and the ice packs. Use every 2 hours for
  reduction of pain and edema.
- Ice massage: Freeze ¾ cup water in Styrofoam cup, break off
  bottom of cup to expose about ¼ inch of frozen ice, and
  slowly in a circular pattern massage the involved painful area
  for about 3 minutes.
- Incomplete tears require a sling for 2 to 3 weeks.

- Ultrasound (pulsed) at 0.5 to 1.0 W/cm^2 over rotator cuff muscles followed by moist heat applications and ROM exercises. Breaks up fibrotic adhesions, reduces muscle spasms, and increases range of motion.

Subacute Phase:

- Crossed interferential current or high-volt galvanism for pain.
- Transverse friction massage: A deep tissue massage at the site of lesion, perpendicular to fiber alignment (subacute phase), to increase fiber mobility without longitudinally stressing the ligaments.
- Gentle manipulation of scapula, humerus, AC joint, sternoclavicular joint, and cervicothoracic spine.
- Passive ROM exercises when pain permits. Strengthen the dynamic shoulder stabilizers to compensate for the stretching of static stabilizers.
- Move to gradually increased active and resistive exercises, then start surgical tubing exercises.
- Any resulting chronic myofascial trigger points should be treated using ischemic compression for 5 to 7 seconds; repeat 3 times.

Surgical Referral:

Should be considered in cases of patients with severe unrelenting pain, after 3 months of conservative treatment without improvement, or in cases involving loss of shoulder function.

NUTRITIONAL MANAGEMENT PROTOCOL (OPTIONS)

Acute Pain and Inflammation:

- Proteolytic enzymes (trypsin, chymotrypsin, bromelin) (3-4 tablets qid in between meals.) Note: Do not give to patients with ulcers!
- Bioflavonoids (quercetin, hesperidin, rutin, etc.) (200 mg mixed bioflavonoids q2h during acute phase).
- Herbals, such as boswellia, ginger, turmeric, cayenne (400 mg, 300 mg, 200 mg, 50 mg, respectively, q2h acute phase).

The above proteolytic enzymes can be obtained in Biozyme (Metagenics, Inc.) or Lyso-lymph Forte (Nutri-West, Inc.). Inflavonoid Intensive Care (Metagenics, Inc.) will provide the above bioflavonoids and herbals. Other manufacturers can provide quality proteolytic enzymes. Consult your product catalogs.

Tissue Healing:

- Amino acids (glycine, L-cystine, L-proline, and L-lysine) (300-400 mg per day each in divided dosages). Supplies the amino acid pool necessary for the structural production of collagen.
- Vitamin C (3000-6000 mg per day in divided dosages).
- Iron (glycinate) (8-12 mg per day in divided dosages).
- Alpha-ketoglutaric acid (15 mg per day in divided dosages).

The above three nutrients are required for the hydroxylation of L-proline to L-hydroxyproline, which is needed for the production of quality collagen.

- Calcium (400 mg tid)
- Vitamin E (200 IU per day)
- Zinc (glycinate) (12-18 mg per day in divided dosages)
- Copper (glycinate) (600-900 μg per day in divided dosages)
- Manganese (glycinate) (4-6 mg per day in divided dosages)

The above provide antioxidant effects and serve as free radical scavengers to help remove cellular debris and promote healing. The zinc, copper, and manganese act as cofactors and catalysts for the potent antioxidant enzyme SOD and are therefore referred to as the *SOD induction complex*. Oral supplementation with SOD can be attempted; however, it has been reported that it is often destroyed in the stomach and intestinal tract before assimilation. SOD can be obtained in Cell Guard (Biotec Foods).

All of the above tissue-healing nutrients can be obtained in the formulary product Collagenics (Metagenics, Inc.).

Other manufacturers make similar formulary products designed to aid in soft tissue repair, such as Rehab Plus Complex (Professional Health Products). Consult the catalog of the reputable venders you use for alternate products.

REFERENCES

1. Balch JF, Balch PA: *Prescription for natural healing*, Wayne, NJ, 1990, Avery Publishing.
2. Bland JH, Cooper SM: Osteoarthritis: a review of the cell biology involved and evidence for reversibility, management rationally related to known genesis and pathophysiology, *Semin Arthritis Rheum* 14(2):106, 1984.
3. Brukner P: *Clinical sports medicine*, New York, 1993, McGraw-Hill.
4. Bucci LR: *Nutrition applied to injury rehabilitation and sports medicine*, Boca Raton, Fla, 1995, CRC Press.

5. Cichoke AJ, Marty L: The use of proteolytic enzymes with soft-tissue athletic injuries, *Am Chiropr*, October 1981, p 32.

6. D'Ambrosio E, et al: Glucosamine sulfate: a controlled clinical investigation in arthrosis, *Pharmatherapeutica* 2(8):504-508, 1981.

7. Davis CD, Greger JL: Longitudinal changes of manganese-dependent superoxide dismutase and other indexes of manganese and iron status in women, *Am J Clin Nutr* 55:747, 1992.

8. Downer AH: *Physical therapy procedures,* ed 4, Springfield, Ill, 1988, Charles C Thomas.

9. Drovanti A, et al: Oral glucosamine sulfate in osteoarthritis: a placebo controlled double-blind investigation, *Clin Ther* 3(4):260-272, 1980.

10. Fauci A, et al: *Harrison's principles of internal medicine,* ed 13, New York, 1994, McGraw-Hill.

11. Gatterman M: *Chiropractic management of spine related disorders,* Baltimore, 1990, Williams & Wilkins.

12. Grabowski RJ: *Current nutritional therapy,* San Antonio, Tex, 1993, Image Press.

13. Hammer W: *Functional soft tissue examination and treatment by manual methods,* Gaithersburg, Md, 1991, Aspen Publishers.

14. Havsteen B: Flavinoids, a class of natural products of high pharmacological potency, *Biochem Pharmacol* 33(24):3933-3939, 1984.

15. Leahy PM, Mock LE: Myofascial release technique and mechanical compromise of peripheral nerves of the upper extremity, *Chiropr Sports Med* 16(4):139-150, 1992.

16. Liebenson C: *Rehabilitation of the spine,* Baltimore, 1996, Williams & Wilkins.

17. Lindahl O, Lindwall L: Double blind study of a *Valerian* preparation, *Pharmacol Biochem Behav* 32(4):10065-10066, 1989.

18. *Manual of medical therapeutics (the Washington manual),* ed 27, Boston, 1992, Little, Brown.

19. *The Merck manual,* ed 16, Rahway, NJ, 1992, Merck Co.

20. Niki E: Interaction of ascorbate and alpha-tocopherol, *Third Conference on Vitamin C* 498:187-189, 1987.

21. Nimmo R: Receptor, effecters and tonus: a new approach, *J Natl Chiropr Assoc,* November 1957.

22. Rakel RE: *Textbook of family practice,* ed 5, Philadelphia, 1995, WB Saunders.

23. Rodgers JA: Rotator cuff disorders, *Am Fam Physician* 54(1):127-134, 1996.

24. Schestack R: *Handbook of physical therapy,* ed 3, New York, 1977, Springer-Verlag.

25. Schneider MJ: Chiropractic management of myofascial and muscular disorders. In Lawrence D, ed: *Advances in chiropractic,* vol 3, St Louis, 1996, Mosby.

26. Schwartz RI, et al: Ascorbate can act as an inducer of collagen pathway because most steps are tightly coupled, *Third Conference on Vitamin C* 498:172-184, 1987.

27. Speroni E, Minghetti A: Neuropharmacological activity of extracts from *Passiflora incarnata, Planta Med* 54(6):488-491, 1988.

28. Taraye JP, Lauressergues H: Advantages of combination of proteolytic enzymes, flavonoids and ascorbic acid in comparison with non-steroid inflammatory drugs, *Arzneimittelforschung* 27(1):1144-1149, 1977.

29. Taylor RB: Manual of family practice, Boston, 1996, Little, Brown.

30. Tierney LM, McPhee SJ, Papadakis MA: *Current medical diagnosis and treatment,* Norwalk, Conn, 1996, Appleton & Lange.

31. Travell JG, Simons DG: *Myofascial pain and dysfunction: the trigger point manual,* vol 2, Baltimore, 1992, Williams & Wilkins.

32. Vear HJ: *Chiropractic standards of practice and quality of care,* Gaithersburg, Md, 1992, Aspen Publishers.

33. Werbach MR: *Nutritional influences on illness,* ed 2, Tarzana, Calif, 1996, Third Line Press.

34. Werbach MR, Murray MT: *Botanical influences on illness,* Tarzana, Calif, 1994, Third Line Press.

35. White AA, Panjabi MM: *Clinical biomechanics of the spine,* Philadelphia, 1990, JB Lippincott.

Biceps Tendon Injury

KARLENE WISE, LEW HUFF, AND DAVID M. BRADY

DEFINITION

A rupture, tear, or inflammatory process that injures the biceps tendon and the transverse ligament that holds it into the bicipital groove of the humerus.

ETIOLOGY

May be due to sports or occupational injury, overuse, overstressing of the biceps muscle, or forceful movement of the arm while the biceps muscle is contracted.

SIGNS AND SYMPTOMS

Biceps tendinitis
Inspection

Heat, redness, and crepitation

Pain

Constant pain or pain with movement

Range of Motion

Decreased ranges of motion in all planes. Pain with muscle contraction, full passive ranges of motion.

Other Manifestations

Tenderness upon palpation of the bicipital groove.

Biceps Strain-Sprain
Inspection

Bulging of muscle near antecubital fossa

Pain

Painful snap often felt at bicipital groove. Pain with movement or stretching of the arm.

Range of Motion

Pain in active ranges of motion. Pain increases with forward flexion of shoulder.

Other Manifestations

Muscle spasms and edema, decreased grip strength, and crepitation.

DIFFERENTIAL DIAGNOSIS

Tendinitis
Strain
Bursitis

X-RAY FINDINGS

Bilateral comparison may show discrepancy in depth of groove
Calcification often seen on radiograph

TREATMENT GOALS

1. Promote soft tissue healing.
2. Relieve pain and prevent recurrence.
3. Increase pain-free ranges of motion.
4. Restore normal strength and stability to joint structure.
5. Quickly change to rehabilitation or restoration of function.

MANAGEMENT PROTOCOL (OPTIONS)

Acute Phase:

- **PRICES:** *p*rotect, *r*est, *i*ce, *c*ompress, *e*levate, and *s*tabilize.
- Ice massage: Freeze ¾ cup water in Styrofoam cup, break off bottom of cup exposing about ¼ inch of frozen ice, and slowly in a circular pattern massage the involved painful area for about 3 minutes.
- Crossed interferential current or high-volt galvanism for pain.
- Sling is worn for 1 to 2 weeks.

Subacute Phase:

- Transverse friction massage: A deep-tissue massage at the site of involvement, stroking perpendicular to the fiber alignment to increase fiber mobility without longitudinal stress. This promotes orientation of fibers and induces hyperemia to hypovascular tissues.
- Moist heat and ultrasound followed by muscle stripping and trigger point therapy to reduce muscle spasms.
- Passive ROM exercises when pain permits. Strengthen the dynamic shoulder stabilizers.
- Ultrasound (pulsed) at 0.5 to 1.0 waves/cm^2 over rotator cuff muscles followed by moist heat applications and ROM exercises. Breaks up fibrotic adhesions, reduces muscle spasms, and increases range of motion.
- Gentle manipulation of scapula, humerus, AC joint, sternoclavicular joint, and cervicothoracic spine. Adjust humerus into internal rotation.
- Shoulder stretching at home followed by ice applications.
- Gradually increase to surgical tubing exercises.

Surgical Referral:

If ruptured, surgical repair may be indicated, followed by therapy and rehabilitation.

NUTRITIONAL MANAGEMENT PROTOCOL (OPTIONS)

Acute Pain and Inflammation:

- Proteolytic enzymes (trypsin, chymotrypsin, bromelin) (3-4 tablets qid in between meals). NOTE: Do not give to patients with ulcers!
- Bioflavonoids (quercetin, hesperidin, rutin, etc.) (200 mg mixed bioflavonoids q2h during acute phase).
- Herbals, such as boswellia, ginger, turmeric, cayenne (400 mg, 300 mg, 200 mg, 50 mg, respectively, q2h acute phase).

The above proteolytic enzymes can be obtained in Biozyme (Metagenics, Inc.) or Lyso-lymph Forte (Nutri-West, Inc.). Inflavonoid Intensive Care (Metagenics, Inc.) will provide the above bioflavonoids and herbals. Other manufacturers can provide quality proteolytic enzymes. Consult your product catalogs.

Tissue Healing:

- Amino acids (glycine, L-cystine, L-proline, and L-lysine) (300-400 mg per day each in divided dosages). Supplies the

amino acid pool necessary for the structural production of collagen.
- Vitamin C (3000-6000 mg per day in divided dosages).
- Iron (glycinate) (8-12 mg per day in divided dosages).
- Alpha-ketoglutaric acid (15 mg per day in divided dosages).

The above three nutrients are required for the hydroxylation of ɪ-proline to ʟ-hydroxyproline, which is needed for the production of quality collagen.
- Calcium (400 mg tid)
- Vitamin E (200 IU per day)
- Zinc (glycinate) (12-18 mg per day in divided dosages)
- Copper (glycinate) (600-900 µg per day in divided dosages)
- Manganese (glycinate) (4-6 mg per day in divided dosages)

The above provide antioxidant effects and serve as free radical scavengers to help remove cellular debris and promote healing. The zinc, copper, and manganese act as cofactors and catalysts for the potent antioxidant enzyme SOD and are therefore referred to as the *SOD induction complex.* Oral supplementation with SOD can be attempted; however, it has been reported that it is often destroyed in the stomach and intestinal tract before assimilation. SOD can be obtained in Cell Guard (Biotec Foods).

All of the above tissue healing nutrients can be obtained in the formulary product Collagenics (Metagenics, Inc.).

Other manufacturers make similar formulary products designed to aid in soft tissue repair, such as Rehab Plus Complex (Professional Health Products). Consult the catalog of the reputable venders you use for alternate products.

REFERENCES

1. Balch JF, Balch PA: *Prescription for natural healing,* Wayne, NJ, 1990, Avery Publishing.
2. Bland JH, Cooper SM: Osteoarthritis: a review of the cell biology involved and evidence for reversibility, management rationally related to known genesis and pathophysiology, *Semin Arthritis Rheum* 14(2):106, 1984.
3. Brukner P: *Clinical sports medicine,* New York, 1993, McGraw-Hill.
4. Bucci LR: *Nutrition applied to injury rehabilitation and sports medicine,* Boca Raton, Fla, 1995, CRC Press.
5. Cichoke AJ, Marty L: The use of proteolytic enzymes with soft-tissue athletic injuries, *Am Chiropr,* October 1981, p 32.

6. Cipriano J: Calcific tendinitis vs chronic bursitis, *Today's Chiropractic,* Sept-Oct 1985, pp 15-16.

7. D'Ambrosio E, et al: Glucosamine sulfate: a controlled clinical investigation in arthrosis, *Pharmatherapeutica* 2(8):504-508, 1981.

8. Davis CD, Greger JL: Longitudinal changes of manganese-dependent superoxide dismutase and other indexes of manganese and iron status in women, *Am J Clin Nutr* 55:747, 1992.

9. Downer AH: *Physical therapy procedures,* ed 4, Springfield, Ill, 1988, Charles C Thomas.

10. Drovanti A, et al: Oral glucosamine sulfate in osteoarthritis: a placebo controlled double-blind investigation, *Clin Ther* 3(4):260-272, 1980.

11. Gatterman M: *Chiropractic management of spine related disorders,* Baltimore, 1990, Williams & Wilkins.

12. Grabowski RJ: *Current nutritional therapy,* San Antonio, Tex, 1993, Image Press.

13. Hammer W: *Functional soft tissue examination and treatment by manual methods,* Gaithersburg, Md, 1991, Aspen Publishers.

14. Hammer W: The use of transverse friction massage in the management of chronic bursitis of the hip and shoulder, *J Manipulative Physiol Ther* 16(2), 1993.

15. Havsteen B: Flavinoids, a class of natural products of high pharmacological potency, *Biochem Pharmacol* 33(24):3933-3939, 1984.

16. Leahy PM, Mock LE: Myofascial release technique and mechanical compromise of peripheral nerves of the upper extremity, *Chiropr Sports Med* 16(4), 139-150, 1992.

17. Liebenson C: *Rehabilitation of the spine,* Baltimore, 1996, Williams & Wilkins.

18. Lindahl O, Lindwall L: Double blind study of a *Valerian* preparation, *Pharmacol Biochem Behav* 32(4):10065-10066, 1989.

19. *The Merck manual,* ed 16, Rahway, NJ, 1992, Merck Co.

20. Niki E: Interaction of ascorbate and alpha-tocopherol, *Third Conference on Vitamin C* 498:187-189, 1987.

21. Nimmo R: Receptor, effecters and tonus: a new approach, *J Natl Chiropr Assoc,* November 1957.

22. Rakel RE: *Conn's current therapy,* Philadelphia, 1996, WB Saunders.

23. Schestack R: *Handbook of physical therapy,* ed 3, New York, 1977, Springer-Verlag.

24. Schneider MJ: Chiropractic management of myofascial and muscular disorders. In Lawrence D, ed: *Advances in chiropractic,* vol 3, St Louis, 1996, Mosby.

25. Schwartz RI, et al: Ascorbate can act as an inducer of collagen pathway because most steps are tightly coupled, *Third Conference on Vitamin C* 498:172-184, 1987.

26. Scully RM, Barnes MR: *Physical therapy,* Philadelphia, 1989, JB Lippincott.
27. Speroni E, Minghetti A: Neuropharmacological activity of extracts from *Passiflora incarnata, Planta Med* 54(6):488-491, 1988.
28. Taraye JP, Lauressergues H: Advantages of combination of proteolytic enzymes, flavonoids and ascorbic acid in comparison with non-steroid inflammatory drugs, *Arzneimittelforschung* 27(1):1144-1149, 1977.
29. Taylor RB: *Manual of family practice,* Boston, 1996, Little, Brown.
30. Travel JG, Simons DG: *Myofascial pain and dysfunction: the trigger point manual,* vol 2, Baltimore, 1992, Williams & Wilkins.
31. Vear HJ: *Chiropractic standards of practice and quality of care,* Gaithersburg, Md, 1992, Aspen Publishers.
32. Werbach MR: *Nutritional influences on illness,* ed 2, Tarzana, Calif, 1996, Third Line Press.
33. Werbach MR, Murray MT: *Botanical influences on illness,* Tarzana, Calif, 1994, Third Line Press.

Adhesive Capsulitis (Frozen Shoulder Syndrome)

KARLENE WISE, LEW HUFF, AND DAVID M. BRADY

DEFINITION

A chronic shoulder condition characterized by limited ranges of motion in all planes and inflammation of the articular synoviae, tendons, joint capsules, and bursa.

ETIOLOGY

Associated with discogenic spondylosis of C5-C7, thoracic kyphosis, and scapulohumeral misalignment. Onset is insidious, and increased prevalence in the nondominant arm is observed. Primarily affects women in the 40- to 60-year age-group. Secondary causes may be rheumatoid arthritis, osteoarthritis, fracture, dislocation, or intraarticular vascular synovitis.

SIGNS AND SYMPTOMS

Inspection

Complete inability to abduct the arm over 30 degrees. There is only scapulothoracic movement noted. Arm often held in internal rotation and adduction.

Palpation

Tenderness upon digital palpation of the deltoid insertion, bicipital groove, and greater tuberosity. Palpable tenderness over the anterior lateral humerus.

Pain Pattern

Onset of pain aggravated by extremes of shoulder joint movement. Pain may be insidious or acute. Night pain may interfere with sleep or awaken the patient. Pain with rest or activity.

Ranges of Motion

Gradual progressive restriction of all joint movements ranging from months to years. Ranges are restricted in all planes. There is a total lack of glenohumeral range of motion. Severely diminished abduction; exquisite pain on external rotation.

Location

Adhesive capsulitis most often affects the left shoulder; bilateral involvement is rare.

Weakness

There is shoulder muscle weakness and soft tissue inflammation.

Radiation of Pain

Pain most frequently radiates to the elbow joint and along the C5 dermatome.

DIFFERENTIAL DIAGNOSIS

Fracture
Contusion
Strain
Referred pain
Subacromial bursitis
Myofascial pain syndrome

ORTHOPEDIC EXAMINATION

Range of motion diminished
Codman's arm drop
Appley scratch test (+)

X-RAY FINDINGS

Negative or possible calcification
Localized osteoporosis
Chronic leads to osteopenia

TREATMENT GOALS

1. Promote soft tissue healing.
2. Relieve pain and prevent recurrence.
3. Increase pain-free ranges of motion.
4. Restore normal strength and stability to joint structure.
5. Quickly change to rehabilitation and restoration of function.

MANAGEMENT PROTOCOL (OPTIONS)

Acute Phase:

- **Forceful manipulation in the acute phase is contraindicated because of risk of tissue damage.**
- Ice massage: Freeze ¾ cup water in Styrofoam cup, break off bottom of cup exposing about ¼ inch of frozen ice, and slowly in a circular pattern massage the involved painful area for about 3 minutes.
- Ultrasound (pulsed) at 0.5 to 1.0 W/cm^2 over rotator cuff muscles followed by moist heat applications and ROM exercises. Breaks up fibrotic adhesions, reduces muscle spasms, and increases range of motion.

Subacute Phase:

- Moist heat and ultrasound followed by muscle stripping and trigger point therapy to reduce muscle spasms.
- Transverse friction massage: A deep-tissue massage at the site of involvement, stroking perpendicular to the fiber alignment to increase fiber mobility without longitudinal stress. This promotes orientation of fibers and induces hyperemia to hypovascular tissues.

- Passive ROM exercises when pain permits. Strengthen the dynamic shoulder stabilizers.
- Gentle manipulation of scapula, humerus, AC joint, sternoclavicular joint, and cervicothoracic spine.
- Scapular mobilization: Physician raises patient's scapula and shoulder girdle up, then back and down, 8 times per visit; follow with ice applications.
- Trigger point therapy to resulting trigger points of shoulder and neck musculature. Apply pressure for 5 to 7 seconds, repeat 3 times.
- Scapular and shoulder proprioceptive neurofasciculation (PNF) stretches.
- Instruct patient in Codman's pendulum exercises and wall walking:

  Codman's exercises: While seated, the patient drops arm and circumducts in clockwise and counterclockwise patterns without resistance. This allows full ranges of motion without stressing the joint. As a progression, Codman's can be done with 1- to 4-lb wrist band weight. Do not have patient hold the weight because this tightens the shoulder muscles and negates any effectiveness of this exercise.

  Wall walking: The patient attempts to use the fingers to "walk" up the wall, increasing the height of abduction at a prescribed rate. Also have patient "walk" in flexion (facing the wall).

- Gradually increase to isometric exercises and surgical tubing exercises.

  Surgical tubing exercises: at a graded level of an increasing number of repetitions and resistance.

NUTRITIONAL MANAGEMENT PROTOCOL (OPTIONS)

Acute Pain and Inflammation:

- Proteolytic enzymes (trypsin, chymotrypsin, bromelin) (3-4 tablets qid in between meals). NOTE: Do not give to patients with ulcers!
- Bioflavonoids (quercetin, hesperidin, rutin, etc.) (200 mg mixed bioflavonoids q2h during acute phase).
- Herbals, such as boswellia, ginger, turmeric, cayenne (400 mg, 300 mg, 200 mg, 50 mg, respectively, q2h acute phase).

The above proteolytic enzymes can be obtained in Biozyme (Metagenics, Inc.) or Lyso-lymph Forte (Nutri-West, Inc.). Inflavonoid Intensive Care (Metagenics, Inc.) will provide the above bioflavonoids and herbals. Other manufacturers can provide quality proteolytic enzymes. Consult your product catalog.

Tissue Healing:

- Amino acids (glycine, L-cystine, L-proline, and L-lysine) (300-400 mg per day each in divided dosages). Supplies the amino acid pool necessary for the structural production of collagen.
- Vitamin C (3000-6000 mg per day in divided dosages).
- Iron (glycinate) (8-12 mg per day in divided dosages).
- Alpha-ketoglutaric acid (15 mg per day in divided dosages).

The above three nutrients are required for the hydroxylation of L-proline to L-hydroxyproline, which is needed for the production of quality collagen.

- Calcium (400 mg tid)
- Vitamin E (200 IU per day)
- Zinc (glycinate) (12-18 mg per day in divided dosages)
- Copper (glycinate) (600-900 µg per day in divided dosages)
- Manganese (glycinate) (4-6 mg per day in divided dosages)

The above provide antioxidant effects and serve as free radical scavengers to help remove cellular debris and promote healing. The zinc, copper, and manganese act as cofactors and catalysts for the potent antioxidant enzyme SOD and are therefore referred to as the *SOD induction complex.* Oral supplementation with SOD can be attempted; however, it has been reported that it is often destroyed in the stomach and intestinal tract before assimilation. SOD can be obtained in Cell Guard (Biotec Foods).

All of the above tissue-healing nutrients can be obtained in the formulary product Collagenics (Metagenics, Inc.).

Other manufacturers make similar formulary products designed to aid in soft tissue repair, such as Rehab Plus Complex (Professional Health Products). Consult the catalog of the reputable venders you use for alternate products.

REFERENCES

1. Balch JF, Balch PA: *Prescription for natural healing,* Wayne, NJ, 1990, Avery Publishing.

2. Bland JH, Cooper SM: Osteoarthritis: a review of the cell biology involved and evidence for reversibility, management rationally related to known genesis and pathophysiology, *Semin Arthritis Rheum* 14(2):106, 1984.

3. Brukner P: *Clinical sports medicine,* New York, 1993, McGraw-Hill.

4. Bucci LR: *Nutrition applied to injury rehabilitation and sports medicine,* Boca Raton, Fla, 1995, CRC Press.

5. Cichoke AJ, Marty L: The use of proteolytic enzymes with soft-tissue athletic injuries, *Am Chiropr,* October 1981, p 32.

6. Cipriano J: Calcific tendinitis vs chronic bursitis, *Today's Chiropractic,* September-October 1985, pp 15-16.

7. D'Ambrosio E, et al: Glucosamine sulfate: a controlled clinical investigation in arthrosis, *Pharmatherapeutica* 2(8):504-508, 1981.

8. Davis CD, Greger JL: Longitudinal changes of manganese-dependent superoxide dismutase and other indexes of manganese and iron status in women, *Am J Clin Nutr* 55:747, 1992.

9. Drovanti A, et al: Oral glucosamine sulfate in osteoarthritis: a placebo controlled double-blind investigation, *Clin Ther* 3(4):260-272, 1980.

10. Ekelund AL, Rydell N: Combination treatment for adhesive capsulitis of the shoulder, *Clin Orthop* 282:105-109, 1992.

11. Fauci A, et al: *Harrison's principles of internal medicine,* ed 13, New York, 1994, McGraw-Hill.

12. Ferguson L: Treating shoulder dysfunction and "frozen shoulders," *Chiropr Techn* 7(3),1995.

13. Grabowski RJ: *Current nutritional therapy,* San Antonio, Tex, 1993, Image Press.

14. Hammer W: *Functional soft tissue examination and treatment by manual methods,* Gaithersburg, Md, 1991, Aspen Publishers.

15. Hammer W: The use of transverse friction massage in the management of chronic bursitis of the hip and shoulder, *J Manipulative Physiol Ther* 16(2), 1993.

16. Havsteen B: Flavinoids, a class of natural products of high pharmacological potency, *Biochem Pharmacol* 33(24):3933-3939, 1984.

17. Leahy PM, Mock LE: Myofascial release technique and mechanical compromise of peripheral nerves of the upper extremity, *Chiropr Sports Med* 6(4):139-150, 1992.

18. Lindahl O, Lindwall L: Double blind study of a *Valerian* preparation, *Pharmacol Biochem Behav* 32(4):10065-10066, 1989.

19. *Manual of medical therapeutics (the Washington manual),* ed 27, Boston, 1992, Little, Brown.

20. Niki E: Interaction of ascorbate and alpha-tocopherol, *Third Conference on Vitamin C* 498:187-189, 1987.

21. Nimmo R: Receptor, effecters and tonus: a new approach, *J Natl Chiropr Assoc,* November 1957.

22. Ogilvie-Harris D Jr, et al: The resistant frozen shoulder: manipulation vs arthroscopic release, *Clin Orthop* 319:238-248, 1995.

23. Polkinghorn BS: Chiropractic treatment of frozen shoulder syndrome (adhesive capsulitis) utilizing mechanical force, manually assisted short lever adjusting procedures, *J Manipulative Physiol Ther* 18(2), 1995.

24. Schneider MJ: Chiropractic management of myofascial and muscular disorders. In Lawrence D, ed: *Advances in chiropractic,* vol 3, St Louis, 1996, Mosby.

25. Schwartz RI, et al: Ascorbate can act as an inducer of collagen pathway because most steps are tightly coupled, *Third Conference on Vitamin C* 498:172-184, 1987.

26. Scully RM, Barnes MR: *Physical therapy,* Philadelphia, 1989, JB Lippincott.

27. Speroni E, Minghetti A: Neuropharmacological activity of extracts from *Passiflora incarnata, Planta Med* 54(6):488-491, 1988.

28. Taraye JP, Lauressergues H: Advantages of combination of proteolytic enzymes, flavonoids and ascorbic acid in comparison with non-steroid inflammatory drugs, *Arzneimittelforschung* 27(1):1144-1149, 1977.

29. Travell JG, Simons DG: *Myofascial pain and dysfunction: the trigger point manual,* vol 2, Baltimore, 1992, Williams & Wilkins.

30. Werbach MR: *Nutritional influences on illness,* ed 2, Tarzana, Calif, 1996, Third Line Press.

31. Werbach MR, Murray MT: *Botanical influences on illness,* Tarzana, Calif, 1994, Third Line Press.

32. White AA, Panjabi MM: *Clinical biomechanics of the spine,* Philadelphia, 1990, JB Lippincott.

Shoulder Tendinitis/Bursitis

Karlene Wise, Lew Huff, and David M. Brady

DEFINITION

An acute or chronic inflammatory disorder of the tendon or bursa of the shoulder often with deposition of calcium salts along the tendons or bursa. The glenohumeral joint has increased range of motion but decreased stability. This, coupled with a poor blood supply, makes it susceptible to injury and inflammation.

ETIOLOGY

May be due to overuse, microtrauma, poor posture, or a functionally weak shoulder muscle. Often referred to as *calcific tendinitis,* which is an inflammation of the capsulotendinous cuff with calcium deposition. Increased incidence in men over 40 years old, especially mechanics, painters, and laborers.

SIGNS AND SYMPTOMS

Tendinitis

Pain Pattern

Acute pain over the lateral aspect of the shoulder joint. Ranges from mild to severe pain on muscle testing and on extreme flexion and abduction.

Palpation

Ranges of motion are diminished with tenderness on digital palpation of tendon insertions.

Ranges of Motion

Painful restriction of extreme flexion and abduction. Resisted shoulder tests cause a variety of painful tendon insertions.

Bursitis (Subacromial, Subdeltoid)
Pain Pattern

Agonizing pain that increases with motion and is generally worse at night. Severe pain develops within a few days of onset.

Palpation

Palpable tenderness over the greater tuberosity, bursa, acromion, and deltoid muscle.

Ranges of Motion

Gross loss of shoulder abduction with little or no loss of internal and external rotation. Diminished active and passive ranges of motion, especially abduction. Often a painful arc of 60 to 130 degrees in bursitis. Resisted shoulder testing is less painful than with tendinitis, if at all.

Clinical Note

With tenderness, positive supraspinatus tendinitis test, and Appley's scratch test, suspect tendinitis. With crepitus, thickening, and positive Dawburn's test, suspect bursitis. Supraspinatus test: Patient seated, abduct arm against resistance while pain is felt over tendon insertion. Appley's scratch test: Patient touches opposite superior angle of scapula, then inferior angle of scapula. Pain or inability represents a positive test. Dawburn's test: Doctor applies pressure just below acromion process, abduct shoulder past 90 degrees with pressure over bursa. Pain or inability to abduct fully represents a positive test.

DIFFERENTIAL DIAGNOSIS

Cervical brachial syndrome
Osteoarthritis, gout

Pyogenic arthritis
Rotator cuff tear

X-RAY FINDINGS

Possible calcium salt deposits

TREATMENT GOALS

1. Promote soft tissue healing.
2. Relieve pain and prevent recurrence.
3. Increase pain-free ranges of motion.
4. Restore normal strength and stability to joint structure.
5. Quickly change to rehabilitation and restoration of function.
6. Identify any shoulder muscle weakness and manipulate associated nerve root level in cervical spine.

MANAGEMENT PROTOCOL (OPTIONS)

Acute Phase:

- Ice massage: freeze ¾ cup water in Styrofoam cup, break off bottom of cup, exposing about ¼ inch of frozen ice, and slowly in a circular pattern massage the involved painful area for about 3 minutes.
- Ultrasound (pulsed) at 0.5 to 1.0 waves/cm^2 over rotator cuff muscles followed by moist heat applications and ROM exercises. Breaks up fibrotic adhesions, reduces muscle spasms, and increases range of motion.

Subacute Phase:

- Moist heat and ultrasound followed by muscle stripping and trigger point therapy to reduce muscle spasms. Other options include short wave diathermy and infrared therapy.
- Gentle manipulation of scapula, humerus, AC joint, sternoclavicular joint, and cervicothoracic spine.
- Passive ROM exercises when pain permits. Strengthen the dynamic shoulder stabilizers to compensate for the stretching of static stabilizers.
- Shoulder shrugs, pull-ups, push-ups, eccentric isotonic exercises as tolerated. Limit overhead exercises (e.g., military press) until external rotators are increased in strength.

NUTRITIONAL MANAGEMENT PROTOCOL (OPTIONS)

Acute Pain and Inflammation:
- Proteolytic enzymes (trypsin, chymotrypsin, bromelin) (3-4 tablets qid in between meals). NOTE: Do not give to patients with ulcers!
- Bioflavonoids (quercetin, hesperidin, rutin, etc.) (200 mg mixed bioflavonoids q2h during acute phase).
- Herbals, such as boswellia, ginger, turmeric, cayenne (400 mg, 300 mg, 200 mg, 50 mg, respectively, q2h acute phase).

The above proteolytic enzymes can be obtained in Biozyme (Metagenics, Inc.) or Lyso-lymph Forte (Nutri-West, Inc.). Inflavonoid Intensive Care (Metagenics, Inc.) will provide the above bioflavonoids and herbals. Other manufacturers can provide quality proteolytic enzymes. Consult your product catalog.

Tissue Healing:
- Amino acids (glycine, L-cystine, L-proline, and L-lysine) (300-400 mg per day each in divided dosages). Supplies the amino acid pool necessary for the structural production of collagen.
- Vitamin C (3000-6000 mg per day in divided dosages).
- Iron (glycinate) (8-12 mg per day in divided dosages).
- Alpha-ketoglutaric acid (15 mg per day in divided dosages).

The above three nutrients are required for the hydroxylation of L-proline to L-hydroxyproline, which is needed for the production of quality collagen.
- Calcium (400 mg tid)
- Vitamin E (200 IU per day)
- Zinc (glycinate) (12-18 mg per day in divided dosages)
- Copper (glycinate) (600-900 μg per day in divided dosages)
- Manganese (glycinate) (4-6 mg per day in divided dosages)

The above provide antioxidant effects and serve as free radical scavengers to help remove cellular debris and promote healing. The zinc, copper, and manganese act as cofactors and catalysts for the potent antioxidant enzyme SOD and are therefore referred to as the *SOD induction complex.* Oral supplementation with SOD can be attempted; however, it has been reported that it is often destroyed in the stomach and intestinal tract before assimilation. SOD can be obtained in Cell Guard (Biotec Foods).

All of the above tissue-healing nutrients can be obtained in the formulary product Collagenics (Metagenics, Inc.).

Other manufacturers make similar formulary products designed to aid in soft tissue repair, such as Rehab Plus Complex (Professional Health Products). Consult the catalog of the reputable venders you use for alternate products.

REFERENCES

1. Balch JF, Balch PA: *Prescription for natural healing,* Wayne, NJ, 1990, Avery Publishing.
2. Bland JH, Cooper SM: Osteoarthritis: a review of the cell biology involved and evidence for reversibility, management rationally related to known genesis and pathophysiology, *Semin Arthritis Rheum* 14(2):106, 1984.
3. Bucci LR: Nutrition applied to injury rehabilitation and sports medicine, Boca Raton, Fla, 1995, CRC Press.
4. Cichoke AJ, Marty L: The use of proteolytic enzymes with soft-tissue athletic injuries, *Am Chiropr,* October 1981, p 32.
5. Cipriano J: Calcific tendinitis vs chronic bursitis, *Today's Chiropractic,* September-October 1985.
6. D'Ambrosio E, et al: Glucosamine sulfate: a controlled clinical investigation in arthrosis, *Pharmatherapeutica* 2(8):504-508, 1981.
7. Davis CD, Greger JL: Longitudinal changes of manganese-dependent superoxide dismutase and other indexes of manganese and iron status in women, *Am J Clin Nutr* 55:747, 1992.
8. Drovanti A, et al: Oral glucosamine sulfate in osteoarthritis: a placebo controlled double-blind investigation, *Clin Ther* 3(4):260-272, 1980.
9. Ekelund AL, Rydell N: Combination treatment for adhesive capsulitis of the shoulder, *Clin Orthop* 282:105-109, 1996.
10. Fauci A, et al: *Harrison's principles of internal medicine,* ed 13, New York, 1994, McGraw-Hill.
11. Grabowski RJ: Current nutritional therapy, San Antonio, Tex, 1993, Image Press.
12. Hammer W: The use of transverse friction massage in the management of chronic bursitis of the hip and shoulder, *J Manipulative Physiol Ther* 16(2), 1993.
13. Havsteen B: Flavinoids, a class of natural products of high pharmacological potency, *Biochem Pharmacol* 33(24):3933-3939, 1984.
14. Lawrence D: *Fundamentals of chiropractic diagnosis and management,* Baltimore, 1991, Williams & Wilkins.
15. Leahy PM, Mock LE: Myofascial release technique and mechanical compromise of peripheral nerves of the upper extremity, *Chiropr Sports Med* 16(4):139-150, 1992.
16. Liebenson C: *Rehabilitation of the spine,* Baltimore, 1996, Williams & Wilkins.

17. Lindahl O, Lindwall L: Double blind study of a *Valerian* preparation, *Pharmacol Biochem Behav* 32(4):10065-10066, 1989.

18. Niki E: Interaction of ascorbate and alpha-tocopherol, *Third Conference on Vitamin C* 498:187-189, 1987.

19. Rakel RE: *Textbook of family practice,* ed 5, Philadelphia, 1996, WB Saunders.

20. Schwartz RI, et al: Ascorbate can act as an inducer of collagen pathway because most steps are tightly coupled, *Third Conference on Vitamin C* 498:172-184, 1987.

21. Speroni E, Minghetti A: Neuropharmacological activity of extracts from *Passiflora incarnata, Planta Med* 54(6):488-491, 1988.

22. Taraye JP, Lauressergues H: Advantages of combination of proteolytic enzymes, flavonoids and ascorbic acid in comparison with non-steroid inflammatory drugs, *Arzneimittelforschung* 27(1):1144-1149, 1977.

23. Tierney LM, McPhee SJ, Papadakis MA: *Current medical diagnosis and treatment,* Norwalk, Conn, 1996, Appleton & Lange.

24. Werbach MR: *Nutritional influences on illness,* ed 2, Tarzana, Calif, 1996, Third Line Press.

25. Werbach MR, Murray MT: *Botanical influences on illness,* Tarzana, Calif, 1994, Third Line Press.

SECTION V

Injuries to the Elbow Joint

Injuries to the Elbow Joint: General Overview

Lateral and Medial Epicondylitis

Olecranon Bursitis

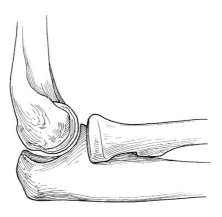

(Modified from Bontrager KL: *Textbook of radiographic positioning and related anatomy*, ed 4, St Louis, 1997, Mosby.)

Injuries to the Elbow Joint: General Overview

LEW HUFF

ELBOW INJURIES

Tennis elbow (lateral epicondylitis) and golfer's elbow (medial epicondylitis) are common injuries of the elbow joint. Although the elbow is not usually a weight-bearing joint, the hinge-and-swivel action of pronation and supination keep it in constant use.

MECHANISM OF PAIN

In lateral epicondylitis, periosteal tearing of the extensor muscle groups occur as they insert in the lateral epicondyle. In medial epicondylitis the periosteal tearing takes place at the insertion of the medial epicondyle.

SITE OF PAIN

Pain is localized to the medial or lateral epicondyle. The origin of the extensor carpi radialis longus and brevis becomes fibrotic with inflammation in lateral epicondylitis. Direct deep palpation over the lateral epicondyle is painful. Pain is intensified with wrist extension.

Pain is localized to the medial epicondyle in golfer's elbow. Deep palpation and wrist flexion increase pain.

EXAMINATION

Examine the strength of the four elbow flexors (biceps brachii, brachialis, brachioradialis, and pronator teres). Also examine the two extensors (triceps brachii and anconeus). Check range of motion and x-rays if appropriate.

RADIATION, REFERRED PAIN

Pain radiates to the ulnar aspect of the forearm, dorsum of the forearm and hand, and posterior brachial area. Referred pain to the seventh cervical segment or to the hand is common.

ACTIVITIES OF DAILY LIVING

Injury to the elbow can interfere with writing, sports activities, occupation, and lifting of heavy objects or twisting motions of the forearm and wrist.

UNINJURED AREA

Examination and radiographic examination for bilateral comparison if appropriate.

REINJURY/FLARE-UP

Restrict aggravating activities, continue care, and start low-impact rehabilitative exercises.

HOME CARE

ROM exercises, passive stretching, surgical tubing exercises, ice applications, or compresses may be appropriate.

WHEN TO DISCHARGE

When patient has reached maximum medical improvement or the need for referral is established.

REFERENCES

1. Clemente C: *Anatomy: a regional atlas of the human body,* ed 3, Baltimore, 1987, Urban & Schwarzenberg.
2. Gatterman M: Chiropractic management of spine related disorders, Baltimore, 1990, Williams & Wilkins.

3. Haldeman S, et al: Guidelines for chiropractic quality assurance & practice parameters, *The Proceedings of the Mercy Center Consensus Conference,* Gaithersburg, Md, 1993, Aspen Publishers.
4. Lawrence D: *Fundamentals of chiropractic diagnosis and management,* Baltimore, 1991, Williams & Wilkins.
5. Schestack R: *Handbook of physical therapy,* ed 3, New York, 1977, Springer-Verlag.
6. Vear HJ: *Chiropractic standards of practice and quality of care,* Gaithersburg, Md, 1992, Aspen Publishers.

Lateral and Medial Epicondylitis

LEW HUFF AND DAVID M. BRADY

DEFINITION

Lateral epicondylitis is known as *tennis elbow,* and medial epicondylitis is known as *golfer's elbow.* They are inflammatory reactions of the lateral and medial epicondyles to a tear of the common flexor tendon insertion in medial epicondylitis and a tear in the extensor insertion in lateral epicondylitis.

ETIOLOGY

May be due to trauma, microtrauma, overuse, chronic strain, or sports or occupational injuries of repetitive stress. The mechanism is a microscopic rupture of the ligaments of the common flexors and extensors of the wrist.

SIGNS AND SYMPTOMS

Pain Pattern

Lateral epicondylitis has painful resisted wrist extension, whereas medial epicondylitis has painful wrist flexion. Pain is aggravated by grasping or overuse and relieved with rest.

Palpation

A tender painful nodule is felt over the lateral or medial epicondyle. Possible atrophy of forearm muscles.

Radiation

Pain may radiate proximally or distally.

Other Manifestations

Loss of grip strength because of pain.

DIFFERENTIAL DIAGNOSIS

Rheumatoid arthritis
Gouty arthritis
Tendinitis
Osteoarthritis of the elbow
Myofascial trigger points of forearm flexors or extensors

ORTHOPEDIC EXAMINATION

Cozen's may be (+)
Mill's may be (+)

X-RAY FINDINGS

Calcium deposits may be seen

TREATMENT GOALS

1. Promote soft tissue healing.
2. Relieve pain and prevent recurrence.
3. Increase pain-free ranges of motion.
4. Restore normal strength and stability to joint structure.
5. Quickly change to rehabilitation or restoration of function.

MANAGEMENT PROTOCOL (OPTIONS)

Acute Phase:
- Ice massage: Freeze ¾ cup water in Styrofoam cup; break off bottom of cup, exposing about ¼ inch of frozen ice; and slowly in a circular pattern massage the involved painful area for about 3 minutes.
- Ultrasound (pulsed) at 0.5 W/cm^2 over site of lesion

followed by moist heat applications and ROM exercises. Breaks up fibrotic adhesions, reduces muscle spasms, and increases range of motion.

Subacute Phase:
- Moist heat and ultrasound followed by muscle stripping and trigger point therapy to reduce muscle spasms of forearm flexors and/or extensors. Other options include short wave diathermy, infrared therapy, interferential, negative low-volt galvanism, and microcurrent.
- Transverse friction massage: A deep-tissue massage at the site of involvement, stroking perpendicular to the fiber alignment to increase fiber mobility without longitudinal stress. This promotes orientation of fibers and induces hyperemia to hypovascular tissues.
- Counterforce bracing is helpful.
- Trigger point therapy to resulting trigger points of forearm flexors and extensors. Apply pressure for 5 to 7 seconds, repeat three times. Muscle stripping with methylsalicylate balm.
- Stretching and strengthening of finger flexors and extensors, supinators, and pronators.
- Adjust subluxations of the radial head, olecranon, and wrist.
- Adjust subluxations of the cervical and thoracic spine and ribs.
- Instruct patient to avoid moisture-filled or pressureless balls in tennis, to avoid off center strikes, and to hit the ball slightly in front of the waist during backhand stroke.

NUTRITIONAL MANAGEMENT PROTOCOL (OPTIONS)

Acute Pain and Inflammation:
- Proteolytic enzymes (trypsin, chymotrypsin, bromelin) (3-4 tablets qid in between meals). NOTE: Do not give to patients with ulcers!
- Bioflavonoids (quercetin, hesperidin, rutin, etc.) (200 mg mixed bioflavonoids q2h during acute phase).
- Herbals, such as boswellia, ginger, turmeric, cayenne (400 mg, 300 mg, 200 mg, 50 mg, respectively, q2h acute phase).

The above proteolytic enzymes can be obtained in Biozyme (Metagenics, Inc.) or Lyso-lymph Forte (Nutri-West, Inc.).

Inflavonoid Intensive Care (Metagenics, Inc.) will provide the above bioflavonoids and herbals. Other manufacturers can provide quality proteolytic enzymes. Consult your product catalog.

Tissue Healing:

- Amino acids (glycine, L-cystine, L-proline, L-lysine) (300-400 mg per day each in divided dosages). Supplies the amino acid pool necessary for the structural production of collagen.
- Vitamin C (3000-6000 mg per day in divided dosages).
- Iron (glycinate) (8-12 mg per day in divided dosages).
- Alpha-ketoglutaric acid (15 mg per day in divided dosages).

The above three nutrients are required for the hydroxylation of L-proline to L-hydroxyproline, which is needed for the production of quality collagen.

- Calcium (400 mg tid)
- Vitamin E (200 IU per day)
- Zinc (glycinate) (12-18 mg per day in divided dosages)
- Copper (glycinate) (600-900 µg per day in divided dosages)
- Manganese (glycinate) (4-6 mg per day in divided dosages)

The above provide antioxidant effects and serve as free radical scavengers to help remove cellular debris and promote healing. The zinc, copper, and manganese act as cofactors and catalysts for the potent antioxidant enzyme SOD and are therefore referred to as the *SOD induction complex.* Oral supplementation with SOD can be attempted; however, it has been reported that it is often destroyed in the stomach and intestinal tract before assimilation. SOD can be obtained in Cell Guard (Biotec Foods).

All of the above tissue-healing nutrients can be obtained in the formulary product Collagenics (Metagenics, Inc.).

Other manufacturers make similar formulary products designed to aid in soft tissue repair, such as Rehab Plus Complex (Professional Health Products). Consult the catalog of the reputable venders you use for alternate products.

REFERENCES

1. Balch JF, Balch PA: *Prescription for natural healing,* Wayne, NJ, 1990, Avery Publishing.
2. Bland JH, Cooper SM: Osteoarthritis: a review of the cell biology involved and evidence for reversibility, management rationally related to known genesis and pathophysiology, *Semin Arthritis Rheum* 14(2):106, 1984.

3. Brukner P: *Clinical sports medicine,* New York, 1993, McGraw-Hill.
4. Bucci LR: *Nutrition applied to injury rehabilitation and sports medicine,* Boca Raton, Fla, 1995, CRC Press.
5. Cichoke AJ, Marty L: The use of proteolytic enzymes with soft-tissue athletic injuries, *Am Chiropr,* October 1981, p 32.
6. D'Ambrosio E, et al: Glucosamine sulfate: a controlled clinical investigation in arthrosis, *Pharmatherapeutica* 2(8):504-508, 1981.
7. Davis CD, Greger JL: Longitudinal changes of manganese-dependent superoxide dismutase and other indexes of manganese and iron status in women, *Am J Clin Nutr* 55:747, 1992.
8. Downer AH: *Physical therapy procedures,* ed 4, Springfield, Ill, 1988, Charles C Thomas.
9. Drovanti A, et al: Oral glucosamine sulfate in osteoarthritis: a placebo controlled double-blind investigation, *Clin Ther* 3(4):260-272, 1980.
10. Fauci A, et al: *Harrison's principles of internal medicine,* ed 13, New York, 1994, McGraw-Hill.
11. Grabowski RJ: *Current nutritional therapy,* San Antonio, Tex, 1993, Image Press.
12. Hammer W: *Functional soft tissue examination and treatment by manual methods,* Gaithersburg, Md, 1991, Aspen Publishers.
13. Havsteen B: Flavinoids, a class of natural products of high pharmacological potency, *Biochem Pharmacol* 33(24):3933-3939, 1984.
14. Lawrence D: *Fundamentals of chiropractic diagnosis and management,* Baltimore, 1991, Williams & Wilkins.
15. Liebenson C: *Rehabilitation of the spine,* Baltimore, 1996, Williams & Wilkins.
16. Lindahl O, Lindwall L: Double blind study of a *Valerian* preparation, *Pharmacol Biochem Behav* 32(4):10065-10066, 1989.
17. *Manual of medical therapeutics (the Washington manual),* ed 27, Boston, 1992, Little, Brown.
18. *The Merck manual,* ed 16, Rahway, NJ, 1992, Merck Co.
19. Niki E: Interaction of ascorbate and alpha-tocopherol, *Third Conference on Vitamin C* 498:187-189, 1987.
20. Rakel RE: *Conn's current therapy,* Philadelphia, 1996, WB Saunders.
21. Rakel RE: *Textbook of family practice,* ed 5, Philadelphia, 1995, WB Saunders.
22. Schestack R: *Handbook of physical therapy,* ed 3, New York, 1977, Springer-Verlag.
23. Schwartz RI, et al: Ascorbate can act as an inducer of collagen pathway because most steps are tightly coupled, *Third Conference on Vitamin C* 498:172-184, 1987.
24. Scully RM, Barnes MR: *Physical therapy,* Philadelphia, 1989, JB Lippincott.
25. Speroni E, Minghetti A: Neuropharmacological activity of extracts from *Passiflora incarnata, Planta Med* 54(6):488-491, 1988.

26. Taraye JP, Lauressergues H: Advantages of combination of proteolytic enzymes, flavonoids and ascorbic acid in comparison with non-steroid inflammatory drugs, *Arzneimittelforschung* 27(1):1144-1149, 1977.

27. Taylor RB: *Manual of family practice,* Boston, 1996, Little, Brown.

28. Tierney LM, McPhee SJ, Papadakis MA: *Current medical diagnosis and treatment,* ed 35, Norwalk, Conn, 1996, Appleton & Lange.

29. Vear HJ: *Chiropractic standards of practice and quality of care,* Gaithersburg, Md, 1992, Aspen Publishers.

30. Werbach MR: *Nutritional influences on illness,* ed 2, Tarzana, Calif, 1996, Third Line Press.

31. Werbach MR, Murray MT: *Botanical influences on illness,* Tarzana, Calif, 1994, Third Line Press.

32. White AA, Panjabi MM: *Clinical biomechanics of the spine,* Philadelphia, 1990, JB Lippincott.

Olecranon Bursitis

Lew Huff and David M. Brady

DEFINITION

An inflammation of the bursa beneath the olecranon process of the elbow; also called *miner's elbow*.

ETIOLOGY

May be due to trauma, overuse, strain, infection, systemic form of arthritis, or entrapment syndrome.

SIGNS AND SYMPTOMS

Location

Pain at the site of the olecranon bursa beneath the olecranon process of the elbow joint.

Inspection

Local rubor, erythema if superficial and inflamed. Difficult arm extension because of pain. Mild edema of elbow.

Palpation

Pain over the olecranon process, increased pain and joint stiffness with movements. Local tenderness on palpation.

Range of Motion

Pain increases with movements, especially extension of the elbow. Painful active and passive ranges of motion. Decreased mobility of affected part.

Timing

Multiple recurrences lasting days or weeks.

Differential

Triceps tendinitis elicits pain on flexion.

DIFFERENTIAL DIAGNOSIS

Triceps tendinitis
Osteoarthritis
Infectious arthritis

ORTHOPEDIC EXAMINATION

Cozen's may be (+)
Mill's may be (+)
Stability tests WNL

X-RAY FINDINGS

No fracture
Possible calcific deposits

TREATMENT GOALS

1. Promote soft tissue healing.
2. Relieve pain and prevent recurrence.
3. Increase pain-free ranges of motion.
4. Restore normal strength and stability to joint structure.
5. Quickly change to rehabilitation and restoration of function.

MANAGEMENT PROTOCOL (OPTIONS)

- Rest the elbow and cease aggravating activities.

Acute Phase:
- Cryotherapy: Ice for the first 24 to 48 hours of onset to prevent contracture. Use mild heat and pulsed ultrasound in subacute phase (48 to 72 hours). Ultrasound causes the resolution of inflammatory exudates and increases blood flow.
- Ice massage: Freeze ¾ cup water in Styrofoam cup; break off bottom of cup, exposing about ¼ inch of frozen ice; and slowly in a circular pattern massage the involved painful area for about 3 minutes.

Subacute Phase:
- Extremity adjusting: Doctor abducts the patient's arm to 90 degrees and internally rotates and extends the forearm while tractioning the humerus proximally and the radius and ulna distally. Perform six times per visit.
- Soft bracing and antiinflammatory medications if indicated.
- With reinjury or flare-up: continue care, restrict activities, and begin rehabilitation exercises.

NUTRITIONAL MANAGEMENT PROTOCOL (OPTIONS)

Acute Pain and Inflammation:
- Proteolytic enzymes (trypsin, chymotrypsin, bromelin) (3-4 tablets qid in between meals). NOTE: Do not give to patients with ulcers!
- Bioflavonoids (quercetin, hesperidin, rutin, etc.) (200 mg mixed bioflavonoids q2h during acute phase).
- Herbals, such as boswellia, ginger, turmeric, cayenne (400 mg, 300 mg, 200 mg, 50 mg, respectively, q2h acute phase).

The above proteolytic enzymes can be obtained in Biozyme (Metagenics, Inc.) or Lyso-lymph Forte (Nutri-West, Inc.). Inflavonoid Intensive Care (Metagenics, Inc.) will provide the above bioflavonoids and herbals. Other manufacturers can provide quality proteolytic enzymes. Consult your product catalog.

HOME CARE PROTOCOL (OPTIONS)

Instruct patient in ROM exercises for the elbow, shoulder, and wrist. ROM exercises should be started as soon as pain allows. Surgical tubing exercises along with active and passive ranges of motion can be started if patient feels no residual pain. ROM exercises can be performed three times per day if tolerated. Instruct patient to avoid heavy lifting.

REFERENCES

1. Balch JF, Balch PA: *Prescription for natural healing,* Wayne, NJ, 1990, Avery Publishing.
2. Brukner P: *Clinical sports medicine,* New York, 1993, McGraw-Hill.
3. Bucci LR: *Nutrition applied to injury rehabilitation and sports medicine,* Boca Raton, Fla, 1995, CRC Press.
4. Cichoke AJ, Marty L: The use of proteolytic enzymes with soft-tissue athletic injuries, *Am Chiropr,* October 1981, p 32.
5. Downer AH: *Physical therapy procedures,* ed 4, Springfield, Ill, Charles C Thomas.
6. Fauci A, et al: *Harrison's principles of internal medicine,* ed 13, New York, 1994, McGraw-Hill.
7. Gatterman M: *Chiropractic management of spine related disorders,* Baltimore, 1990, Williams & Wilkins.
8. Grabowski RJ: *Current nutritional therapy,* San Antonio, Tex, 1993, Image Press.
9. Hammer W: *Functional soft tissue examination and treatment by manual methods,* Gaithersburg, Md, 1991, Aspen Publishers.
10. Hammer W: The use of transverse friction massage in the management of chronic bursitis of the hip and shoulder, *J Manipulative Physiol Ther* 16(2), 1993.
11. Havsteen B: Flavinoids, a class of natural products of high pharmacological potency, *Biochem Pharmacol* 33(24):3933-3939, 1984.
12. Liebenson C: *Rehabilitation of the spine,* Baltimore, 1996, Williams & Wilkins.
13. *Manual of medical therapeutics (the Washington manual),* ed 27, Boston, 1992, Little, Brown.
14. *The Merck manual,* ed 16, Rahway, NJ, 1992, Merck Co.
15. Rakel RE: *Conn's current therapy,* Philadelphia, 1996, WB Saunders.
16. Rakel RE: *Textbook of family practice,* ed 5, Philadelphia, 1995, WB Saunders.
17. Schestack R: *Handbook of physical therapy,* ed 3, New York, 1977, Springer-Verlag.
18. Scully RM, Barnes MR: *Physical therapy,* Philadelphia, 1989, JB Lippincott.
19. Taraye JP, Lauressergues H: Advantages of combination of proteolytic enzymes, flavonoids and ascorbic acid in comparison with non-steroid inflammatory drugs, *Arzneimittelforschung* 27(1):1144-1149, 1977.
20. Taylor RB: *Manual of family practice,* Boston, 1996, Little, Brown.

21. Tierney LM, McPhee SJ, Papadakis MA: *Current medical diagnosis and treatment,* ed 35, Norwalk, Conn, 1996, Appleton & Lange.
22. Vear HJ: *Chiropractic standards of practice and quality of care,* Gaithersburg, Md, 1992, Aspen Publishers.
23. Werbach MR: *Nutritional influences on illness,* ed 2, Tarzana, Calif, 1996, Third Line Press.
24. Werbach MR, Murray MT: *Botanical influences on illness,* Tarzana, Calif, 1994, Third Line Press.

SECTION VI

Injuries to the Wrist Joint

Injuries to the Wrist Joint: General Overview

Carpal Tunnel Syndrome

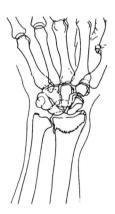

(Modified from Bontrager KL: *Textbook of radiographic positioning and related anatomy,* ed 4, St Louis, 1997, Mosby.)

Injuries to the Wrist Joint: General Overview

Lew Huff

WRIST INJURIES

The wrist is prone to injuries caused by sports, occupation, or daily activities. Although not a weight-bearing joint at most times, it is extremely flexible and under constant use.

SITE OF PAIN

Pain involving ligaments is superficial in nature and well localized. About 90% of wrist sprains are flexion sprains with no fracture. In wrist fracture, diffuse swelling occurs with ecchymosis and skin temperature elevation.

EXAMINATION

Examine the surrounding bones and tendon insertions. Visualize the range of motion in all planes. A complete rupture may have less pain or no pain because a ruptured ligament has complete loss of continuity and the fibers are no longer intact and therefore cannot be stressed. Painless hypermobility is seen in chronic ligamentous rupture.

RADIATION, REFERRED PAIN

Pain radiates to the elbow, shoulder girdle, or neck.

ACTIVITIES OF DAILY LIVING

Injury to the wrist joints can interfere with grasping, typing, computer work, writing, and other activities involving the hand and wrist.

UNINJURED AREA

Examination and radiographic examination for bilateral comparison, if appropriate.

REINJURY/FLARE-UP

Restrict aggravating activities, continue care, and start low-impact rehabilitative exercises.

HOME CARE

ROM exercises and passive stretching. Surgical tubing exercises, ice applications, or compresses may be appropriate.

WHEN TO DISCHARGE

When patient has reached maximum medical improvement or the need for referral is established.

REFERRAL

If fracture, dislocation, or neurological complications are present. Daily treatment exceeding 2 weeks may signal the need for a second opinion or referral. Treatment exceeding 4 weeks or temporary disability for longer than 4 weeks with no objective signs of improvement or worsening of the condition within the first 2 weeks may signal the need for a second opinion or referral. Suspected fracture, bone pathology, systemic disease, or infection signals the need for referral.[4]

REFERENCES

1. Clemente C: *Anatomy: a regional atlas of the human body,* ed 3, Baltimore, 1987, Urban & Schwarzenberg.

2. Gatterman M: *Chiropractic management of spine related disorders,* Baltimore, 1990, Williams & Wilkins.
3. Haldeman S, et al: Guidelines for chiropractic quality assurance & practice parameters, *The Proceedings of the Mercy Center Consensus Conference,* Gaithersburg, Md, 1993, Aspen Publishers.
4. Hansen DT: *Chiropractic standards of practice and utilization guidelines in the care and treatment of injured workers,* 1988, Washington State Department of Labor & Industries.
5. Lawrence D: *Fundamentals of chiropractic diagnosis and management,* Baltimore, 1991, Williams & Wilkins.
6. Schestack R: *Handbook of physical therapy,* ed 3, New York, 1977, Springer-Verlag.
7. Vear HJ: *Chiropractic standards of practice and quality of care,* Gaithersburg, Md, 1992, Aspen Publishers.

Carpal Tunnel Syndrome

STEVEN FOSTER, LEW HUFF, AND DAVID M. BRADY

DEFINITION

A neurologic disorder of the wrist and hand, characterized by pain and loss of sensation along the course of the median nerve. True carpal tunnel syndrome is nerve entrapment at or distal to the wrist. Carpal tunnel syndrome is the most common entrapment syndrome.

ETIOLOGY

Compression of the median nerve between the carpal bones and the flexor retinaculum resulting from carpal subluxation, mal-healed fracture, tenosynovitis, tumor, congenital malformation, and secondary to pregnancy, diabetes, rheumatoid arthritis, sarcoidosis, or amyloidosis. Carpal tunnel syndrome may be associated with menstrual cycle and menopause. Often described as a combination of joint laxity syndrome and subluxation of the capitate and lunate bones of the wrist. There is an increased incidence in females over males.

SIGNS AND SYMPTOMS

Pain Pattern

Episodic and often nocturnal pain and paresthesia of the hand. Pain described as sharp and burning with numbness and tingling associated with wrist and hand weakness. Pain is exacerbated by manual activity.

Neurological Manifestations

Weakness or atrophy of the abductor pollicis brevis muscles. Burning pain with numbness, tingling sensations, and weakness. Loss of light touch and pain sensations. Loss of grip strength. Feeling of pins and needles in hands and wrist.[25] Decreased pain sensation and numbness in the thumb, index finger, and middle finger.

Location

Pain over the lateral aspect of the hand, usually over the distribution of the median nerve (thumb, index finger, and thenar eminence).

Radiation

Pain may radiate up the forearm and into the shoulder joint and neck areas.

Aggravating Factors

Heat to wrist may aggravate during acute phases. Repeated finger flexion.

Palliative

Rubbing wrist, shaking wrists, dangling wrist over the side of the bed.

DIFFERENTIAL DIAGNOSIS

Brachial neuritis
Trauma, fracture
Tenosynovitis
C6 nerve root compression
Referred pain from myofascial trigger points
Tunnel of Guyon entrapment
TOS

ORTHOPEDIC/NEUROLOGICAL EXAMINATION

Phalen's, prayer sign
Tinel's, nerve conduction

RESULTS (OF ORTHOPEDIC/NEUROLOGICAL EXAMINATION)

(+) findings of Phalen's, Tinel's
Delayed nerve conduction velocity

SPECIAL TESTS (WHEN NECESSARY)

Electromyography, x-ray
MRI, NCV

Clinical Note

TOS or ulnar nerve compression may cause decreased sensation of the little finger and the ulnar aspect of the ring finger along with intrinsic muscle weakness, as opposed to the median distribution of carpal tunnel syndrome.[2]

TREATMENT GOALS

1. Promote soft tissue healing.
2. Relieve pain and prevent recurrence.
3. Increase pain-free ranges of motion.
4. Restore normal strength and stability to joint structure.
5. Quickly change to rehabilitation and restoration of function.

MANAGEMENT PROTOCOL (OPTIONS)

Rest involved area.
Acute Phase:
- Volar cock-up splinting or taping of wrist, especially at night to decrease edema. Soft cast with zinc oxide. Elastic wrist support as needed.
- Cryotherapy: Ice for the first 24 to 48 hours of onset to prevent contracture and reduce edema.

- Apply ice packs for 15 to 20 minutes with dry towel between the patient and the ice packs. Use every 2 hours for reduction of pain and edema.
- Ice massage: Freeze ¾ cup water in Styrofoam cup; break off bottom of cup, exposing about ¼ inch of frozen ice; and slowly in a circular pattern massage the involved painful area for about 3 minutes.
- Ultrasound (pulsed) 20% at 0.5 W/cm^2 under water for 5 minutes. Ultrasound causes the resolution of inflammatory exudates and increases blood flow.

Subacute Phase:

- High-volt galvanic and interferential may be used to decrease inflammatory process and edema.
- Microcurrent: Positive polarity during acute phase. Increases protein synthesis to promote healing. Some modulation of pain and inflammation.
- Scan and treat myofascial trigger points in the forearm flexor and/or extensor musculature by compressing each trigger point 5 to 7 seconds and repeating this procedure three times, or use active release technique (ART) procedures.[17]
- Transverse friction massage: A deep-tissue massage at the site of involvement, stroking perpendicular to the fiber alignment to increase fiber mobility without longitudinal stress. This promotes orientation of fibers and induces hyperemia to hypovascular tissues. In addition, transverse friction massage has a mechanical influence on tissue maturation.
- Use gentle mobilization techniques, manipulation, and joint traction.
- Extremity adjusting: Adjust posterior radius, elbow extension technique, and wrist. Wrist adjustment: Reduce subluxation of lunate and capitate; traction wrist in direction of subluxation to gap the joint; with thumb over the bone, perform a slight thrust to adjust carpals. Follow with adjustment of cervical spine.
- Rehabilitation: Have patient squeeze racquetball or putty with wrist in neutral position.

NUTRITIONAL MANAGEMENT PROTOCOL (OPTIONS)

Acute Pain and Inflammation:
- Proteolytic enzymes (trypsin, chymotrypsin, bromelin) (3-4 tablets qid in between meals). NOTE: Do not give to patients with ulcers!
- Bioflavonoids (quercetin, hesperidin, rutin, etc.) (200 mg mixed bioflavonoids q2h during acute phase).
- Herbals, such as boswellia, ginger, turmeric, cayenne (400 mg, 300 mg, 200 mg, 50 mg, respectively, q2h acute phase).
- The above proteolytic enzymes can be obtained in Biozyme (Metagenics, Inc.) or Lyso-lymph Forte (Nutri-West, Inc.). Inflavonoid Intensive Care (Metagenics, Inc.) will provide the above bioflavonoids and herbals. Other manufacturers can provide quality proteolytic enzymes. Consult your product catalog.

Carpal Tunnel Syndrome:
- Pyridoxine (vitamin B_6) (100 mg bid for 8 to 12 weeks)
- B complex vitamins (50-100 mg bid for 8 to 12 weeks)

HOME CARE PROTOCOL (OPTIONS)

- Avoid heavy lifting with involved wrist.
- Use a cervical pillow at night.
- Elevate wrist and use ice packs to decrease edema.

REFERENCES

1. Balch JF, Balch PA: *Prescription for natural healing,* Wayne, NJ, 1990, Avery Publishing.
2. Bracker M, Ralph L: Problem-oriented diagnosis: the numb arm and hand, *Am Fam Phys* 51(1), 1995.
3. Brukner P: *Clinical sports medicine,* New York, 1993, McGraw-Hill.
4. Bucci LR: *Nutrition applied to injury rehabilitation and sports medicine,* Boca Raton, Fla, 1995, CRC Press.
5. Cichoke AJ, Marty L: The use of proteolytic enzymes with soft-tissue athletic injuries, *Am Chiropr,* October 1981, p 32.
6. Downer AH: *Physical therapy procedures,* ed 4, Springfield, Ill, 1988, Charles C Thomas.
7. Driskell JA, et al: Effectiveness of pyridoxine hydrochloride treatment on carpal tunnel patients, *Nutr Rep Int* 34:1031-140, 1986.
8. Ellis J, et al: Clinical results of a cross-over treatment with pyridoxine and placebo of the carpal tunnel syndrome, *Am J Clin Nutr* 32:2040-2046, 1979.

9. Ellis J, et al: Therapy with vitamin B$_6$ with and without surgery for treatment of patients having the idiopathic carpal tunnel syndrome, *Res Commun Chem Pathol Pharmacol* 33(2):331, 1981.

10. Ellis JM, Folkers K: Clinical aspects of treatment of carpal tunnel syndrome with vitamin B$_6$, *Ann NY Acad Sci* 585:302-320, 1990.

11. Fauci A, et al: *Harrison's principles of internal medicine,* ed 13, New York, 1994, McGraw-Hill.

12. Fuhr JE, et al: Vitamin B$_6$ levels in patients with carpal tunnel syndrome, *Arch Surg* 124:1329-1330, 1989.

13. Grabowski RJ: *Current nutritional therapy,* San Antonio, Tex, 1993, Image Press.

14. Hammer W: *Functional soft tissue examination and treatment by manual methods,* Gaithersburg, Md, 1991, Aspen Publishers.

15. Havsteen B: Flavinoids, a class of natural products of high pharmacological potency, *Biochem Pharmacol* 33(24):3933-3939, 1984.

16. Kasdan ML, Janes C: Carpal tunnel syndrome and vitamin B$_6$, *Plast Reconstr Surg* 79(3):156-162, 1987.

17. Lawrence D: *Fundamentals of chiropractic diagnosis and management,* Baltimore, 1991, Williams & Wilkins.

18. Leahy PM, Mock LE: Myofascial release technique and mechanical compromise of peripheral nerves of the upper extremity, *Chiropr Sports Med* 16(4):139-150, 1992.

19. Liebenson C: *Rehabilitation of the spine,* Baltimore, 1996, Williams & Wilkins.

20. *Manual of medical therapeutics (the Washington manual),* ed 27, Boston, 1992, Little, Brown.

21. Mariano K, et al: Double crush syndrome: chiropractic care for an entrapment neuropathy, *J Manipulative Physiol Ther* 14(4):262-266, 1991.

22. *The Merck manual,* ed 16, Rahway, NJ, 1992, Merck Co.

23. Niki E: Interaction of ascorbate and alpha-tocopherol, *Third Conference on Vitamin C* 498:187-189, 1987.

24. Nimmo R: Receptor, effecters and tonus: a new approach, *J Natl Chiropr Assoc,* November 1957.

25. Petruska G: Carpal tunnel syndrome: a new perspective that blends active and passive care, *J Sports Chiropr Rehab* 11(2):57-60, 1997.

26. Rakel RE: *Conn's current therapy,* Philadelphia, 1996, WB Saunders.

27. Rakel RE: *Textbook of family practice,* ed 5, Philadelphia, 1995, WB Saunders.

28. Schestack R: *Handbook of physical therapy,* ed 3, New York, 1977, Springer-Verlag.

29. Schneider MJ: Chiropractic management of myofascial and muscular disorders. In Lawrence D, ed: *Advances in chiropractic,* vol 3, St Louis, 1996, Mosby.

30. Scully RM, Barnes MR: *Physical therapy,* Philadelphia, 1989, JB Lippincott.
31. Stransky M, et al: Treatment of carpal tunnel syndrome with vitamin B_6: a double-blind study, *South Med J* 82(7):841-842, 1989.
32. Taraye JP, Lauressergues H: Advantages of combination of proteolytic enzymes, flavonoids and ascorbic acid in comparison with non-steroid inflammatory drugs, *Arzneimittelforschung* 27(1):1144-1149, 1977.
33. Taylor RB: *Manual of family practice,* Boston, 1996, Little, Brown.
34. Tierney LM, McPhee SJ, Papadakis MA: *Current medical diagnosis and treatment,* Norwalk, Conn, 1996, Appleton & Lange.
35. Travell JG, Simons DG: *Myofascial pain and dysfunction: the trigger point manual,* vol 2, Baltimore, 1992, Williams & Wilkins.
36. Vear HJ: *Chiropractic standards of practice and quality of care,* Gaithersburg, Md, 1992, Aspen Publishers.
37. Werbach MR: *Nutritional influences on illness,* ed 2, Tarzana, Calif, 1996, Third Line Press.
38. Werbach MR, Murray MT: *Botanical influences on illness,* Tarzana, Calif, 1994, Third Line Press.
39. White AA, Panjabi MM: *Clinical biomechanics of the spine,* Philadelphia, 1990, JB Lippincott.

SECTION VII

Low Back Pain Syndromes

Injuries to the Lumbar Spine: General Overview

Lumbar Facet Syndrome

Lumbar Disk Herniation

Lumbosacral Strain/Sprain

Sciatic Neuralgia

Piriformis Syndrome

Spondylolisthesis

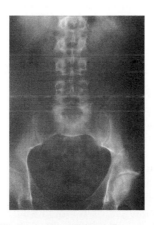

(From Bergmann TF, Davis PT: *Mechanically assisted manual techniques: distraction procedures*, St Louis, 1997, Mosby.)

Injuries to the Lumbar Spine: General Overview

Lew Huff

LUMBAR SPINE INJURIES (Fig. 2)

The lumbar spine may be susceptible to injuries caused by chronic trauma, microtrauma, excessive weight bearing resulting from obesity, decreased disk height, and increased lumbosacral lordosis. Degenerative changes and faulty posture are other contributing factors.

SITE OF PAIN

Pain may be localized to the lumbar paraspinal muscles, lumbar vertebrae, sacroiliac joints, sacrum, or gluteals. Pain may be intensified by active or passive ranges of motion or weight bearing.

EXAMINATION

Deep palpation may reveal edema, pinpoint tenderness, myospasms, nodules, adhesions, and trigger points.

Full passive ranges of motion with restricted active ranges of motion may indicate muscle weakness as a cause.

Pain on resistive ranges of motion may indicate a strain, whereas pain with passive ranges of motion may indicate ligamentous involvement.

With restriction of passive ROM, look for bony or soft tissue blockage.

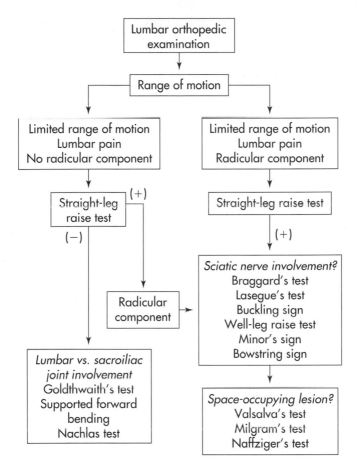

FIG. 2 Examination and diagnosis flow diagram.

RADIATION, REFERRED PAIN

Pain may radiate to the upper thighs, groin, hip, buttocks, and often the leg or foot. Possible referred pain to the sacroiliac joints or gluteals. Radiation may be aggravated by lumbar extension, flexion or rotation, prolonged sitting, and repetitive movements. Numbness and tingling of distal dermatomal patterns may be seen.

ACTIVITIES OF DAILY LIVING

Patient may experience low back pain relieved by motion, diffuse morning stiffness, antalgic gait and posture, diminished mobility, and pain upon rising from bed or a seated position.

TIME FRAMES OF CARE

NOTE: The need for all phases of care and the time frames suggested are highly dependent on the *severity of the initial injury and the level of dysfunction.* Correctional care and rehabilitation are stages used only if clinical signs warrant the need for continued care.

Acute Care

Appropriate when pain is felt at rest and aggravated by activity; it is often felt over a diffuse area. Movements are restricted by pain and guarding. Goals are to promote anatomical rest, decrease myospasm, diminish inflammatory reactions, alleviate pain to a tolerable level, and improve overall function.

Acute injuries may be superimposed on degenerative conditions, anomalies, or prior trauma that may slow or complicate the healing process.

Clinical Note

In general, some evidence of measurable clinical improvement (objective or subjective) should be noted within eight visits or 2 to 4 weeks to justify continued care.[10]

Active/Correctional Care

Characterized by little or no pain at rest, pain increases with activity. Pain is generally localized at this stage. Goals are to further reduce symptoms, improve function, and return patient to preclinical status.

Rehabilitation

Goals are to restore strength and endurance, increase physical work capacity, and improve function to preinjury status. Continue rehabilitation to maximum medical improvement, whether or not preinjury status has been achieved. Rehabilitation should include therapeutic exercises and activities of daily living training. Active ROM exercises help disperse edema and prevent the formation of adhesions. ROM exercises should not be performed in planes that stress the joint.

Clinical Notes

Proceed to rehabilitation as quickly as possible to avoid or minimize dependency on passive forms of treatment.[4]

Short duration of signs or symptoms may signal a quick response to manipulation.[4]

AHCPR guidelines state that conservative care is warranted with low back pain without radiculopathy in the first month of signs and symptoms. After 1 month of manipulation, stop and reevaluate the patient for appropriateness of continued care.[1]

Relief of discomfort can be accomplished most safely with nonprescription medications and/or spinal manipulation.[1]

After 3 months of follow-up examinations, the clinician should request a consultation for unimproved patients. The consultation should be multidisciplinary, including specialists for the spine, the psyche, and functional and occupational rehabilitation.[9]

Lab work: Management over the first 4 weeks: all laboratory evaluation, including plain radiographs, are generally useless at this stage unless clinical signs suggest a specific disease.[9]

Bed rest: Although some activity modification may be necessary during the acute phase, bed rest more than 4 days is not helpful and may further debilitate the patient.[1]

Therapy over the first 4 weeks deemphasizes prolonged bed rest. If used, bed rest should be prescribed for 2 days at a time to a maximum of 4 days for low back pain and 7 days for neck pain.[9]

Bed rest for 2 to 7 days is worse than a placebo or ordinary activity and is not as effective as alternative treatments for relief of pain, rate of recovery, and return to daily activities and work.[11]

Aerobics: Low-stress aerobic activities can be started safely in the first 2 weeks of symptoms to help avoid debilitation; exercises to condition trunk muscles are commonly delayed at least 2 weeks.[1]

Surgery: Within the first 3 months of low back pain symptoms, only patients with evidence of serious spinal pathology or severe debilitating symptoms of sciatica and physiological evidence of specific nerve root compression on imaging studies can expect to benefit from surgery.[1]

Lifestyle Adaptations

To modify social and recreational activities, to diminish work environmental risk factors, and to adapt to psychological factors related to the disorder.

REINJURY/FLARE-UP

Restrict aggravating activities, continue care, and start low-impact rehabilitative exercises.

HOME CARE

ROM exercises, passive stretching, stretching under the shower, and the use of pillows while sleeping may be emphasized. Ice applications or compresses may be appropriate. Avoid heavy lifting and assess for the need of a heel lift.

WHEN TO DISCHARGE

When patient has reached maximum medical improvement or the need for referral is established.

REFERRAL

If fracture, dislocation, or neurological complications are present. Daily treatment exceeding 2 weeks may signal the need for a second opinion or referral. Treatment exceeding 4 weeks, temporary disability for longer than 4 weeks with no objective signs of improvement, or worsening of the condition within the first 2 weeks may signal the need for a second opinion or referral.

Suspected fracture, bone pathology, spinal motion instability, contraindication for spinal manipulation, systemic disease, or infection signals the need for referral.[5]

REFERENCES

1. Bigos S, et al: Acute low back problems in adults, *AHCPR Clinical Practice Guidelines No 14*, AHCPR Pub No 95-0642, Rockville, Md, 1994, US Dept of Health and Human Services.
2. Clemente C: *Anatomy: a regional atlas of the human body*, Baltimore, ed 3, 1987, Urban & Schwarzenberg.
3. Gatterman M: *Chiropractic management of spine related disorders*, Baltimore, 1990, Williams & Wilkins.
4. Haldeman S, et al: Guidelines for chiropractic quality assurance & practice parameters, *The Proceedings of the Mercy Center Consensus Conference*, Gaithersburg, Md, 1993, Aspen Publishers.
5. Hansen DT: *Chiropractic standards of practice and utilization guidelines in the care and treatment of injured workers*, 1988, Washington State Department of Labor & Industries.
6. Lawrence D: *Fundamentals of chiropractic diagnosis and management*, Baltimore, 1991, Williams & Wilkins.
7. Manga P, et al: *The effectiveness and cost effectiveness of chiropractic management of low-back pain*, 1993, Ontario Ministry of Health.
8. Schestack R: *Handbook of physical therapy*, ed 3, New York, 1977, Springer-Verlag.
9. Spitzer WO, et al: Scientific approach to the assessment and management of activity-related spinal disorders: a monograph for clinicians, report of the Quebec Task Force on Spinal Disorders, *Spine* 12(7s), 1987.
10. Vear HJ: *Chiropractic standards of practice and quality of care*, Gaithersburg, Md, 1992, Aspen Publishers.
11. Waddel G, et al: *Low back pain evidence review*, London, 1996, Royal College of General Practitioners.

Lumbar Facet Syndrome

KEVIN PRINGLE, LEW HUFF, STEVEN FOSTER,
DAVID M. BRADY, AND JASON FLANAGAN

DEFINITION

A rotational and compression injury of the richly innervated articulating facets of the lumbar spine, characterized by local and/or referred pain arising from the zygapophyseal joints. Also referred to as *posterior joint syndrome* or *acute locked back.*

ETIOLOGY

Causes may include trauma, microtrauma, excessive weight bearing resulting from obesity, decreased disk height, and increased lumbosacral lordosis. Degenerative changes and faulty posture are other contributing factors. Mechanism may be a tear or pinch of the facet capsule caused by a hyperextension or hyperflexion injury.

SIGNS AND SYMPTOMS

Pain Pattern

Low back pain at rest that is relieved with motion. Aggravated by lumbar extension and rotation, prolonged sitting, and repetitive movements. Diffuse morning stiffness and sacroiliac joint pain.

Radiation

Radiation to the upper thighs, groin, hip, buttocks, and often the leg. Pain is generally not below the knees. Possible referred pain to sacroiliac joint or posterior superior iliac spine.

Quality

Sharp, well defined, superficial, and unilateral. Morning stiffness is common.

Palliative

Lying supine with knees flexed to chest opens facets and may reduce pain. Forward flexion of the spine reduces pain.

Aggravating Factors

Extension of the spine, prolonged sitting, repetitive motion, and weather changes may aggravate.

Sensory Changes

Minor sensory changes are often noted: minor numbness or weakness associated with pain.

Palpation

Tenderness on palpation of lumbar spinous processes and transverse processes.

Other Findings

Diffuse morning stiffness, sacroiliac joint pain, guarded movements and muscle spasms. Neurological examination is essentially negative. Unilateral hypertrophy of a facet can impinge on the foramen producing nerve root entrapment. Facet syndrome may predispose patient to disk herniation as the joint complex degenerates.

DIFFERENTIAL DIAGNOSIS

Disk herniation, strain-sprains, mechanical instability (pain with motion, relieved with rest)

ORTHOPEDIC TESTING

Straight leg raise, Goldthwait's sign may be (+)
(+) Kemp's test for low back pain, not radiculopathy

Dejerine's triad may be (+)
Spinous percussion tenderness

RADIOGRAPHIC FINDINGS

Sclerosis of facets; no osteophytes; stress films may reveal abnormal joint locking. Chronic facet changes may be noted. McNab's line and Hadley's line may be positive for imbrication. (See Fig. 2.)

TREATMENT GOALS

1. Promote soft tissue healing.
2. Relieve pain and prevent recurrence.
3. Increase pain-free ranges of motion.
4. Restore normal strength and stability to joint structure.
5. Quickly change to rehabilitation and restoration of function.

Clinical Notes

Proceed to rehabilitation as quickly as possible to avoid or minimize dependency on passive forms of treatment.[20]

Short duration of signs or symptoms may signal a quick response to manipulation.[20]

The number of prior episodes may increase the number of treatments to restore pain-free ranges of motion.

AHCPR guidelines state that conservative care is warranted with low back pain without radiculopathy in the first month of signs and symptoms. After 1 month of manipulation, stop and reevaluate the patient for appropriateness of continued care.[5]

AHCPR guidelines state that, in absence of red flags, imaging studies and further diagnostic testing are not helpful during the first 4 weeks of low back pain.[5]

AHCPR guidelines state that low-stress aerobics may be started within 2 weeks in low back pain patients if tolerated.[5]

MANAGEMENT PROTOCOL (OPTIONS)

Acute Phase:

- Apply ice packs for 15 to 20 minutes with a dry towel between the patient and the ice packs. Use every 2 hours for reduction of pain and edema.
- Ice massage: Freeze ¾ cup water in Styrofoam cup; break off bottom of cup, exposing about ¼ inch of frozen ice; and slowly in a circular pattern massage the involved painful area for about 3 minutes.
- High-volt galvanic and interferential may be used to decrease inflammatory process and edema. Sinusoidal current to paravertebral muscles and alternating heat and cold therapy is beneficial.[44]
- Ultrasound (pulsed) at 0.5 W/cm^2 for 5 to 7 minutes. Ultrasound causes the resolution of inflammatory exudates and increases blood flow.

Subacute or Chronic Phase:

- Moist hot packs heated to 270° F with 2 dry towels between hot packs and patient, applied for 20 minutes to reduce muscle spasms and increase circulation.
- TENS: frequency 50 to 100 Hz, pulse width set at 20 to 60 ms, time 23 hours, set below the motoric threshold to block pain.
- Short wave diathermy: heat source is placed 18 inches from body part, treatment time is 20 minutes, use one towel between heat source and patient.
- Manipulation is beneficial.[14,17,19,25,26,28]

Clinical Notes

On the evidence, particularly the most scientifically valid clinical studies, spinal manipulation applied by chiropractors is shown to be more effective than alternative treatments for low back pain. Many medical therapies are of questionable validity or are clearly inadequate. Our reading of the literature suggests that chiropractic manipulation is safer than medical management of low back pain.[31]

Within the first 6 weeks of onset, manipulation can provide short-term improvement in pain and activity levels and higher patient satisfaction. The risks of manipulation are very low in skilled hands.[51]

The Rand Study of 1991 suggests an adequate trial of manipulation is a course of 12 manipulations given over a period of up to 4 weeks, after which, in the absence of documented improvement, spinal manipulation is no longer indicated.[45]

- Flexion/distraction and traction may be beneficial.[44]
- Lumbar distraction technique: Patient supine, legs drawn to chest. Clinician places forearm across the knees for stabilization and places the opposite hand covering the sacral region. While pushing forward on the knees, clinician lifts the sacrum in a rocking motion to gap the joint spaces.
- Corrective exercises: Pelvic flattening, mat exercises to correct anterior pelvic tilt. Strengthen abdominal muscles and flatten the lumbar curve while balancing the agonist with the antagonistic groups.[17]
- McKenzie lumbar extensor strengthening and stabilization exercises help reduce edema and pain, improve range of motion, and stimulate healing. These exercises improve hydration of the IV disks, which is important in reversing the acidic pH of the nucleus. The acidic pH is implicated as a cause of pain.[26]

Clinical Note

There is some evidence that exercise programs and physical reconditioning can improve pain and functional levels in patients with chronic low back pain, and theoretical arguments exist for starting this by 6 weeks.[51]

- Stretching exercises for the low back, abdominals, and hamstrings.
- Weight reduction is beneficial in the obese.
- Administration and utilization of an "outcome assessment" questionnaire, such as the Oswestry Low Back Disability Index for chronic low back pain and the Roland-Morris Disability Index for acute low back pain, is strongly

recommended to gauge patient progress, suggest alterations in treatment protocol, and determine the level of disability, if any[15,35] (see Appendix C).

NUTRITIONAL MANAGEMENT PROTOCOL (OPTIONS)

Acute Pain and Inflammation:
- Proteolytic enzymes (trypsin, chymotrypsin, bromelin) (3-4 tablets qid in between meals). NOTE: Do not give to patients with ulcers!
- Bioflavonoids (quercetin, hesperidin, rutin, etc.) (200 mg mixed bioflavonoids q2h during acute phase).
- Herbals, such as boswellia, ginger, turmeric, cayenne (400 mg, 300 mg, 200 mg, 50 mg, respectively, q2h acute phase).

The above proteolytic enzymes can be obtained in Biozyme (Metagenics, Inc.) or Lyso-lymph Forte (Nutri-West, Inc.). Inflavonoid Intensive Care (Metagenics, Inc.) will provide the above bioflavonoids and herbals. Other manufactures can provide quality proteolytic enzymes. Consult your product catalog.

Tissue Healing:
- Amino acids (glycine, L-cystine, L-proline, and L-lysine) (300-400 mg per day each in divided dosages). Supplies the amino acid pool necessary for the structural production of collagen.
- Glucosamine sulfate (1500 mg per day in divided dosages). Supplies the needed nutrients for the production of healthy ground substance of the articular cartilage.
- Vitamin C (3000-6000 mg per day in divided dosages).
- Iron (glycinate) (8-12 mg per day in divided dosages)
- Alpha-ketoglutaric acid (15 mg per day in divided dosages).

The above three nutrients are required for the hydroxylation of L-proline to L-hydroxyproline, which is needed for the production of quality collagen.
- Calcium (400 mg tid)
- Vitamin E (200 IU per day)
- Zinc (glycinate) (12-18 mg per day in divided dosages)
- Copper (glycinate) (600-900 µg per day in divided dosages)
- Manganese (glycinate) (4-6 mg per day in divided dosages)

The above provide antioxidant effects and serve as free radical scavengers to help remove cellular debris and promote healing. The zinc, copper, and manganese act as cofactors and catalysts for the potent antioxidant enzyme SOD and are therefore referred to as the *SOD induction complex.* Oral supplementation with SOD can be attempted; however, it has been reported that it is often destroyed in the stomach and intestinal tract before assimilation. SOD can be obtained in Cell Guard (Biotec Foods).

All of the above tissue-healing nutrients can be obtained in the formulary product Collagenics (Metagenics, Inc.), with the exception of the glucosamine sulfate. For glucosamine sulfate, the sister product Collagenics Intensive Care (IC) must be used. However, this product does not contain the amino acid pool contained in the Collagenics. Other manufacturers make similar formulary products designed to aid in soft tissue repair, such as Rehab Plus (Professional Health Products). Consult the catalog of the reputable vendors you use for alternative products.

HOME CARE PROTOCOL (OPTIONS)

Instruct patient to:
- Wear low back support when needed.
- Avoid heavy lifting until authorized by chiropractor.
- Wear heel lift, which may be helpful.
- Perform posture and stretching/strengthening exercises as instructed by chiropractor.

REFERENCES

1. Atlas SJ: The Quebec Task Force classification for spinal disorders and the severity, treatment, and outcomes of sciatica and lumbar spinal stenosis, *Spine* 21(24):2885-2892, 1996.
2. Back to back support: British issue clinical standards similar to US guidelines, *J Am Chiropr Assoc* 32(3), 1995.
3. Balch JF, Balch PA: *Prescription for natural healing,* Wayne, NJ, 1990, Avery Publishing.
4. Banks S: Lumbar facet syndrome: spinographic assessment of treatment by spinal manipulative therapy, *J Manipulative Physiol Ther* 6:175-180, 1983.
5. Bigos S, et al: *Acute low back problems in adults,* AHCPR Clinical Practice Guidelines No 14, AHCPR Pub No 95-0642, Rockville, Md, 1994, US Dept of Health and Human Services.
6. Bland JH, Cooper SM: Osteoarthritis: a review of the cell biology involved and evidence for reversibility, management rationally related to known genesis and pathophysiology, *Semin Arthritis Rheum* 14(2):106, 1984.

7. Brukner P: *Clinical sports medicine,* New York, 1993, McGraw-Hill.

8. Bucci LR: *Nutrition applied to injury rehabilitation and sports medicine,* Boca Raton, Fla, 1995, CRC Press.

9. Cailliet R: *Low back pain syndrome,* ed 5, Philadelphia, 1995, FA Davis.

10. Cichoke AJ, Marty L: The use of proteolytic enzymes with soft-tissue athletic injuries, *Am Chiropr,* October 1981, p 32.

11. D'Ambrosio E, et al: Glucosamine sulfate: a controlled clinical investigation in arthrosis, *Pharmatherapeutica* 2(8):504-508, 1981.

12. Davis CD, Greger JL: Longitudinal changes of manganese-dependent superoxide dismutase and other indexes of manganese and iron status in women, *Am J Clin Nutr* 55:747, 1992.

13. Drovanti A, et al: Oral glucosamine sulfate in osteoarthritis: a placebo controlled double-blind investigation, *Clin Ther* 3(1):260-272, 1980.

14. Elswick CC: Facet syndrome, *J Chiropr Res Clin Invest* 6(4), 1991.

15. Fairbank JC, et al: The Oswestry Low Back Pain Disability Questionnaire, *Physiotherapy* 55(8):271-273, 1980.

16. Fauci A, et al: *Harrison's principles of internal medicine,* ed 13, New York, 1994, McGraw-Hill.

17. Gatterman M: *Chiropractic management of spine related disorders,* Baltimore, 1990, Williams & Wilkins.

18. Grabowski RJ: *Current nutritional therapy,* San Antonio, Tex, 1993, Image Press.

19. Haldeman S: *Principles and practice of chiropractic,* ed 2, Norwalk, Conn, 1992, Appleton & Lange.

20. Haldeman S, et al: Guidelines for chiropractic quality assurance & practice parameters, *The Proceedings of the Mercy Center Consensus Conference,* Gaithersburg, Md, 1993, Aspen Publishers.

21. Hammer W: *Functional soft tissue examination and treatment by manual methods,* Gaithersburg, Md, 1991, Aspen Publishers.

22. Hansen D, et al: Implementation of chiropractic guidelines: a prospective pilot study, *Transactions of the Consortium for Chiropractic Research,* June 1993.

23. Havsteen B: Flavinoids, a class of natural products of high pharmacological potency, *Biochem Pharmacol* 33(24):3933-3939, 1984.

24. Helbig T, Lee C: The lumbar facet syndrome, *Spine* 13(1):61-64, 1988.

25. Hooper PD: *Physical modalities: a primer for chiropractic,* Baltimore, 1996, Williams & Wilkins.

26. Hourigan CL, Bassett JM: Facet syndrome: clinical signs, symptoms, diagnosis and treatment, *J Manipulative Physiol Ther* 12(4):293-297, 1989.

27. Jarvis K: The guidelines in practice: the grass roots impact of the AHCPR document, *J Am Chiropr Assoc,* February 1995.

28. Kirkaldy-Willis WH: *Managing low back pain,* ed 2, Edinburgh, 1988, Churchill Livingstone.

29. Lawrence D: *Fundamentals of chiropractic diagnosis and management,* Baltimore, 1991, Williams & Wilkins.

30. Lindahl O, Lindwall L: Double blind study of a *Valerian* preparation, *Pharmacol Biochem Behav* 49(4):10065-10066, 1989.

31. Manga P, et al: *The effectiveness and cost effectiveness of chiropractic management of low-back pain,* 1993, Ontario Ministry of Health.

32. *Manual of medical therapeutics (the Washington manual),* ed 27, Boston, 1992, Little, Brown.

33. *The Merck manual,* ed 16, Rahway, NJ, 1992, Merck Co.

34. Mooney V, Leggett S: Back pain: which exercises can help, which can harm? *Consultant* 36(12), 1996.

35. Morris RM: A study of the natural history of back pain. Parts 1 and 2: development of a reliable and sensitive measure of disability in low back pain, *Spine* 8:141-150, 1983.

36. Niki E: Interaction of ascorbate and alpha-tocopherol, *Third Conference on Vitamin C* 498:187-189, 1987.

37. Phillips R: Impact of guidelines on health policy: health care policy formation—Backpain Outcome Assessment Team (BOAT), *Transactions of the Consortium for Chiropractic Research,* June 1993.

38. Rakel RE: *Conn's current therapy,* Philadelphia, 1996, WB Saunders.

39. Rakel RE: *Textbook of family practice,* ed 5, Philadelphia, 1995, WB Saunders.

40. Rossignol M, et al: Should the gap be filled between guidelines and actual practice for management of low back pain in primary care? The Quebec experience, *Spine* 21(24):2893-2898, 1996.

41. Schneider MJ: Chiropractic management of myofascial and muscular disorders. In Lawrence D, ed: *Advances in chiropractic,* vol 3, St Louis, 1996, Mosby.

42. Schwartz RI, et al: Ascorbate can act as an inducer of collagen pathway because most steps are tightly coupled, *Third Conference on Vitamin C* 498:172-184, 1987.

43. Schwarzer A, et al: Clinical features of patients with pain stemming from the lumbar zygapophyseal joints: is the lumbar facet syndrome a clinical entity? *Spine* 19(10):1132-1137, 1994.

44. Scully RM, Barnes MR: *Physical therapy,* Philadelphia, 1989, JB Lippincott.

45. Shekelle PG, et al: *The appropriateness of spinal manipulation for low back pain. Indications and ratings by an all-chiropractic expert panel,* Santa Monica, Calif, 1991, Rand.

46. Speroni E, Minghetti A: Neuropharmacological activity of extracts from *Passiflora incarnata, Planta Med* 54(6):488-491, 1988.

47. Spitzer WO, et al: Scientific approach to the assessment and management of activity-related spinal disorders: a monograph for clinicians, report of the Quebec Task Force on Spinal Disorders, *Spine* 12(7s), 1987.

48. Sprovieri J: Federal guidelines endorse manipulation, discourage surgery, *DO* 36(6), 1995.
49. Taraye JP, Lauressergues H: Advantages of combination of proteo-lytic enzymes, flavonoids and ascorbic acid in comparison with non-steroid inflammatory drugs, *Arzneimittelforschung* 27(1):1144-1149, 1977.
50. Tierney LM, McPhee SJ, Papadakis MA: *Current medical diagnosis and treatment,* Norwalk, Conn, 1996, Appleton & Lange.
51. Waddel G, et al: *Low back pain evidence review,* London, 1996, Royal College of General Practitioners.
52. Werbach MR: *Nutritional influences on illness,* ed 2, Tarzana, Calif, 1996, Third Line Press.
53. Werbach MR, Murray MT: *Botanical influences on illness,* Tarzana, Calif, 1994, Third Line Press.
54. White AA, Panjabi MM: *Clinical biomechanics of the spine,* Philadelphia, 1990, JB Lippincott.

Lumbar Disk Herniation

KEVIN PRINGLE, STEVEN FOSTER, LEW HUFF,
JASON FLANAGAN, AND DAVID M. BRADY

DEFINITION

A condition of disk protrusion into and beyond the annulus fibrosis, which may cause nerve root compression and neurological signs.

Nuclear protrusion is a localized protrusion of the nuclear material into the spinal canal resulting from thinned but not ruptured annulus fibers.

Nuclear herniation occurs when material has torn through the annulus fibrosis and is a free fragment.

ETIOLOGY

May be due to degenerative changes in the disk and spine, sudden trauma, gradual microtrauma, or a combination of the latter two. Mechanism is rotational or compression injuries that produce circumferential and radial tears in the annulus, leading to herniation. Increased incidence among the 30- to 50-year-old age-group and the elderly when the nucleus is fibrotic.

SIGNS AND SYMPTOMS

History

History of low back pain and/or leg pain over months or years.

Quality

Acute severe low back pain and leg pain. Back pain often disappears with onset of leg pain. Leg pain often predominates over back pain.

Aggravating Factors

Pain increases with forward flexion, coughing, and sneezing.

Relieving Factors

Pain is often relieved when recumbent with knees flexed. Extension of back may relieve pain.

Neurological Findings

Hypoesthesia over affected dermatome. Muscle weakness of quadriceps, dorsiflexors of ankles and toes, or plantar flexors may be present. Diminished or absent deep tendon reflexes. The above may or may not be present. **Complications: may include bladder and bowel dysfunction and cauda equina syndrome, which are surgical emergencies.**

Inspection

Diminished lumbar lordosis, antalgic posturing. Minor's sign may be noted. Myospasms may be present over the lumbosacral paraspinals and gluteals. Classic presentation is antalgic posture with pain running down the leg into the foot. Patient may have limited forward flexion of the lumbosacral spine.

Orthopedic Findings

(+) SLR, Kemp's, Lasague, bowstring. Well leg sign may or may not be (+). Decreased ranges of motion with increased pain on forward flexion. With small central herniation, lower limb signs may be absent.

Other Findings

Muscle guarding, morning stiffness, muscle atrophy. Loss of sensation occurs first.

DIFFERENTIAL DIAGNOSIS

Facet syndrome with pain referred to groin
Myofascial pain syndrome

ORTHOPEDIC EXAMINATION

Bilateral straight leg raise (+)
Well leg raise (+)/(−)
Valsalva's maneuver (+)
Decreased flexion of spine
Decreased lateral bending
Kemp's test (+)

RADIOGRAPHIC FINDINGS

Normal with incidental DJD findings. AHCPR guidelines suggest the need for plain films only if red flags exist, which include radicular signs. (See Fig. 2.)

MRI FINDINGS

May be (+) for herniation

TREATMENT GOALS

1. Promote soft tissue healing.
2. Relieve pain and prevent recurrence.
3. Increase pain-free ranges of motion.
4. Restore normal strength and stability to joint structure.
5. Quickly change to rehabilitation or restoration of function.

Clinical Notes

Proceed to rehabilitation as quickly as possible to avoid or minimize dependency on passive forms of treatment.[19]

Short duration of signs or symptoms may signal a quick response to manipulation.[19]

The number of prior episodes may increase the number of treatments to restore pain-free ranges of motion.[19]

AHCPR guidelines state that conservative care is warranted with low back pain without radiculopathy in the first month of signs and symptoms. After 1 month of manipulation, stop and reevaluate the patient for appropriateness of continued care.[4]

AHCPR guidelines state that, in absence of red flags, imaging studies and further diagnostic testing are not helpful during the first 4 weeks of low back pain.[4]

AHCPR guidelines state that low-stress aerobics may started within 2 weeks in low back pain patients.[4]

MANAGEMENT PROTOCOL (OPTIONS)

- Conservative Care Rationale:
  - Symptoms are not too severe.
  - The patient is young without spinal degeneration.
  - The occurrence is recent.
  - The patient is in otherwise good health.[27]
- Stress the importance of short-term bed rest with knees flexed. Prolonged bed rest and inactivity are discouraged. Eliminate all aggravating movements or endeavors.[8,27]

Acute Phase:

- Cold packs, ice massage, and interferential for pain and edema. Interferential can be attached with two electrodes in the lumbosacral region and two on the plantar surface of the foot.[16]
- TENS of low frequency and high intensity of less than 10 Hz creates an analgesic affect and increases the production of endorphins. Electrical stimulation increases the levels of dopamine, epinephrine, and serotonin while diminishing nerve action potentials of A delta fibers, which are pain mediators.[8]

Subacute Phase:

- Other modalities and procedures include trigger point therapy, acupuncture, high-volt galvanic therapy, and ultrasound therapy.
- Short period of spinal traction followed by a well-fitted lumbosacral support. Intermittent traction may be used when past the acute phase. Flexion/distraction technique when past the acute phase. Bracing may be accomplished with a flexible metal or plastic stay.[16]
- *Spinal adjusting/manipulation* is indicated after the first 24 to 48 hours.[8,18,26,27] Side posture manipulation is considered by some as safe and effective.[9] Hubka et al advocate flexion-distraction and extension manipulation.[24]

Clinical Notes

On the evidence, particularly the most scientifically valid clinical studies, spinal manipulation applied by chiropractors is shown to be more effective than alternative treatments for low back pain. Many medical therapies are of questionable validity or are clearly inadequate. Our reading of the literature suggests that chiropractic manipulation is safer than medical management of low back pain.[29]

Within the first 6 weeks of onset, manipulation can provide short-term improvement in pain and activity levels and higher patient satisfaction. The risks of manipulation are very low in skilled hands.[52]

The Rand Study of 1991 suggests an adequate trial of manipulation is a course of 12 manipulations given over a period of up to 4 weeks, after which, in the absence of documented improvement, spinal manipulation is no longer indicated.[46]

- **Contraindications for manipulation** include peripheralization of symptoms and a patient with a history of having lifted, twisted, or moved, a heavy object. If the lesion occurs above L1-L2 disk space, the possibility of UMN signs exists, which include saddle anesthesia, tonic bladder, and positive Babinski's reflex. Examine for sphincter incontinence and bowel and bladder dysfunction. *This is a red flag for immediate referral.*
- Rehabilitation: Use repetitive flexion and extension exercises and determine which is palliative. Have patient perform exercises with instructions to cease if peripheralization of symptoms occurs. Extension exercises help maintain correction of spinal biomechanics. Follow with 15 minutes of ice to decrease pain and edema.
- McKenzie extension exercises are beneficial.[16,42] McKenzie lumbar extensor strengthening and stabilization exercises help reduce edema and pain, improve range of motion, and stimulate healing. These exercises improve hydration of the IV disks, which is important in reversing the acidic pH of the nucleus. The acidic pH is implicated as a cause of pain.[32]

Clinical Note

There is some evidence that exercise programs and physical reconditioning can improve pain and functional levels in patients with chronic low back pain, and theoretical arguments exist for starting this by 6 weeks.[52]

- Administration and utilization of an "outcome assessment" questionnaire, such as the Oswestry Low Back Disability Index for chronic low back pain and the Roland-Morris Disability Index for acute low back pain, is strongly recommended to gauge patient progress, suggest alterations in treatment protocol, and determine level of disability, if any[14,33] (see Appendix C).

NUTRITIONAL MANAGEMENT PROTOCOL (OPTIONS)

Acute Pain and Inflammation:
- Proteolytic enzymes (trypsin, chymotrypsin, bromelin) (3-4 tablets qid in between meals). NOTE: Do not give to patients with ulcers!
- Bioflavonoids (quercetin, hesperidin, rutin, etc.) (200 mg mixed bioflavonoids q2h during acute phase).
- Herbals, such as boswellia, ginger, turmeric, cayenne (400 mg, 300 mg, 200 mg, 50 mg, respectively, q2h acute phase).

The above proteolytic enzymes can be obtained in Biozyme (Metagenics, Inc.) or Lyso-lymph Forte (Nutri-West, Inc.). Inflavonoid Intensive Care (Metagenics, Inc.) will provide the above bioflavonoids and herbals. Other manufacturers can provide quality proteolytic enzymes. Consult your product catalog.

Tissue Healing:
- Amino acids (glycine, L-cystine, L-proline, and L-lysine) (300-400 mg per day each in divided dosages). Supplies the amino acid pool necessary for the structural production of collagen.
- Glucosamine sulfate (1500 mg per day in divided dosages). Supplies the needed nutrients for the production of healthy ground substance.
- Vitamin C (3000-6000 mg per day in divided dosages).

- Iron (glycinate) (8-12 mg per day in divided dosages).
- Alpha-ketoglutaric acid (15 mg per day in divided dosages).

The above three nutrients are required for the hydroxylation of L-proline to L-hydroxyproline, which is needed for the production of quality collagen.

- Calcium (400 mg tid)
- Vitamin E (200 IU per day)
- Zinc (glycinate) (12-18 mg per day in divided dosages)
- Copper (glycinate) (600-900 µg per day in divided dosages)
- Manganese (glycinate) (4-6 mg per day in divided dosages)

The above provide antioxidant effects and serve as free radical scavengers to help remove cellular debris and promote healing. The zinc, copper, and manganese act as cofactors and catalysts for the potent antioxidant enzyme SOD and are therefore referred to as the *SOD induction complex.* Oral supplementation with SOD can be attempted; however, it has been reported that it is often destroyed in the stomach and intestinal tract before assimilation. SOD can be obtained in Cell Guard (Biotec Foods).

All of the above tissue-healing nutrients can be obtained in the formulary product Collagenics (Metagenics, Inc.), with the exception of the glucosamine sulfate. For glucosamine sulfate, the sister product Collagenics Intensive Care (IC) must be used. However, this product does not contain the amino acid pool contained in the Collagenics. Other manufacturers make similar formulary products designed to aid in soft tissue repair, such as Rehab Plus (Professional Health Products). Consult the catalog of the reputable vendors you use for alternative products.

HOME CARE PROTOCOL (OPTIONS)

Short-term bed rest, ice pack applications, home electrical stimulation, and traction when available.

REFERENCES

1. Atlas SJ: The Quebec Task Force classification for spinal disorders and the severity, treatment, and outcomes of sciatica and lumbar spinal stenosis, *Spine* 21(24):2885-2892, 1996.
2. Back to back support: British issue clinical standards similar to US guidelines, *J Am Chiropr Assoc* 32(3), 1995.
3. Balch JF, Balch PA: *Prescription for natural healing,* Wayne, NJ, 1990, Avery Publishing.

4. Bigos S, et al: *Acute low back problems in adults,* AHCPR Clinical Practice Guidelines No 14, AHCPR Pub No 95-0642, Rockville, Md, 1994, US Dept of Health and Human Services.

5. Bland JH, Cooper SM: Osteoarthritis: a review of the cell biology involved and evidence for reversibility, management rationally related to known genesis and pathophysiology, *Semin Arthritis Rheum* 14(2):106, 1984.

6. Brukner P: *Clinical sports medicine,* New York, 1993, McGraw-Hill.

7. Bucci LR: *Nutrition applied to injury rehabilitation and sports medicine,* Boca Raton, Fla, 1995, CRC Press.

8. Cailliet R: *Low back pain syndrome,* Philadelphia, 1995, FA Davis.

9. Cassidy D: Side posture manipulation for lumbar intervertebral disk herniation, *J Manipulative Physiol Ther* 16(2):96-103, 1993.

10. Cichoke AJ, Marty L: The use of proteolytic enzymes with soft-tissue athletic injuries, *Am Chiropr,* October 1981, p 32.

11. D'Ambrosio E, et al: Glucosamine sulfate: a controlled clinical investigation in arthrosis, *Pharmatherapeutica* 2(8):504-508, 1981.

12. Davis CD, Greger JL: Longitudinal changes of manganese-dependent superoxide dismutase and other indexes of manganese and iron status in women, *Am J Clin Nutr* 55:747, 1992.

13. Drovanti A, et al: Oral glucosamine sulfate in osteoarthritis: a placebo controlled double-blind investigation, *Clin Ther* 3(4):260-272, 1980.

14. Fairbank JC, et al: The Oswestry Low Back Pain Disability Questionnaire, *Physiotherapy* 66(8):271-273, 1980.

15. Fauci A, et al: *Harrison's principles of internal medicine,* ed 13, New York, 1994, McGraw-Hill.

16. Gatterman M: *Chiropractic management of spine related disorders,* Baltimore, 1990, Williams & Wilkins.

17. Grabowski RJ: *Current nutritional therapy,* San Antonio, Tex, 1993, Image Press.

18. Haldeman S: *Principles and practice of chiropractic,* ed 2, Norwalk, Conn, 1992, Appleton & Lange.

19. Haldeman S, et al: Guidelines for chiropractic quality assurance & practice parameters, *The Proceedings of the Mercy Center Consensus Conference,* Gaithersburg, Md, 1993, Aspen Publishers.

20. Hammer W: *Functional soft tissue examination and treatment by manual methods,* Gaithersburg, Md, 1991, Aspen Publishers.

21. Hansen D, et al: Implementation of chiropractic guidelines: a prospective pilot study, *Transactions of the Consortium for Chiropractic Research,* June 1993.

22. Havsteen B: Flavinoids, a class of natural products of high pharmacological potency, *Biochem Pharmacol* 33(24):3933-3939, 1984.

23. Hooper PD: *Physical modalities: a primer for chiropractic,* Baltimore, 1996, Williams & Wilkins.

24. Hubka M, et al: Lumbar intervertebral disc herniation: chiropractic management using flexion, extension, and rotational manipulative therapy, *Chiropr Techn* 3(1), 1991.

25. Jarvis K: The guidelines in practice: the grass roots impact of the AHCPR document, *J Am Chiropr Assoc*, February 1995.

26. Kirkaldy-Willis WH: *Managing low back pain,* ed 2, Edinburgh, 1988, Churchill Livingstone.

27. Lawrence D: *Fundamentals of chiropractic diagnosis and management,* Baltimore, 1991, Williams & Wilkins.

28. Lindahl O, Lindwall L: Double blind study of a *Valerian* preparation, *Pharmacol Biochem Behav* 49(4):10065-10066, 1989.

29. Manga P, et al: *The effectiveness and cost effectiveness of chiropractic management of low-back pain,* 1993, Ontario Ministry of Health.

30. *Manual of medical therapeutics (the Washington manual),* ed 27, Boston, 1992, Little, Brown.

31. *The Merck manual,* ed 16, Rahway, NJ, 1992, Merck Co.

32. Mooney V, Leggett S: Back pain: which exercises can help, which can harm? *Consultant* 36(12), 1996.

33. Morris RM: A study of the natural history of back pain. Parts 1 and 2: development of a reliable and sensitive measure of disability in low back pain, *Spine* 8:141-150, 1983.

34. New clinical perspectives on lumbar disc herniation, *Spinal Manipulation* 5(4):1-3, 1990.

35. Niki E: Interaction of ascorbate and alpha-tocopherol, *Third Conference on Vitamin C* 498:187-189, 1987.

36. Phillips R: Impact of guidelines on health policy: health care policy formation—Backpain Outcome Assessment Team (BOAT), *Transactions of the Consortium for Chiropractic Research,* June 1993.

37. Quon J, et al: Lumbar intervertebral disc herniation: treatment by rotational manipulation, *J Manipulative Physiol Ther* 12:220-227, 1989.

38. Rakel RE: *Conn's current therapy,* Philadelphia, 1996, WB Saunders.

39. Rakel RE: *Textbook of family practice,* ed 5, Philadelphia, 1995, WB Saunders.

40. Richards G, et al: Low force chiropractic care of two patients with sciatic neuropathy and lumbar disc herniation, *Am J Chiropr Med* 3(1):25-32, 1990.

41. Rossignol M, et al: Should the gap be filled between guidelines and actual practice for management of low back pain in primary care? The Quebec experience, *Spine* 21(24):2885-2892, 1996.

42. Saal JA: Natural history and nonoperative treatment of lumbar herniation, *Spine* 21:(24S):2S-9S, 1996.

43. Sanders M, Stein K: Conservative management of herniated nucleus pulposis: treatment approaches, *J Manipulative Physiol Ther* 11(4):309-313, 1988.

44. Schwartz RI, et al: Ascorbate can act as an inducer of collagen pathway because most steps are tightly coupled, *Third Conference on Vitamin C* 498:172-184, 1987.
45. Scully RM, Barnes MR: *Physical therapy,* Philadelphia, 1989, JB Lippincott.
46. Shekelle PG, et al: *The appropriateness of spinal manipulation for low back pain. Indications and ratings by an all-chiropractic expert panel,* Santa Monica, Calif, 1991, Rand.
47. Speroni E, Minghetti A: Neuropharmacological activity of extracts from *Passiflora incarnata, Planta Med* 54(6):488-491, 1988.
48. Spitzer WO, et al: Scientific approach to the assessment and management of activity-related spinal disorders: a monograph for clinicians, report of the Quebec Task Force on Spinal Disorders, *Spine* 12(7s), 1987.
49. Sprovieri J: Federal guidelines endorse manipulation, discourage surgery, *DO* 36(6), 1995.
50. Taraye JP, Lauressergues H: Advantages of combination of proteolytic enzymes, flavonoids and ascorbic acid in comparison with non-steroid inflammatory drugs, *Arzneimittelforschung* 27(1):1144-1149,1977.
51. Tierney LM, McPhee SJ, Papadakis MA: *Current medical diagnosis and treatment,* Norwalk, Conn, 1996, Appleton & Lange.
52. Waddel G, et al: *Low back pain evidence review,* London, 1996, Royal College of General Practitioners.
53. Werbach MR: *Nutritional influences on illness,* ed 2, Tarzana, Calif, 1996, Third Line Press.
54. Werbach MR, Murray MT: *Botanical influences on illness,* Tarzana, Calif, 1994, Third Line Press.
55. White AA, Panjabi MM: *Clinical biomechanics of the spine,* Philadelphia, 1990, JB Lippincott.

Lumbosacral
Strain-Sprain

LEW HUFF, JASON FLANAGAN, AND DAVID M. BRADY

DEFINITION

A combination stretch, rupture, or separation injury of the muscles and supporting ligaments of the lumbosacral spine. A stretching and tearing of spinal muscles and their attachments as a result of uncontrolled movements or direct trauma. Minor muscle strains may result from overuse or repetitive tasks.

ETIOLOGY

May be due to work or sports injuries, car accidents, continuous use, or microtrauma. Contributing factors can be leg length inequality, muscle imbalance, or excessive foot pronation.

SIGNS AND SYMPTOMS

Pain Pattern

Immediate transitory pain followed by pain-free intervals, which leads to stiffness, spasm, and diminished mobility. Pain ranges from sharp and intense to a dull ache and gnawing. Pain is localized to the lumbosacral region, there is no pain below the knee. Pain increases on muscle resistance.

Muscle Spasms

Frequently patient has difficulty rising from bed or a seated position because of pain from muscle spasms. There may be reversal of lumbar lordosis caused by multifidus spasms.

Gait and Posture

The gait is slow and guarded, the posture antalgic.

Ranges of Motion

Restricted in all planes. Joint stiffness occurs, and unilateral spasm may result in a functional scoliosis. Forward flexion may increase the pain. Strains are painful with active and isometric movements, whereas sprains are painful in active and passive ranges of motion.

Palpation

Palpable tenderness over the involved muscles, spinous tips, and transverse processes. Edema that decreases with rest. Diffuse tenderness over the paravertebral muscles and joint fixation occur.

Radiation

Pain may radiate to thoracic spine or buttocks.

Timing

Mild strains may take 7 to 10 days to heal.
Mild sprains may take 1 to 4 weeks to heal.
Moderate strains may take 2 to 4 weeks to heal.
Moderate sprains may take 1 month to 1 year to heal.
Severe strains-sprains may need surgical repair.

DIFFERENTIAL DIAGNOSIS

Facet syndrome
Lumbar instability
Metastatic lesions
Facet trophism

ORTHOPEDIC EXAMINATION

Bilateral straight leg raise
O'Donahue's

Well leg raise
Neri's bowing

ORTHOPEDIC RESULTS

All tests above (+) in acute phase for pain, but not radiculopathy
(+) Barry's sign
NOTE: all orthopedic tests are usually benign.

NEUROLOGICAL EXAMINATION

Pinwheel
Cottonswab
DTRs
Muscle strength
(All usually within normal limits)

X-RAY RESULTS

Flattened lumbosacral curve as a result of myospasms possible.
(See Fig. 2.)

TREATMENT GOALS

1. Promote soft tissue healing.
2. Relieve pain and prevent recurrence.
3. Increase pain-free ranges of motion.
4. Restore normal strength and stability to joint structure.
5. Quickly change to rehabilitation or restoration of function.

Clinical Notes

Proceed to rehabilitation as quickly as possible to avoid or
minimize dependency on passive forms of treatment.[17]

Short duration of signs or symptoms may signal a quick response
to manipulation.[17]

The number of prior episodes may increase the number of
treatments to restore pain-free ranges of motion.[17]

AHCPR guidelines state that conservative care is warranted with low back pain without radiculopathy in the first month of signs and symptoms. After 1 month of manipulation, stop and reevaluate the patient for appropriateness of continued care.[4]

AHCPR guidelines state that, in absence of red flags, imaging studies and further diagnostic testing are not helpful during the first 4 weeks of low back pain.[4]

AHCPR guidelines state that low-stress aerobics may be started within 2 weeks in low back pain patients.[4]

MANAGEMENT PROTOCOL (OPTIONS)

Acute Phase:
- Ice packs to promote vasoconstriction to decrease inflammation, pain, edema, and muscle spasms. Ice packs over affected area for 20 minutes with dry towel between ice packs and subject.
- Interferential for pain and edema management.
- High-frequency TENS used in a crossing IF pattern. Frequency 80 to 150 Hz, continuous, 15 minutes with no muscle contraction. Used for pain control and increasing levels of endorphins and enkephalins.[21]
- Short-term use of a lumbosacral support (3 to 7 days depending on the severity of the injury).[24]
- *Do not traction* during acute phase.

Subacute Phase:
- Manipulation: Determine joint locking and manipulate. Manipulation helps increase the pain-free ranges of motion, prevent fibrotic adhesion, decrease pain, and increase facet joint play. Moist hot packs, ultrasound, and galvanic and electrical muscle stimulation may be used. **Do not manipulate** if there is joint effusion or significant active joint inflammation.

Clinical Notes

On the evidence, particularly the most scientifically valid clinical studies, spinal manipulation applied by chiropractors is shown to be more effective than alternative treatments for low back pain. Many medical therapies are of questionable validity or are clearly inadequate. Our reading of the literature suggests that chiropractic manipulation is safer than medical management of low back pain.[26]

Within the first 6 weeks of onset, manipulation can provide short-term improvement in pain and activity levels and higher patient satisfaction. The risks of manipulation are very low in skilled hands.[48]

The Rand Study of 1991 suggests an adequate trial of manipulation is a course of 12 manipulations given over a period of up to 4 weeks, after which, in the absence of documented improvement, spinal manipulation is no longer indicated.[40]

- Other modalities may include whirlpool and hot soaks in tub at home to reduce muscle spasm and tension and improve flexibility.
- Moist hot packs for 15 to 20 minutes over affected area to induce vasodilation, decrease pain, and reduce muscle spasms.
- Low-frequency "acupuncture-like" TENS. Frequency 1 to 5 Hz, continuous, 30 minutes, intensity to muscle contraction. Used to diminish pain and increase the production of endorphins and enkephalins.[21]
- Electrical muscle stimulation with alternating, sinusoidal current. Frequency 80 to 150 Hz, continuous, 15 minutes with muscle contraction to reduce myospasms.[21]
- Muscle work, including trigger point therapy, myofascial release, spray and stretch techniques, and massage, to recondition muscles and prevent fibrotic adhesions.
- Begin active reconditioning program within 4 weeks or at chiropractor's determination of patient tolerance.[24]
- Stretching exercises may begin after the acute inflammatory phase. *Acute inflammatory phase* defined as 1 week or until patient has no pain at rest and can perform unstressed daily activities.[24]
- Exercises:
  1. Abdominal exercises to strengthen agonist/antagonist.

2. Stretch low back, abdominals, and hamstrings to recondition injured muscles and prevent fibrotic adhesions.
3. McKenzie extension exercises are beneficial.[24] McKenzie lumbar extensor strengthening and stabilization exercises help reduce edema and pain, improve range of motion, and stimulate healing.[29]

___

Clinical Note

There is some evidence that exercise programs and physical reconditioning can improve pain and functional levels in patients with chronic low back pain, and theoretical arguments exist for starting this by 6 weeks.[48]

___

- Administration and utilization of an "outcome assessment" questionnaire, such as the Oswestry Low Back Disability Index for chronic low back pain and the Roland-Morris Disability Index for acute low back pain, is strongly recommended to gauge patient progress, suggest alterations in treatment protocol, and determine the level of disability, if any[12,30] (see Appendix C).

Healing Time:
1. Uncomplicated spinal injuries should resolve within 6 weeks. More time may be required for moderate to severe traumatic injuries or prolapsed disk with neuropathy.[48]
2. Lawrence suggests that minor strain-sprain injuries resolve in 1 to 2 weeks, moderate strain-sprains resolve in 3 to 4 weeks, and injuries beyond moderate may require 5 to 10 weeks. Severe strain-sprain injuries may require surgery and postoperative rehabilitation.[37] If no satisfactory recovery is met within the initial 3 weeks of treatment, reevaluate for further complications.

NUTRITIONAL MANAGEMENT PROTOCOL (OPTIONS)

Acute Pain and Inflammation:
- Proteolytic enzymes (trypsin, chymotrypsin, bromelin) (3-4 tablets qid in between meals). NOTE: Do not give to patients with ulcers!

- Bioflavonoids (quercetin, hesperidin, rutin, etc.) (200 mg mixed bioflavonoids q2h during acute phase).
- Herbals, such as boswellia, ginger, turmeric, cayenne (400 mg, 300 mg, 200 mg, 50 mg, respectively, q2h acute phase).

The above proteolytic enzymes can be obtained in Biozyme (Metagenics, Inc.) or Lyso-lymph Forte (Nutri-West, Inc.). Inflavonoid Intensive Care (Metagenics, Inc.) will provide the above bioflavonoids and herbals.

Acute Myospasms:

- Valerian root *(Valeriana officinalis)* (100 mg q4h)
- Passion flower *(Passiflora incarnata)* (100-200 mg q4h)
- Magnesium (citrate) (100 mg q4h)
- Calcium (lactate) (50 mg q4h)

Many vendors offer formulary products with the above elements, including Valerian Daytime/Calmicin Plus (Murdock Madaus Schwabe) and Myoplex/Myoplex PM (Metagenics, Inc.).

Tissue Healing:

- Amino acids (glycine, L-cystine, L-proline, and L-lysine) (300-400 mg per day each in divided dosages). Supplies the amino acid pool necessary for the structural production of collagen.
- Glucosamine sulfate (1500 mg per day in divided dosages). Supplies the needed nutrients for the production of healthy ground substance of the IV disk and articular cartilage.
- Vitamin C (3000-6000 mg per day in divided dosages).
- Iron (glycinate) (8-12 mg per day in divided dosages).
- Alpha-ketoglutaric acid (15 mg per day in divided dosages).

The above three nutrients are required for the hydroxylation of L-proline to L-hydroxyproline, which is needed for the production of quality collagen.

- Calcium (400 mg tid)
- Vitamin E (200 IU per day)
- Zinc (glycinate) (12-18 mg per day in divided dosages)
- Copper (glycinate) (600-900 μg per day in divided dosages)
- Manganese (glycinate) (4-6 mg per day in divided dosages)

The above provide antioxidant effects and serve as free radical scavengers to help remove cellular debris and promote healing. The zinc, copper, and manganese act as cofactors and catalysts for the potent antioxidant enzyme SOD and are therefore referred to as the *SOD induction complex.* Oral supplementation with SOD can be attempted; however, it has been reported that it is often destroyed in the stomach and intestinal tract before assimilation. SOD can be obtained in Cell Guard (Biotec Foods).

All of the above tissue-healing nutrients can be obtained in the formulary product Collagenics (Metagenics, Inc.), with the exception of the glucosamine sulfate. For glucosamine sulfate, the sister product Collagenics Intensive Care (IC) must be used; however, this product does not contain the amino acid pool contained in the Collagenics. Other manufacturers make similar formulary products designed to aid in soft tissue repair, such as Rehab Plus (Professional Health Products). Consult the catalog of the reputable vendors you use for alternate products.

HOME CARE PROTOCOL (OPTIONS)

Acute and Chronic:
Instruct patient to:
- Get adequate rest on a firm mattress.
- Use a lumbosacral support during activities that stress the spine.
- Avoid heavy lifting or bending postures.
- Avoid soft furniture, deep sofas, and high heels.
- Learn weight reduction programs and perform posture exercises.
- Sleep supine with pillows under the knees or on the side with pillows between the legs.

REFERENCES

1. Atlas SJ: The Quebec Task Force classification for spinal disorders and the severity, treatment, and outcomes of sciatica and lumbar spinal stenosis, *Spine* 21(24):2885-2892, 1996.
2. Back to back support: British issue clinical standards similar to US guidelines, *J Am Chiropr Assoc* 32(3), 1995.
3. Balch JF, Balch PA: *Prescription for natural healing,* Wayne, NJ, 1990, Avery Publishing.
4. Bigos S, et al: *Acute low back problems in adults,* AHCPR Clinical Practice Guidelines No 14, AHCPR Pub No 95-0642, Rockville, Md, 1994, US Dept of Health and Human Services.
5. Bland JH, Cooper SM: Osteoarthritis: a review of the cell biology involved and evidence for reversibility, management rationally related to known genesis and pathophysiology, *Semin Arthritis Rheum* 14(2):106, 1984.
6. Brukner P: *Clinical sports medicine,* New York, 1993, McGraw-Hill.

7. Bucci LR: *Nutrition applied to injury rehabilitation and sports medicine,* Boca Raton, Fla, 1995, CRC Press.

8. Cichoke AJ, Marty L: The use of proteolytic enzymes with soft-tissue athletic injuries, *Am Chiropr,* October 1981, p 32.

9. D'Ambrosio E, et al: Glucosamine sulfate: a controlled clinical investigation in arthrosis, *Pharmatherapeutica* 2(8):504-508, 1981.

10. Davis CD, Greger JL: Longitudinal changes of manganese-dependent superoxide dismutase and other indexes of manganese and iron status in women, *Am J Clin Nutr* 55:747, 1992.

11. Drovanti A, et al: Oral glucosamine sulfate in osteoarthritis: a placebo controlled double-blind investigation, *Clin Ther* 3(4):260-272, 1980.

12. Fairbank JC, et al: The Oswestry Low Back Pain Disability Index Questionnaire, *Physiotherapy* 66(8):271-273, 1980.

13. Fauci A, et al: *Harrison's principles of internal medicine,* ed 13, New York, 1994, McGraw-Hill.

14. Gatterman M: *Chiropractic management of spine related disorders,* Baltimore, 1990, Williams & Wilkins.

15. Glass J: Acute lumbar strain: clinical signs and prognosis, *Bull Europ Chiropr Union* 27(2):39-43, 1979.

16. Grabowski RJ: *Current nutritional therapy,* San Antonio, Tex, 1993, Image Press.

17. Haldeman S, et al: Guidelines for chiropractic quality assurance & practice parameters, *The Proceedings of the Mercy Center Consensus Conference,* Gaithersburg, Md, 1993, Aspen Publishers.

18. Hammer W: *Functional soft tissue examination and treatment by manual methods,* Gaithersburg, Md, 1991, Aspen Publishers.

19. Hansen D, et al: Implementation of chiropractic guidelines: a prospective pilot study, *Transactions of the Consortium for Chiropractic Research,* June 1993.

20. Havsteen B: Flavinoids, a class of natural products of high pharmacological potency, *Biochem Pharmacol* 33(24):3933-3939, 1984.

21. Hooper PD: *Physical modalities: a primer for chiropractic,* Baltimore, 1996, Williams & Wilkins.

22. Jarvis K: The guidelines in practice: the grass roots impact of the AHCPR document, *J Am Chiropr Assoc* 32(2):39-40, 1995.

23. Lawrence D: *Fundamentals of chiropractic diagnosis and management,* Baltimore, 1991, Williams & Wilkins.

24. Liebenson C: *Rehabilitation of the spine,* Baltimore, 1996, Williams & Wilkins.

25. Lindahl O, Lindwall L: Double blind study of a *Valerian* preparation, *Pharmacol Biochem Behav* 32(4):10065-10066, 1989.

26. Manga P, et al: *The effectiveness and cost effectiveness of chiropractic management of low-back pain,* 1993, Ontario Ministry of Health.

27. *Manual of medical therapeutics (the Washington manual)*, ed 27, Boston, 1992, Little, Brown.

28. *The Merck manual*, ed 16, Rahway, NJ, 1992, Merck Co.

29. Mooney V, Leggett S: Back pain: which exercises can help, which can harm? *Consultant* 36(12), 1996.

30. Morris RM: A study of the natural history of back pain. Parts 1 and 2: development of a reliable and sensitive measure of disability in low back pain, *Spine* 8:141 150, 1983.

31. Niki E: Interaction of ascorbate and alpha-tocopherol, *Third Conference on Vitamin C* 498:187-189, 1987.

32. Nimmo R: Receptor, effecters and tonus: a new approach, *J Natl Chiropr Assoc*, November 1957.

33. Phillips R: Impact of guidelines on health policy: health care policy formation—Backpain Outcome Assessment Team (BOAT), *Transactions of the Consortium for Chiropractic Research*, June 1993.

34. Rakel RE: *Conn's current therapy*, Philadelphia, 1996, WB Saunders.

35. Rakel RE: *Textbook of family practice*, ed 5, Philadelphia, 1995, WB Saunders.

36. Rossignol M, et al: Should the gap be filled between guidelines and actual practice for management of low back pain in primary care? The Quebec experience, *Spine* 21(24), 1996.

37. Schneider MJ: Chiropractic management of myofascial and muscular disorders. In Lawrence D, ed: *Advances in chiropractic*, vol 3, St Louis, 1996, Mosby.

38. Schwartz RI, et al: Ascorbate can act as an inducer of collagen pathway because most steps are tightly coupled, *Third Conference on Vitamin C* 498:172-184, 1987.

39. Scully RM, Barnes MR: *Physical therapy*, Philadelphia, 1989, JB Lippincott.

40. Shekelle PG, et al: *The appropriateness of spinal manipulation for low back pain. Indications and ratings by an all-chiropractic expert panel*, Santa Monica, Calif, 1991, Rand.

41. Speroni E, Minghetti A: Neuropharmacological activity of extracts from *Passiflora Incarnata*, *Planta Med* 54(6):488-491, 1988.

42. Spitzer WO, et al: Scientific approach to the assessment and management of activity-related spinal disorders: a monograph for clinicians, report of the Quebec Task Force on Spinal Disorders, *Spine* 12(7s), 1987.

43. Sprovieri J: Federal guidelines endorse manipulation, discourage surgery, *DO* 36(6), 1995.

44. Taraye JP, Lauressergues H: Advantages of combination of proteolytic enzymes, flavonoids and ascorbic acid in comparison with non-steroid inflammatory drugs, *Arzneimittelforschung* 27(1):1144-1149, 1977.

45. Tierney LM, McPhee SJ, Papadakis MA: *Current medical diagnosis and treatment,* Norwalk, Conn, 1996, Appleton & Lange.
46. Travell JG, Simons DG: *Myofascial pain and dysfunction: the trigger point manual,* 1992, Baltimore, 1992, Williams & Wilkins.
47. US Agency for Health Care Policy and Research, Dec 8, 1994.
48. Waddel G, et al: *Low back pain evidence review,* London, 1996, Royal College of General Practitioners.
49. Werbach MR: *Nutritional influences on illness,* ed 2, Tarzana, Calif, 1996, Third Line Press.
50. Werbach MR, Murray MT: *Botanical influences on illness,* Tarzana, Calif, 1994, Third Line Press.
51. White AA, Panjabi MM: *Clinical biomechanics of the spine,* Philadelphia, 1990, JB Lippincott.

Sciatic Neuralgia

Lew Huff, Jason Flanagan, and David M. Brady

DEFINITION

A low back pain condition characterized by pain radiating down the posterolateral leg, unilaterally or bilaterally along the distribution of the sciatic nerve.

ETIOLOGY

May be due to peripheral nerve compression, IV disk herniation, degenerative joint disease, sports or occupational injuries, fractures, infection, spinal tumor, back strain, or spondylolisthesis. Spinal stenosis is an uncommon form of sciatica that mimics vascular disease by simulating intermittent claudication.

SIGNS AND SYMPTOMS

Pain Pattern

Increased pain and paresthesia along dermatomal patterns of sciatic nerve roots. Antalgic gait noted.

Palpation

Digital palpation of the popliteal fossa and gluteals reveals pain and tenderness. Piriformis spasm present in 80% of cases.

Radiation

Shooting pain down the posterolateral leg, which may radiate to or below the knee.

Neurological Manifestations

Motor weakness, diminished reflexes, sensory loss, muscle atrophy possible.

DIFFERENTIAL DIAGNOSIS

Osteoarthritis
Referred pain
Fracture
Myofascial pain syndrome
Piriformis syndrome

ORTHOPEDIC EXAMINATION

Valsalva's maneuver
Straight leg raise

NEUROLOGICAL EXAMINATION

Toe, heel walk
Pinwheel
Cottonswab
Reflexes
Motor testing

TEST RESULTS

(+) straight leg raise 50%
(+) well leg raise possible
Diminished reflex, sensory, and/or motor changes may be present

X-RAY FINDINGS

Bony defects
DJD
Sacral instability

Clinical Note

Piriformis syndrome is often misdiagnosed when it presents as sciatic pain and numbness down the leg. Diagnosis may be made by rectal or transvaginal palpation of the piriformis muscle and by the presence of trigger point tenderness of the muscle adjacent to the sacrum.[35]

(See Fig. 2.)

TREATMENT GOALS

1. Promote soft tissue healing.
2. Relieve pain and prevent recurrence.
3. Increase pain-free ranges of motion.
4. Restore normal strength and stability to joint structure.
5. Quickly change to rehabilitation and restoration of function.

Clinical Notes

Proceed to rehabilitation as quickly as possible to avoid or minimize dependency on passive forms of treatment.[14]

Short duration of signs or symptoms may signal a quick response to manipulation.[14]

The number of prior episodes may increase the number of treatments to restore pain-free ranges of motion.[14]

AHCPR guidelines state that low-stress aerobics may be started within 2 weeks in low back pain patients.[4]

AHCPR guidelines state that with or without surgery, 80% of sciatica patients will recover.[4]

MANAGEMENT PROTOCOL (OPTIONS)

Acute Phase:

- Ice packs to promote vasoconstriction to decrease inflammation, pain, edema, and muscle spasms. Ice packs over affected area for 20 minutes with dry towel between ice packs and subject. Ice, ultrasound, and galvanism may be used. Interferential current for pain and edema management.

- Bed rest no longer than 3 to 5 days to decrease inflammation. Antiinflammatories and bracing may be needed. Each additional day of bed rest may produce weeks of rehabilitation. Back support used no longer than 10 to 14 days.
- High-frequency TENS used in a crossing IF pattern. Frequency 80 to 150 Hz, continuous, 15 minutes with no muscle contraction. Used for pain control and increasing levels of endorphins and enkephalins.
- Stretching exercises may begin after the acute inflammatory phase. *Acute inflammatory phase* is defined as 1 week or until patient has no pain at rest and can perform unstressed daily activities.[21]
- **Do not traction** during acute phase of treatment.

Subacute Phase:

- Manipulation: Determine joint locking and manipulate. Manipulation helps increase the pain-free ranges of motion, prevent fibrotic adhesion, decrease pain, and increase facet joint play. **Do not manipulate** if there is joint effusion or significant active joint inflammation.

Clinical Notes

On the evidence, particularly the most scientifically valid clinical studies, spinal manipulation applied by chiropractors is shown to be more effective than alternative treatments for low back pain. Many medical therapies are of questionable validity or are clearly inadequate. Our reading of the literature suggests that chiropractic manipulation is safer than medical management of low back pain.[22]

Within the first 6 weeks of onset, manipulation can provide short-term improvement in pain and activity levels and higher patient satisfaction. The risks of manipulation are very low in skilled hands.[41]

The Rand Study of 1991 suggests an adequate trial of manipulation is a course of 12 manipulations given over a period of up to

4 weeks, after which, in the absence of documented improvement, spinal manipulation is no longer indicated.[34]

- Ultrasound may be used.
- Moist hot packs for 15 to 20 minutes over affected area to induce vasodilation, decrease pain, and reduce muscle spasms.
- Low-frequency "acupuncture-like" TENS. Frequency 1 to 5 Hz, continuous, 30 minutes, intensity to muscle contraction. Used to diminish pain and increase the production of endorphins and enkephalins.[18]
- Electrical muscle stimulation with alternating, sinusoidal current. Frequency 80 to 150 Hz, continuous, 15 minutes with muscle contraction to reduce myospasms.[18]
- Muscle work, including trigger point therapy, myofascial release, spray and stretch techniques, and massage, to recondition muscles and prevent fibrotic adhesions. Screen piriformis musculature closely.
- Exercises:
  1. Rehabilitation may begin within 4 to 6 weeks.
  2. Abdominal exercises to strengthen agonist/antagonist.
  3. Stretch low back, abdominals, and hamstrings to recondition injured muscles and prevent fibrotic adhesions.
  4. Surgical tubing and ROM exercises are beneficial.
  5. McKenzie extension exercises are beneficial.[11,25] McKenzie lumbar extensor strengthening and stabilization exercises help reduce edema and pain, improve range of motion, and stimulate healing.[26]

Clinical Note

There is some evidence that exercise programs and physical reconditioning can improve pain and functional levels in patients with chronic low back pain, and theoretical arguments exist for starting this by 6 weeks.[41]

- Administration and utilization of an "outcome assessment" questionnaire, such as the Oswestry Low Back Disability

Index for chronic low back pain and the Roland-Morris Disability Index for acute low back pain, is strongly recommended to gauge patient progress, suggest alterations in treatment protocol, and determine the level of disability, if any[9,26] (see Appendix C).

NUTRITIONAL MANAGEMENT PROTOCOL (OPTIONS)

Acute Pain and Inflammation:
- Proteolytic enzymes (trypsin, chymotrypsin, bromelin) (3-4 tablets qid in between meals). NOTE: Do not give to patients with ulcers!
- Bioflavonoids (quercetin, hesperidin, rutin, etc.) (200 mg mixed bioflavonoids q2h during acute phase).
- Herbals, such as boswellia, ginger, turmeric, cayenne (400 mg, 300 mg, 200 mg, 50 mg, respectively, q2h acute phase).

The above proteolytic enzymes can be obtained in Biozyme (Metagenics, Inc.) or Lyso-lymph Forte (Nutri-West, Inc.). Inflavonoid Intensive Care (Metagenics, Inc.) will provide the above bioflavonoids and herbals. Other manufactures can provide quality proteolytic enzymes. Consult your product catalog.

If myospasm is present:
- Valerian root *(Valeriana officinalis)* (100 mg q4h)
- Passion flower *(Passiflora incarnata)* (100-200 mg q4h)
- Magnesium (citrate) (100 mg q4h)
- Calcium (lactate) (50 mg q4h)

Many vendors offer formulary products with the above elements, including Valerian Daytime/Calmicin Plus (Murdock Madaus Schwabe) and Myoplex/Myoplex PM (Metagenics, Inc.).

HOME CARE PROTOCOL (OPTIONS)

Acute and Chronic:
Instruct patient to:
- Get adequate rest on a firm mattress.
- Use a lumbosacral support during activities that stress the spine.
- Avoid heavy lifting or bending postures. Avoid soft furniture, deep sofas, and high heels.
- Learn weight reduction programs, and perform posture exercises.

- Sleep supine with pillows under the knees or on the side with pillows between the legs.

REFERENCES

1. Atlas SJ: The Quebec Task Force classification for spinal disorders and the severity, treatment, and outcomes of sciatica and lumbar spinal stenosis, *Spine* 21(24):2885-2892, 1996.
2. Back to back support: British issue clinical standards similar to US guidelines, *J Am Chiropr Assoc* 32(3), 1995.
3. Balch JF, Balch PA: *Prescription for natural healing*, Wayne, NJ, 1990, Avery Publishing.
4. Bigos S, et al: *Acute low back problems in adults*, AHCPR Clinical Practice Guidelines No 14, AHCPR Pub No 95-0642, Rockville, Md, 1994, US Dept of Health and Human Services.
5. Brukner P: *Clinical sports medicine*, New York, 1993, McGraw-Hill.
6. Bucci LR: *Nutrition applied to injury rehabilitation and sports medicine*, Boca Raton, Fla, 1995, CRC Press.
7. Cailliet R: *Low back pain syndrome*, Philadelphia, 1995, FA Davis.
8. Cichoke AJ, Marty L: The use of proteolytic enzymes with soft-tissue athletic injuries, *Am Chiropr*, October 1981, p 32.
9. Fairbank JC, et al: The Oswestry Low Back Pain Disability Index Questionnaire, *Physiotherapy* 66(8):271-273, 1980.
10. Fauci A, et al: *Harrison's principles of internal medicine*, ed 13, New York, 1994, McGraw-Hill.
11. Gatterman M: *Chiropractic management of spine related disorders*, Baltimore, 1990, Williams & Wilkins.
12. Grabowski RJ: *Current nutritional therapy*, San Antonio, Tex, 1993, Image Press.
13. Haldeman S: *Principles and practice of chiropractic*, ed 2, Norwalk, Conn, 1992, Appleton & Lange.
14. Haldeman S, et al: Guidelines for chiropractic quality assurance & practice parameters, *The Proceedings of the Mercy Center Consensus Conference*, Gaithersburg, Md, 1993, Aspen Publishers.
15. Hammer W: *Functional soft tissue examination and treatment by manual methods*, Gaithersburg, Md, 1991, Aspen Publishers.
16. Hansen D, et al: Implementation of chiropractic guidelines: a prospective pilot study, *Transactions of the Consortium for Chiropractic Research*, June 1993.
17. Havsteen B: Flavinoids, a class of natural products of high pharmacological potency, *Biochem Pharmacol* 33(24):3933-3939, 1984.
18. Hooper PD: *Physical modalities: a primer for chiropractic*, Baltimore, 1996, Williams & Wilkins.
19. Jarvis K: The guidelines in practice: the grass roots impact of the AHCPR document, *J Am Chiropr Assoc*, February 1995.

20. Lawrence D: *Fundamentals of chiropractic diagnosis and management,* Baltimore, 1991, Williams & Wilkins.

21. Liebenson C: *Rehabilitation of the spine,* Baltimore, 1996, Williams & Wilkins.

22. Manga P, et al: *The effectiveness and cost effectiveness of chiropractic management of low-back pain,* 1993, Ontario Ministry of Health.

23. *Manual of medical therapeutics (the Washington manual),* ed 27, Boston, 1992, Little, Brown.

24. *The Merck manual,* ed 16, Rahway, NJ, 1992, Merck Co.

25. Mooney V, Leggett S: Back pain: which exercises can help, which can harm? *Consultant* 36(12), 1996.

26. Morris RM: A study of the natural history of back pain. Parts 1 and 2: development of a reliable and sensitive measure of disability in low back pain, *Spine* 8:141-150, 1983.

27. Nimmo R: Receptor, effecters and tonus: a new approach, *J Natl Chiropr Assoc,* November 1957.

28. Phillips R: Impact of guidelines on health policy: health care policy formation—Backpain Outcome Assessment Team (BOAT), *Transactions of the Consortium for Chiropractic Research,* June 1993.

29. Rakel RE: *Conn's current therapy,* Philadelphia, 1996, WB Saunders.

30. Rakel RE: *Textbook of family practice,* ed 5, Philadelphia, 1995, WB Saunders.

31. Rossignol M, et al: Should the gap be filled between guidelines and actual practice for management of low back pain in primary care? The Quebec experience, *Spine* 21(24), 1996.

32. Schneider MJ: Chiropractic management of myofascial and muscular disorders. In Lawrence D, ed: *Advances in chiropractic,* vol 3, St Louis, 1996, Mosby.

33. Scully RM, Barnes MR: *Physical therapy,* Philadelphia, 1989, JB Lippincott.

34. Shekelle PG, et al: *The appropriateness of spinal manipulation for low back pain. Indications and ratings by an all-chiropractic expert panel,* Santa Monica, Calif, 1991, Rand.

35. Singler R: Misdiagnosing piriformis syndrome as sciatica, *Cortlandt Letters,* August 1996.

36. Spitzer WO, et al: Scientific approach to the assessment and management of activity-related spinal disorders: a monograph for clinicians, report of the Quebec Task Force on Spinal Disorders, *Spine* 12(7s), 1987.

37. Sprovieri J: Federal guidelines endorse manipulation, discourage surgery, *DO* 36(6), 1995.

38. Taraye JP, Lauressergues H: Advantages of combination of proteolytic enzymes, flavonoids and ascorbic acid in comparison with non-steroid inflammatory drugs, *Arzneimittelforschung* 27(1):1144-1149,1977.

39. Tierney LM, McPhee SJ, Papadakis MA: *Current medical diagnosis and treatment,* Norwalk, Conn, 1996, Appleton & Lange.
40. Travell JG, Simons DG: *Myofascial pain and dysfunction: the trigger point manual,* vol 2, Baltimore, 1992, Williams & Wilkins.
41. Waddel G, et al: *Low back pain evidence review,* London, 1996, Royal College of General Practitioners.
42. Werbach MR: *Nutritional influences on illness,* ed 2, Tarzana, Calif, 1996, Third Line Press.
43. Werbach MR, Murray MT: *Botanical influences on illness,* Tarzana, Calif, 1994, Third Line Press.
44. White AA, Panjabi MM: *Clinical biomechanics of the spine,* Philadelphia, 1990, JB Lippincott.

Piriformis Syndrome

URSULA FUNDERBURK, LEW HUFF, AND DAVID M. BRADY

DEFINITION

A low back pain condition described as a compression or irritation of the sciatic nerve by a contracted or stretched piriformis muscle. The syndrome is 6 times more common in females than in males.

ETIOLOGY

Trauma to the sacroiliac joint produces a ligamentous sprain, leading to piriformis syndrome. Irritation of the sciatic nerve sheath is caused by biochemical agents released from an inflamed piriformis muscle, where the two structures meet at the greater sciatic foramen. Prolonged sitting, buttock trauma, leg length discrepancy, and hip flexor tightness are among other causative factors.[16]

SIGNS AND SYMPTOMS

Pain Pattern

Pain and paresthesia may travel the course of the sciatic nerve. Either deep boring or dull ache down the posterior thigh to the knee occasionally extending to the foot occur.

Palpation

Digital palpation reveals trigger points and spasms at the site of the piriformis muscle. Gluteals may be tender, and tightness and stiffness of the hamstrings and low back might occur. Deep pressure over affected piriformis reproduces sciatic pain.

Range of Motion

Internal rotation of hip with knees flexed is painful.

Orthopedic

(+) straight leg raise with pain intensified by simultaneous internal rotation of the leg and relieved by external rotation (piriformis test).

Neurological Findings

Absence of true neurological findings. Radiation pattern mimics sciatica.

Other Manifestations

Symptoms are almost identical to lumbar disk syndrome. CT, MRI, x-ray, myelography, and electromyography are of limited diagnostic value.

DIFFERENTIAL DIAGNOSIS

Sciatica
Referred pain
Fracture
Myofascial pain syndrome
Intevertebral disk syndrome (IVD syndrome)

ORTHOPEDIC EXAMINATION

Valsalva's maneuver (−)
Straight leg raise (+/−)

NEUROLOGICAL EXAMINATION

Toe, heel walk (−)
Pinwheel (−)

Cottonswab (−)
Reflexes (−)
Motor (−)

X-RAY FINDINGS

Unremarkable

Clinical Notes

Piriformis syndrome is often misdiagnosed when it presents as sciatic pain and numbness down the leg. Diagnosis may be made by rectal or transvaginal palpation of the piriformis muscle and by the presence of trigger point tenderness of the muscle adjacent to the sacrum.[20]

Testing the piriformis muscle: Patient prone, knees flexed at 90 degrees, the tibia are allowed to fall laterally, causing the hips to rotate internally. Clinician stands at caudal end of table, comparing each side for the amount of internal rotation. Decreased rotation internally concurrent with other findings may indicate tight piriformis.

TREATMENT GOALS

1. Promote soft tissue healing.
2. Relieve pain and prevent recurrence.
3. Increase pain-free ranges of motion.

MANAGEMENT PROTOCOL (OPTIONS)

Acute Phase:
- Ice packs to promote vasoconstriction to decrease inflammation, pain, edema, and muscle spasms. Ice packs over affected area for 20 minutes with dry towel between ice packs and subject. Ice, ultrasound (pulsed), and galvanism may be used. Interferential current for pain and edema management. Success has been reported with the use of ultrasound.[22]

Subacute Phase:
- Moist hot packs to affected area for 10 minutes to relax the muscle and increase blood flow, ultrasound-electrical muscle stimulation combination: acute (pulsed), chronic (continuous). Combination therapy facilitates healing, decreases pain and spasm.
- Muscle work, including trigger point therapy, myofascial release, spray and stretch techniques, and massage, to recondition muscles and prevent fibrotic adhesions. Screen piriformis musculature closely for spasms and tender points.
- Manipulation: Determine joint locking and manipulate. Manipulation helps increase the pain-free ranges of motion, prevent fibrotic adhesion, decrease pain, and increase facet joint play. Manipulation of the sacrum and ilium subluxations.[8,13,18]

Clinical Notes

On the evidence, particularly the most scientifically valid clinical studies, spinal manipulation applied by chiropractors is shown to be more effective than alternative treatments for low back pain. Many medical therapies are of questionable validity or are clearly inadequate. Our reading of the literature suggests that chiropractic manipulation is safer than medical management of low back pain.[12]

The Rand Study of 1991 suggests an adequate trial of manipulation is a course of 12 manipulations given over a period of up to 4 weeks, after which, in the absence of documented improvement, spinal manipulation is no longer indicated.[18]

- Piriformis stretch: Patient supine, midback flattened against the floor, bend knee to waist level, cross the affected leg over the other leg, gently pull the affected leg over the unaffected leg and toward the floor, hold for 10 to 15 seconds. Fifteen repetitions twice a day.
- Postisometric relaxation (PIR) stretch technique: *Step 1:* Record the length of piriformis bilaterally. *Step 2:* Place the

patient supine with the knee flexed to chest and internally rotated. It is preferable if the knee is turned in to the point of hypertonicity. Instruct the patient to take a deep breath and hold, contracting the muscle against your resistance of no more than 80%. Have the patient hold the contraction for 3 to 5 seconds, blow the air out, and relax the muscle. Repeat three cycles.

- McKenzie extension exercises are beneficial. McKenzie lumbar extensor strengthening and stabilization exercises help reduce edema and pain, improve range of motion, and stimulate healing.[14]

Clinical Note

There is some evidence that exercise programs and physical reconditioning can improve pain and functional levels in patients with chronic low back pain, and theoretical arguments exist for starting this by 6 weeks.[24]

- Administration and utilization of an "outcome assessment" questionnaire, such as the Oswestry Low Back Disability Index for chronic low back pain and the Roland-Morris Disability Index for acute low back pain, is strongly recommended to gauge patient progress, suggest alterations in treatment protocol, and determine the level of disability, if any[2,14] (see Appendix C).

NUTRITIONAL MANAGEMENT PROTOCOL (OPTIONS)

Acute Muscle Spasm:
- Valerian root *(Valeriana officinalis)* (100 mg q4h)
- Passion flower *(Passiflora incarnata)* (100-200 mg q4h)
- Magnesium (citrate) (100 mg q4h)
- Calcium (lactate) (50 mg q4h)

Many vendors offer formulary products with the above elements, including Valerian Daytime/Calmicin Plus (Murdock Madaus Schwabe) and Myoplex/Myoplex PM (Metagenics, Inc.).

HOME CARE PROTOCOL (OPTIONS)

Acute and Chronic:

Instruct patient to:

- Get adequate rest on a firm mattress.
- Avoid heavy lifting or bending postures.
- Sleep supine with pillows under the knees or on the side with pillows between the legs.
- Perform piriformis stretch as per chiropractor's instruction.

REFERENCES

1. Balch JF, Balch PA: *Prescription for natural healing,* Wayne, NJ, 1990, Avery Publishing.
2. Fairbank JC, et al: The Oswestry Low Back Pain Disability Questionnaire, *Physiotherapy* 66(8):271-273, 1980.
3. Gatterman M: *Chiropractic management of spine related disorders,* Baltimore, 1990, Williams & Wilkins
4. Grabowski RJ: *Current nutritional therapy,* San Antonio, Tex, 1993, Image Press.
5. Huber H: The piriformis syndrome: a possible cause of sciatica, *Schweiz Rundsch Med Prax* 79(9):235-236, 1990.
6. Johansson J: Piriformis syndrome: a case study, *Osteopathic Annals* 14(5):21-23, 1987.
7. Kirkaldy-Willis W, Hill R: A more precise diagnosis for low-back pain, *Spine* 4:102-108, 1979.
8. Lamb KL: Sacroiliac joint dysfunction with associated piriformis syndrome mimicking intervertebral disc syndrome resulting in failed low back surgery, *Chiropr Techn* 9(3), 1997.
9. Lawrence D: *Fundamentals of chiropractic diagnosis and management,* Baltimore, 1991, Williams & Wilkins.
10. Liebenson C: *Rehabilitation of the spine,* Baltimore, 1996, Williams & Wilkins.
11. Lindahl O, Lindwall L: Double blind study of a *Valerian* preparation, *Pharmacol Biochem Behav* 32(4):10065-10066, 1989.
12. Manga P, et al: *The effectiveness and cost effectiveness of chiropractic management of low-back pain,* 1993, Ontario Ministry of Health.
13. Mooney V, Leggett S: Back pain: which exercises can help, which can harm? *Consultant* 36(12), 1996.
14. Morris RM: A study of the natural history of back pain. Parts 1 and 2: development of a reliable and sensitive measure of disability in low back pain, *Spine* 8:141-150, 1983.
15. Myers K, et al: Sciatica of muscular origin in recreational runner: a case report, *Chiropr Sports Med* 5(2), 1991.

16. Nimmo R: Receptor, effecters and tonus: a new approach, *J Natl Chiropr Assoc,* November 1957.

17. Rich B, Mckeag D: When sciatica is not disk disease: detecting piriformis syndromes in active patients, *Phys Sports Med* 20(10):105-115, 1992.

18. Shekelle PG, et al: *The appropriateness of spinal manipulation for low back pain. Indications and ratings by an all-chiropractic expert panel,* Santa Monica, Calif, 1991, Rand.

19. Simons D, Travell J: Myofascial origins of low back pain: 3 pelvic and lower extremity muscles, *Postgrad Med* 73(2):99-108, 1983.

20. Singler R: Misdiagnosing piriformis syndrome as sciatica, *Cortlandt Letters,* August 1996.

21. Speroni E, Minghetti A: Neuropharmacological activity of extracts from *Passiflora incarnata, Planta Med* 54(6):488-491, 1988.

22. Steiner C, et al: Piriformis syndrome: pathogenesis, diagnosis, and treatment, *J Am Osteopath Assoc* 87(4):318-323, 1987.

23. Travell JG, Simons DG: *Myofascial pain and dysfunction: the trigger point manual,* vol 2, Baltimore, 1992, Williams & Wilkins.

24. Waddel G, et al: *Low back pain evidence review,* London, 1996, Royal College of General Practitioners.

25. Werbach MR: *Nutritional influences on illness,* ed 2, Tarzana, Calif, 1996, Third Line Press.

26. Werbach MR, Murray MT: *Botanical influences on illness,* Tarzana, Calif, 1994, Third Line Press.

Spondylolisthesis

Jeffrey Weiss

DEFINITION

An anterior displacement of a vertebral body in relation to the segment immediately below. The displacement is the result of loss in continuity or elongation of the pars interarticularis. A loss in continuity without slippage is called *spondylolysis*.

ETIOLOGY

Dysplastic: Inadequate development of the posterior elements without slippage is called *spondylolysis*.

Isthmic: A break of the pars interarticularis as a result of a fatigue fracture (most common), acute trauma (rare), or repeated microtrauma leading to elongation.

Degenerative: A break in the pars interarticularis as a result of erosive pressure from the superior articular facet below and the inferior articular facet above.

Traumatic: A break in the neural arch as a result of acute trauma to any area other than the pars interarticularis.

Pathologic: Destructive lesion to the pars interarticularis as a result of dysplasia, carcinoma, metastasis, Paget's disease, or others.

SIGNS AND SYMPTOMS

Palpation

Paraspinal muscle spasms. Hamstring tightness. Possible protrusion of spinous process. Chronic muscle spasms or myofascitis is common.

Pain Pattern

Pain may increase with activity, upright posture, or hyper-extension of the lumbar spine.[6] Spondylolisthesis may be asymptomatic.

Grading of Spondylolisthesis

Grade I: 0% to 25% slippage
Grade II: 25% to 50% slippage
Grade III: 50% to 75% slippage
Grade IV: 75% to 100% slippage
Grade V: Complete slippage of vertebral body in relation to the
  segment below.

ORTHOPEDIC EXAMINATION

Negative unless acute inflammation or trauma

NEUROLOGICAL EXAMINATION

Hypo or hyper DTRs possible; in rare cases, paresthesia over lumbar root dermatome patterns

LABORATORY EXAMINATION

Negative

RADIOGRAPHIC FINDINGS

Spondylolysis: lucent defect in the pars interarticularis. Spondy-lolisthesis: lucent defect of pars with forward slippage. Will appear as collar on the "Scotty Dog": A-P spot film gives better view of L5-S1 disk space.

Flexion/extension views will help rule out instability. If over 25% migration or progressive neurological involvement, refer for surgical consult. Compression/distraction views can be used if flexion/extension views do not demonstrate instability.

TREATMENT GOALS

1. Relieve pain and prevent recurrence.
2. Increase pain-free ranges of motion.

3. Restore normal strength and stability to joint structure.
4. Quickly change to rehabilitation and restoration of function.

Clinical Note

Spinal manipulative therapy is not contraindicated in the presence of spondylolisthesis if specific to the site of joint hypomobility and if the underlying spondylolisthesis is stable.[6]

MANAGEMENT PROTOCOL (OPTIONS)

Acute Stage:
- Interferential, TENS, ultrasound (pulsed), galvanic-positive pole, and cryotherapy may be used to diminish pain and muscle spasms in acute phase. Treatment during the acute phase or with demonstrable antalgia should consist of daily treatments for the first week, then diminish the number of visits as tolerated.

Chronic Phase:
- Sine wave, diathermy, galvanic-negative pole, and ultrasound may be used to diminish pain and spasms.
- *Manipulation:*
  1. Confine manipulation to the adjacent joints, and avoid the involved joint.
  2. Manipulate the sacroiliac joints if needed.
  3. Flexion-distraction technique is beneficial.
  4. Sacral pull (bilateral knee to chest):
     a. Bring both knees up to patient's chest.
     b. Place arm between patient's leg and palm of hand on sacrum; noncontact arm rests across patient's knees.
     c. Pull anterior and superior on sacrum and hold 15 seconds or to patient tolerance.

Clinical Notes

On the evidence, particularly the most scientifically valid clinical studies, spinal manipulation applied by chiropractors is shown to be more effective than alternative treatments for low back pain. Many medical therapies are of questionable validity or are clearly inadequate. Our reading of the literaturesuggests that chiropractic manipulation is safer than medical management of low back pain.[18]

Within the first 6 weeks of onset, manipulation can provide short-term improvement in pain and activity levels and higher patient satisfaction. The risks of manipulation are very low in skilled hands.[32]

- *Exercise Therapy:* Various exercise techniques may be used to stretch and strengthen the surrounding musculature.
  1. Knee to chest—single and double
  2. Pelvic tilt
  3. Bridging stabilization
  4. Iliopsoas stretch: kneeling stretch (lunge)
  5. Cat back
  6. Forward trunk kneeling prayer position stretch
  7. Quadruped alternate arm and leg stabilization—cross crawl
  8. Adductor stretch—Indian sitting
  9. Hamstring stretch
     a. Medial—rotate foot laterally
     b. Neutral—straight
     c. Lateral—rotate foot medially
     d. Door jam stretch
  10. Gastrocnemius/soleus stretch
      a. Wall push
         (1) Gastrocnemius—involved leg straight
         (2) Soleus—involved leg bent
      b. Foot on ledge (heels hangs over ledge)

Clinical Note

There is some evidence that exercise programs and physical reconditioning can improve pain and functional levels in patients with chronic low back pain, and theoretical arguments for starting this by 6 weeks.[32]

- Administration and utilization of an "outcome assessment" questionnaire, such as the Oswestry Low Back Disability Index for chronic low back pain and the Roland-Morris Disability Index for acute low back pain, is strongly recommended to gauge patient progress, suggest alterations in treatment protocol, and determine the level of disability, if any[7,22] (see Appendix C).

REFERENCES

1. Atlas SJ: The Quebec Task Force classification for spinal disorders and the severity, treatment, and outcomes of sciatica and lumbar spinal stenosis, *Spine* 21(24):2885-2892, 1996.
2. Back to back support: British issue clinical standards similar to US guidelines, *J Am Chiropr Assoc* 32(3), 1995.
3. Bigos S, et al: *Acute low back problems in adults,* AHCPR Clinical Practice Guidelines No 14, AHCPR Pub No 95-0642, Rockville, Md, 1994, US Dept of Health and Human Services.
4. Brukner P: *Clinical sports medicine,* New York, 1993, McGraw-Hill.
5. Cailliet R: *Low back pain syndrome,* Philadelphia, 1995, FA Davis.
6. Day MO: Spondylolytic spondylolisthesis in an elite athlete, *Chiropr Sports Med* 5(4):91-97, 1991.
7. Fairbank JC, et al: The Oswestry Low Back Pain Disability Questionnaire, *Physiotherapy* 66(8):271-273, 1980.
8. Fauci A, et al: *Harrison's principles of internal medicine,* ed 13, New York, 1994, McGraw-Hill.
9. Gatterman M: *Chiropractic management of spine related disorders,* Baltimore, 1990, Williams & Wilkins.
10. Haldeman S: *Principles and practice of chiropractic,* ed 2, Norwalk, Conn, 1992, Appleton & Lange.
11. Haldeman S, et al: Guidelines for chiropractic quality assurance & practice parameters, *The Proceedings of the Mercy Center Consensus Conference,* Gaithersburg, Md, 1993, Aspen Publishers.
12. Hammer W: *Functional soft tissue examination and treatment by manual methods,* Gaithersburg, Md, 1991, Aspen Publishers.
13. Hansen D, et al: Implementation of chiropractic guidelines: a prospective pilot study, *Transactions of the Consortium for Chiropractic Research,* June 1993.
14. Hooper PD: *Physical modalities: a primer for chiropractic,* Baltimore, 1996, Williams & Wilkins.
15. Jarvis K: The guidelines in practice: the grass roots impact of the AHCPR document, *J Am Chiropr Assoc,* February 1995.
16. Lawrence D: *Fundamentals of chiropractic diagnosis and management,* Baltimore, 1991, Williams & Wilkins.

17. Liebenson C: *Rehabilitation of the spine,* Baltimore, 1996, Williams & Wilkins.

18. Manga P, et al: *The effectiveness and cost effectiveness of chiropractic management of low-back pain,* 1993, Ontario Ministry of Health.

19. *Manual of medical therapeutics (the Washington manual),* ed 27, Boston, 1992, Little, Brown.

20. *The Merck manual,* ed 16, Rahway, NJ, 1992, Merck Co.

21. Mooney V, Leggett S: Back pain: which exercises can help, which can harm? *Consultant* 36(12), 1996.

22. Morris RM: A study of the natural history of back pain. Parts 1 and 2: development of a reliable and sensitive measure of disability in low back pain, *Spine* 8:141-150, 1983.

23. Phillips R: Impact of guidelines on health policy: health care policy formation–Backpain Outcome Assessment Team (BOAT), *Transactions of the Consortium for Chiropractic Research,* June 1993.

24. Rakel RE: *Conn's current therapy,* Philadelphia, 1996, WB Saunders.

25. Rakel RE: *Textbook of family practice,* ed 5, Philadelphia, 1995, WB Saunders.

26. Rossignol M, et al: Should the gap be filled between guidelines and actual practice for management of low back pain in primary care? The Quebec experience, *Spine* 21(24), 1996.

27. Scully RM, Barnes MR: *Physical therapy,* Philadelphia, 1989, JB Lippincott.

28. Shekelle PG, et al: *The appropriateness of spinal manipulation for low back pain. Indications and ratings by an all-chiropractic expert panel,* Santa Monica, Calif, 1991, Rand.

29. Spitzer WO, et al: Scientific approach to the assessment and management of activity-related spinal disorders: a monograph for clinicians, report of the Quebec Task Force on Spinal Disorders, *Spine* 12(7s), 1987.

30. Tierney LM, McPhee SJ, Papadakis MA: *Current medical diagnosis and treatment,* Norwalk, Conn, 1996, Appleton & Lange.

31. Ventura J, Justice B: Need for multiple diagnosis in the presence of spondylolisthesis, *J Manipulative Physiol Ther* 11(1):41-42, 1988.

32. Waddel G, et al: *Low back pain evidence review,* London, 1996, Royal College of General Practitioners.

33. White AA, Panjabi MM: *Clinical biomechanics of the spine,* Philadelphia, 1990, JB Lippincott.

34. Wyatt I, Schwartz MP: Spondylolytic spondylolisthesis: surgical lesion or normal variant? *J Am Chiropr Assoc* 32(4):67-70, 1995.

35. Yochum TR, Rowe LJ: *Essentials of skeletal radiology,* ed 2, Baltimore, 1995, Williams & Wilkins.

SECTION VIII

Scoliosis

Scoliosis

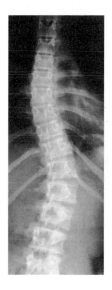

(Courtesy Lisette Logan, MRT, Brampton, Ontario, Canada.)

Scoliosis

Brian Dannenfelser, Lew Huff, and David M. Brady

DEFINITION

A genetic or acquired condition of the spine, characterized by exaggerated lateral deviation of the spine. May or may not be painful. Scoliosis is 7 times more common in females.

ETIOLOGY

Infantile: From birth to age 3, usually resolves spontaneously and is more common in males. Left thoracic curvature is common.

Juvenile: Ages 4 to 10, affects females more often than males and can progress to adult form. Right thoracic curvature is common.

Adult: Ages 10 to skeletal maturity, increase of double major curves, physical therapy and exercise may arrest the progression.

COMPLICATIONS

Scoliosis may be progressive, and if curvature exceeds 60 degrees, it may lead to cardiac and pulmonary complications and IV foraminal encroachment.

SIGNS AND SYMPTOMS

Inspection

Spinous processes rotate into the concavity of the curve. Loss of normal height. Posture analysis may reveal low occiput, low shoulder, pelvic obliquity, or increased musculature tonus on one side.

Curve Patterns

Left major: T11 to L5; usually lumbar left curve. Progressive after skeletal maturity. Curve may increase 5 to 8 degrees with pregnancy.

Right major: T4 to L1; associated with rib deformities. A curve more than 60 degrees may lead to cardiac or pulmonary problems.

Double major: Usually a right thoracic curve and a left lumbar curve.

Thoracolumbar: T4 to L4; may be left or right; no classic pattern; less rib deformity, but flank deformity and crease pattern of the skin may be present.

Nonstructural variation (postural): Disappears when patient lies down.

Compensatory: May be due to tilted pelvis or leg length discrepancy.

Structural (idiopathic): Congenital malformation; musculoskeletal, traumatic, or mesenchymal disorder.

Transient structural (sciatic): Disk herniation leads to nerve pressure and subsequent muscle spasm. Symptoms do not disappear when the patient lies down, and spinous processes do not rotate into the concavity.

Examination

Inspect for rotational prominence of ribs or flank. Look for high shoulder, pelvic tilting, leg length inequality, or other biomechanical faults. Postural analysis and Adam's test may confirm observation. Scoliometer may be used to confirm. Determine if curve is structural or functional. Scoliosis screening should be conducted at an early age, especially with female adolescents.

Radiographic Analysis

Cobb's analysis should be performed. Skeletal maturation is intimately associated with curve progression. Ascertain need for lateral flexion views to determine flexibility of the curve.

TREATMENT GOALS

1. Relieve pain and prevent progression.
2. Increase pain-free ranges of motion.
3. Restore normal strength and stability to joint structures.
4. Quickly change to rehabilitation and restoration of function.

MANAGEMENT PROTOCOL (OPTIONS)

- *Manipulation:*
  1. Approach from the convexity of the curve.
  2. Spinal adjusting may increase the size of the IVF and restore function to the immobilized joints along with diminishing pain.
- *Contraindications:*
  1. Manipulation is contraindicated in hypermobile segments.
  2. Curves in excess of 50 degrees should be managed with a multidisciplinary approach.

Clinical Note

Siragusa states that, after chiropractic care, curves were reduced by 50% and 13%, respectively, in two clinical trials. Sallahian states that, after 3 months of active chiropractic care, curves were shown to have been reversed by 16 degrees.[16,18]

- Electrical muscle stimulation with alternating, sinusoidal current. Frequency 80 to 150 Hz, continuous, 15 minutes with muscle contraction to reduce myospasms.[6] Use muscle stimulator up to 24 hours per day. Good results with children under 12 years of age.
  1. May help halt progression.
  2. Appears to be equal to bracing in slowing progression.
  3. Higher compliance than bracing therapy.
- TENS: Frequency 50 to 100 Hz, pulse width set at 20 to 60 ms, time 23 hours, set below the motoric threshold to block pain.

- Exercise Therapy:
  1. Supine, prone, and crawling exercises
  2. Dry swimming exercises
  3. Cross-stretching exercises
  4. Derotation exercises
  5. Knapp exercises
- Muscle reeducation: Stretch tight muscles and balance the agonist with the antagonist. Use weight lifting bilaterally.
- Bracing:
  1. Seldom recommend for curves greater than 50 degrees or less than 20 degrees.
  2. May cause persistent vomiting.
  3. Poor compliance with most children.
  4. Milwaukee brace on younger patients 23.5 hours per day.
  5. Body casting from hips to shoulders (severe cases).
  6. Corset with adjustable frames.
- Orthotics:
  1. Orthotics to correct leg length discrepancy.
  2. Determine actual leg length inequality.
  3. Apply 5:2 rule:
     a. For every 5 mm of PI or EX correction, femoral head raises 2 mm.
     b. For every 5 mm of AS or IN correction, femoral head lowers 2 mm.

NUTRITIONAL MANAGEMENT PROTOCOL (OPTIONS)

Acute Muscle Spasm:
- Valerian root *(Valeriana officinalis)* (100 mg q4h)
- Passion flower *(Passiflora incarnata)* (100-200 mg q4h)
- Magnesium (citrate) (100 mg q4h)
- Calcium (lactate) (50 mg q4h)

Many vendors offer formulary products with the above elements, including Valerian Daytime/Calmicin Plus (Murdock Madaus Schwabe) and Myoplex/Myoplex PM (Metagenics, Inc.).

HOME CARE PROTOCOL (OPTIONS)

- Weight lifting as instructed by doctor.
- Stretching exercises.
- Daily rest periods.

REFERENCES

1. Balch JF, Balch PA: *Prescription for natural healing,* Wayne, NJ, 1990, Avery Publishing.

2. Brukner P: *Clinical sports medicine,* New York, 1993, McGraw-Hill.

3. Fauci A, et al: *Harrison's principles of internal medicine,* ed 13, New York, 1994, McGraw-Hill.

4. Gatterman M: *Chiropractic management of spine related disorders,* Baltimore, 1990, Williams & Wilkins.

5. Grabowski RJ: *Current nutritional therapy,* San Antonio, Tex, 1993, Image Press.

6. Hammer W: *Functional soft tissue examination and treatment by manual methods,* Gaithersburg, Md, 1991, Aspen Publishers.

7. Hooper PD: *Physical modalities: a primer for chiropractic,* Baltimore, 1996, Williams & Wilkins.

8. Lawrence D: *Fundamentals of chiropractic diagnosis and management,* Baltimore, 1991, Williams & Wilkins.

9. Liebenson C: *Rehabilitation of the spine,* Baltimore, 1996, Williams & Wilkins.

10. Lindahl O, Lindwall L: Double blind study of a *Valerian* preparation, *Pharmacol Biochem Behav* 32(4):10065-10066,1989.

11. *Manual of medical therapeutics (the Washington manual),* ed 27, Boston, 1992, Little, Brown.

12. Maurer K: Physical exam best way to detect scoliosis, *Family Practice News,* 6300-7073, December 1996.

13. *The Merck manual,* ed 16, Rahway, NJ, 1992, Merck Co.

14. Rakel RE: *Conn's current therapy,* Philadelphia, 1996, WB Saunders.

15. Rakel RE: *Textbook of family practice,* ed 5, Philadelphia, 1995, WB Saunders.

16. Sallahian C: Reduction of scoliosis in an adult male utilizing specific chiropractic spinal manipulation: a case report, *J Chiropr Res Clin Invest* 7(2):42-45, 1991.

17. Scully RM, Barnes MR: *Physical therapy,* Philadelphia, 1989, JB Lippincott.

18. Siragusa J: Scoliosis as a variation of the vertebral subluxation complex and its reduction under chiropractic care, *Proceedings of the National Conference on Chiropractic and Pediatrics,* November 1992, pp 49-59.

19. Speroni E, Minghetti A: Neuropharmacological activity of extracts from *Passiflora incarnata, Planta Med* 54(6):488-491, 1988.

20. Tierney LM, McPhee SJ, Papadakis MA: *Current medical diagnosis and treatment,* Norwalk, Conn, 1996, Appleton & Lange.

21. Werbach MR: *Nutritional influences on illness,* ed 2, Tarzana, Calif, 1996, Third Line Press.

22. Werbach MR, Murray MT: *Botanical influences on illness,* Tarzana, Calif, 1994, Third Line Press.
23. White AA, Panjabi MM: *Clinical biomechanics of the spine,* Philadelphia, 1990, JB Lippincott.

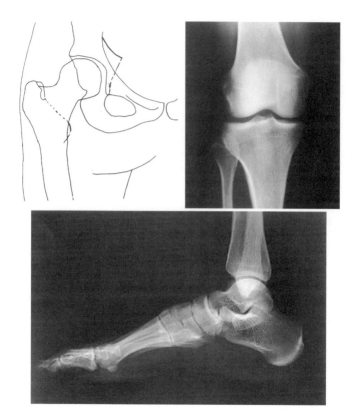

(Top left) Modified from Bontranger KL: *Textbook of radiographic positioning and related anatomy,* ed 4, St Louis, 1997, Mosby. *(Top right and bottom)* Modified from Ballinger PW: *Merrill's atlas of radiographic positioning and radiologic procedures,* ed 8, St Louis, 1995, Mosby.

SECTION IX

Lower Extremity Injuries and Pain Syndromes

Injuries to the Hip Joint: General Overview

LEW HUFF

HIP INJURIES

The hip joint is similar to the shoulder joint but far more stable, with strong ligaments and a deeper socket holding the joint securely. Stronger muscles surrounding the hip add to the stability. Coxa vara deformity (inward angulation of the femur head) leads to DJD development.

SITE OF PAIN

With DJD of the hip, the site of pain is the groin or trochanteric region. In trochanteric bursitis the onset is insidious and pain is felt over the lateral hip region above the trochanteric bursa. The large iliopectineal bursas over the anterior hip region may be responsible for anterior hip pain.

EXAMINATION

Examine the gait to determine the need for a crutch or walker. Examine leg length to determine the need for heel lifts. Rule out hip pathology with Patrick's test (fabere sign) and by putting the hip joint through ranges of motion. Observe for contraindications for physical medicine modalities, such as metal implants, thermal nerve deficiencies, and vascular disease.

RADIATION, REFERRED PAIN

Examine the joints and musculature above and below the hip joint to rule out referred pain patterns mimicking a hip disorder.

Hip pain is referred to the knee (L2, L3) or the anterior thigh. Trochanteric bursitis can refer pain to the L5 dermatome, thigh, knee, and/or lower leg.

ACTIVITIES OF DAILY LIVING

A patient with a hip disorder can have difficulty raising from a bed or chair, climbing stairs, dressing, or walking long distances.

UNINJURED AREA

Examination and radiographic examination for bilateral comparison, when necessary.

REINJURY/FLARE-UP

Restrict aggravating activities, and continue care and rehabilitative exercises.

HOME CARE

ROM exercises, passive stretching, heat applications before activities, and ice after ROM exercises may be beneficial.

WHEN TO DISCHARGE

When patient has reached maximum medical improvement or the need for referral is established.

REFERRAL

If fracture, dislocation, or neurologic complications are present. Daily treatment exceeding 2 weeks may signal the need for a second opinion or referral. Treatment exceeding 4 weeks or temporary disability for longer than 4 weeks with no objective signs of improvement, or worsening of the condition within the first 2 weeks, may signal the need for a second opinion or referral.

Suspected fracture, bone pathology, contraindication for manipulation, systemic disease, or infection signals the need for referral.

REFERENCES

1. Clemente C: *Anatomy: a regional atlas of the human body,* ed 3, Baltimore, 1987, Urban & Schwarzenberg.
2. Gatterman M: *Chiropractic management of spine related disorders,* Baltimore, 1990, Williams & Wilkins.
3. Haldeman S, et al: Guidelines for chiropractic quality assurance & practice parameters, *The Proceedings of the Mercy Center Consensus Conference,* Gaithersburg, Md, 1993, Aspen Publishers.
4. Hansen DT: *Chiropractic standards of practice and utilization guidelines in the care and treatment of injured workers,* 1988, Washington State Department of Labor & Industries.
5. Lawrence D: *Fundamentals of chiropractic diagnosis and management,* Baltimore, 1991, Williams & Wilkins.
6. Schestack R: *Handbook of physical therapy,* ed 3, New York, 1977, Springer-Verlag.
7. Vear HJ: *Chiropractic standards of practice and quality of care,* Gaithersburg, Md, 1992, Aspen Publishers.

Osteoarthritis of the Hip Joint

Brian Dannenfelser, Lew Huff, and David M. Brady

DEFINITION

A degenerative process of the hip joint, involving the articulation between the femur and the innominate bone (a ball-and-socket joint) formed when the femur head fits into the acetabulum. DJD of the hip is the most disabling form of osteoarthritis.

ETIOLOGY

Causes may include a shallow acetabulum, slipped capital femoral epiphysis, Legg-Calvé-Perthes disease, or abnormal biomechanical stresses. Coxa vara deformity (inward angulation of the femur head) leads to DJD of the hip joint in many cases.

SIGNS AND SYMPTOMS

Pain Pattern

Pain is often felt at the groin or trochanteric area. Pain increases with motion and weight bearing. Joint stiffness subsides within a few minutes of motion. Morning stiffness may last a few minutes. Nocturnal pain is present in late stages. Hip stiffness may worsen with osteoarthritis of the hip.

Radiation

Pain radiates to the lateral side of the leg.

Ranges of Motion

Diminished ranges of motion, especially in abduction and internal rotation. Straight leg raise testing is seldom limited.

Guidelines for Diagnosis

Hip pain and 2 of 3: Erythrocyte sedimentation rate (ESR) <20 mm/hr, femoral and acetabular osteophytes, and narrowing of joint space.

Palpation

Palpable pinpoint tenderness over the greater trochanter. Crepitus felt with joint movement. Muscle atrophy of quads may denote severe stage of osteoarthritis.

Other Manifestations

Patient with hip disorder may have difficulty raising from bed or chair, climbing stairs, walking long distances, or dressing. Inspection of gait may reveal antalgic gait, adductor lurch, or Trendelenburg gait.

DIFFERENTIAL DIAGNOSIS

Hip bursitis
Hip strain

ORTHOPEDIC FINDINGS

Hibb's
Telescoping
Patrick (FABERE)

LABORATORY FINDINGS

Look for ESR <20 mm/hr

X-RAY FINDINGS

Spurring, lipping
Decreased joint space
Bony enlargement

TREATMENT GOALS

1. Promote soft tissue healing.
2. Relieve pain and prevent recurrence.
3. Increase pain-free ranges of motion.
4. Restore maximal strength and stability to joint structure.
5. Quickly change to rehabilitation or restoration of function.
6. Severe cases may need to be evaluated for total joint replacement.

MANAGEMENT PROTOCOL

- Examine the gait and determine need for crutch or walker.
- Examine the joints and muscles above and below to rule out referred pain patterns.
- Examine leg length to determine the need for heel lifts or pelvic manipulative correction.
- Observe for contraindications, such as vascular disease, metal implants, open epiphyseal plates, thermal nerve deficiencies, or encapsulated swelling.

Options

Acute Phase:
- Ice packs to promote vasoconstriction and decrease inflammation, pain, edema, and muscle spasms. Ice packs over affected area for 20 minutes with dry towel between ice packs and subject.
- Interferential for pain and edema management.
- Ultrasound (pulsed) at 0.5 W/cm^2 for 5 minutes. Ultrasound causes the resolution of inflammatory exudates and increases blood flow.

Subacute or Chronic Phase:
- Moist hot packs heated to 270° F with two dry towels between hot packs and patient, applied for 20 minutes to reduce muscle spasms and increase circulation.
- Short wave diathermy: Heat source is placed 18 inches form

body part, treatment time is 20 minutes, use one towel between heat source and patient.

- Transverse friction massage: A deep tissue massage at the site of involvement, stroking perpendicular to the fiber alignment to increase fiber mobility without longitudinal stress. This promotes orientation of fibers and induces hyperemia to hypovascular tissues. In addition, transverse friction massage has a mechanical influence on tissue maturation. Hip may feel worse for the first few days, then improvement will be seen.[15]
- Treat any associated myofascial trigger points in the pelvic region, low back, or leg muscles using 5 to 7 seconds of ischemic compression. Repeat 3 times each visit.
- Adjust hip and lumbosacral regions. Stretch tensor fascia lata and gluteals. Apply heat and do active exercises in all planes. Joint mobilization for capsular stretching and prolonged stretching of hip joint musculature.
- In early hip disease use active, passive, and assisted ROM exercises. A personalized exercise program should be developed. Add aquatics and/or aerobic walking exercises. Exercise program is designed to preserve at least 30 degrees of flexion and full hip extension and to strengthen the hip abductors and extensors.
- Determine the need for ambulatory devices, such as cane, crutch, or walker.

Surgical Referral:

In late stages ir patient cannot tolerate the pain, or if activities of daily living are impossible, total joint replacement should be considered.

NUTRITIONAL MANAGEMENT PROTOCOL (OPTIONS)

DJD–Osteoarthritis:

- Glucosamine sulfate (1500 mg per day in divided dosages)
- Vitamin C (3000-6000 mg per day in divided dosages)
- Iron (glycinate) (8-12 mg per day in divided dosages)
- Alpha-ketoglutaric acid (15 mg per day in divided dosages)

The above three nutrients are required for the hydroxylation of L-proline to L-hydroxyproline, which is needed for the production of quality collagen. The glucosamine sulfate is needed for proper ground substance production.

- Calcium (400 mg tid)
- Vitamin E (200 IU per day)
- Zinc (glycinate) (12-18 mg per day divided dosages)
- Copper (glycinate) (600-900 µg per day in divided dosages)
- Manganese (glycinate) (4-6 mg per day in divided dosages)

The above provide antioxidant effect and serve as free radical scavengers to help remove cellular debris and promote healing. The zinc, copper, and manganese act as cofactors and catalysts for the potent antioxidant enzyme SOD and are therefore referred to as the *SOD induction complex*. Oral supplementation with SOD can be attempted; however, it has been reported that it is often destroyed in the stomach and intestinal tract before assimilation. SOD can be obtained in Cell Guard (Biotec Foods).

All of the above tissue-healing nutrients can be obtained in the formulary product Collagenics Intensive Care (Metagenics, Inc.).

HOME CARE PROTOCOL (OPTIONS)

Instruct patient to do the following:

- Learn about weight loss programs (possibly use low carbohydrate diet; e.g., "The Zone").
- Apply moist heat to hips before exercise program.
- Perform hydrotherapy (swimming exercises).
- Do moderate walking and bicycle exercises.
- Perform ROM exercises while supine (modified Patrick [FABERE]).
- Use ice compresses, elevate the joint, and take rest periods.
- Use crutch or walker if needed.
- Live in a single-story home.
- Avoid stair climbing.
- Raise toilet seats, install wall bars.

REFERENCES

1. American College of Rheumatology issues management guidelines for OA of the hip and knee, *Am Fam Physician,* 53(3):985, 1996.
2. Balch JF, Balch PA: *Prescription for natural healing,* Wayne, NJ, 1990, Avery Publishing.
3. Bland JH, Cooper SM: Osteoarthritis: a review of the cell biology involved and evidence for reversibility, management rationally related to known genesis and pathophysiology, *Semin Arthritis Rheum* 14(2):106, 1984.

4. Bolton P, Bolton S: Is there a role for the chiropractor in the treatment and management of rheumatism? A clinical perspective, *J Austral Chiropr Assoc* 16(1):19-22, 1986.

5. Brukner P: *Clinical sports medicine,* New York, 1993, McGraw-Hill.

6. Bucci LR: *Nutrition applied to injury rehabilitation and sports medicine,* Boca Raton, Fla, 1995, CRC Press.

7. Clemen M: Delivering effective force adjustments on patients with degenerative spinal conditions, *Int Rev Chiropr* 44:27-35, 1988.

8. D'Ambrosio E, et al: Glucosamine sulfate: a controlled clinical investigation in arthrosis, *Pharmatherapeutica* 2(8):504-508, 1981.

9. Davis CD, Greger JL: Longitudinal changes of manganese-dependent superoxide dismutase and other indexes of manganese and iron status in women, *Am J Clin Nutr* 55:747, 1992.

10. Drovanti A, et al: Oral glucosamine sulfate in osteoarthritis: a placebo controlled double-blind investigation, *Clin Ther* 3(4):260-272, 1980.

11. Fauci A, et al: *Harrison's principles of internal medicine,* ed 13, New York, 1994, McGraw-Hill.

12. Gatterman M: *Chiropractic management of spine related disorders,* Baltimore, 1990, Williams & Wilkins.

13. Grabowski RJ: *Current nutritional therapy,* San Antonio, Tex, 1993, Image Press.

14. Hammer W: *Functional soft tissue examination and treatment by manual methods,* Gaithersburg, Md, 1991, Aspen Publishers.

15. Hammer W: The use of transverse friction massage in the management of chronic bursitis of the hip or shoulder, *J Manipulative Physiol Ther* 16(2), 1990.

16. Hochberg MC, et al: Guidelines for the medical management of osteoarthritis. Part 1: osteoarthritis of the hip, *Arthritis Rheum* 38:1535-1540, 1995.

17. Kamimura M: Anti-inflammatory activity of vitamin E, *J Vitaminol* 18(4):204-209, 1972.

18. Liebenson C: *Rehabilitation of the spine,* Baltimore, 1996, Williams & Wilkins.

19. *Manual of medical therapeutics (the Washington manual),* ed 27, Boston, 1992, Little, Brown.

20. *The Merck manual,* ed 16, Rahway, NJ, 1992, Merck Co.

21. New management guidelines in osteoarthritis of the hip, *Consultant,* February 1996.

22. Niki E: Interaction of ascorbate and alpha-tocopherol, *Third Conference on Vitamin C* 498:187-189, 1987.

23. Nimmo R: Receptor, effecters and tonus: a new approach, *J Natl Chiropr Assoc,* November 1957.

24. Rakel RE: *Conn's current therapy,* Philadelphia, 1996, WB Saunders.

25. Rakel RE: *Textbook of family practice,* ed 5, Philadelphia, 1995, WB Saunders.
26. Schneider MJ: Chiropractic management of myofascial and muscular disorders. In Lawrence D, ed: *Advances in chiropractic,* vol 3, St Louis, 1996, Mosby.
27. Schwartz RI, et al: Ascorbate can act as an inducer of collagen pathway because most steps are tightly coupled, *Third Conference on Vitamin C* 498:172-184, 1987.
28. Scully RM, Barnes MR: *Physical therapy,* Philadelphia, 1989, JB Lippincott.
29. Tierney LM, McPhee SJ, Papadakis MA: *Current medical diagnosis and treatment,* ed 35, Norwalk, Conn, 1996, Appleton & Lange.
30. Travell JG, Simons DG: *Myofascial pain and dysfunction: the trigger point manual,* vol 2, Baltimore, 1992, Williams & Wilkins.
31. Weaver K: Magnesium and its role in vascular reactivity and coagulation, *Contemp Nutr* 12(3), 1987.
32. Werbach MR: *Nutritional influences on illness,* ed 2, Tarzana, Calif, 1996, Third Line Press.
33. Werbach MR, Murray MT: *Botanical influences on illness,* Tarzana, Calif, 1994, Third Line Press.
34. White AA, Panjabi MM: *Clinical biomechanics of the spine,* Philadelphia, 1990, JB Lippincott.

Injuries to the Knee and Foreleg: General Overview

Lew Huff

KNEE INJURIES

The knee joint is the largest joint of the body. It is a very complicated joint in that it bears all the body weight yet allows a high degree of freedom of movement.

PATELLOFEMORAL PAIN SYNDROME

A condition of painful patella that can occur with or without the presence of pathologic changes to the patella.

SHIN SPLINTS

Also termed *tibial tendinitis* or *tendinoperiositis*, this is a loosely defined condition of pain, tightness, and inflammation of the anterior or posterior muscle groups and fascia of the foreleg.

COMPARTMENT SYNDROME

A condition of increased pressure within one of the four compartments of the lower leg, leading to motor and sensory disturbances.

SITE OF PAIN

Knee Sprain

Ligamentous sprain is generally superficial and well localized. The primary site of pain is localized to the site of tearing, with the exception of an anterior cruciate ligament tear, which causes a generalized knee pain. Hypertrophy of the medial and lateral fat pads of the knee with pain just medial and lateral to the patellar tendon is also noted in acute ACL tears. Approximately 70% of acute swelling cases of the knee are related to anterior cruciate injury and require immediate surgery. A medial meniscus tear manifests tenderness over the medial joint space.

Patellofemoral Syndrome

Aching patellar pain and stiffness relieved by activity. Tenderness and pain over the joint line and the anteromedial or anterolateral aspect of the knee.

Shin Splints

Extreme palpable tenderness over the medial tibia, anterolateral tibia, or posteromedial tibia. Pain and myospasms and hypertonicity of calf muscles, tibialis anterior, gastrocnemius, or soleus muscles. Pain described as a deep, dull ache and throbbing.

Compartment Syndrome

Painful tight sensation in the calf. Extreme tenderness within the compartment. Extreme pain upon passive stretching of the involved muscles.

EXAMINATION

Knee Sprain

Examine the fat pads, meniscus, collateral ligaments, patella, patellar heights, infrapatellar bursa, and tibial tubercle. If anterior glide is painful, the anterior cruciate is implicated. If posterior glide is painful, the posterior cruciate is implicated. Gross hypermobility on valgus stress suggests rupture of the medial capsule and medial collateral ligament. Varus stress will reproduce pain from a lateral collateral ligament injury. In generalized swelling there is intraarticular hemorrhage, synovitis, and synovial thickening, and the knee remains partially flexed to accommodate the swelling. Other areas of swelling include bursal swelling, which is localized, most frequently over the prepatellar bursa in bursitis. Infrapatellar bursitis manifests swelling over the tibial tubercle, whereas in pes anserine bursitis there is swelling over the medial tibial tubercle. A Baker's cyst causes swelling over the popliteal fossa area.

Patellofemoral Pain Syndrome

Examine painful fat pads, meniscus, collateral ligaments, patella, infrapatellar bursa, and tibial tubercle. Examine for patella pain with weight bearing, active motion, or running. Observe patient ascending and descending stairs. Palpate for possible tenderness over the anterior, medial, or lateral aspect of the patella; the joint space; and over the iliotibial band. Test for movie sign by having patient sit with knees flexed for a prolonged period of time. Check for patellar grinding and tracking abnormalities.

Shin Splints

Examine tibia, tibialis anterior, gastrocnemius, and peroneals. Evaluate pulses and tendon reflexes. Palpate surrounding muscle groups and evaluate ranges of motion and pain on weight bearing or with stressful activities.

Compartment Syndrome

Examine for edema, extreme pain, or passive stretch of the involved muscle groups. Palpate the pulses and check for sensory loss or paresthesias. Observe for footdrop.

RADIATION, REFERRED PAIN

Knee Pain

Referred pain is common to L3, L4.

ACTIVITIES OF DAILY LIVING

A patient with a knee injury can have difficulty walking, climbing stairs, running, or rising from a bed or chair. A patient with patellar pain syndrome, shin splints, or compartment syndrome will also have difficulty walking, climbing stairs, running, and performing other activities of daily living.

NOTE: The following applies to all of the above conditions.

UNINJURED AREA

Examination and radiographic examination for bilateral comparison if necessary.

REINJURY/FLARE-UP

Restrict aggravating activities, continue care, and start low-impact rehabilitative exercises.

HOME CARE

ROM exercises, passive stretching, surgical tubing exercises, ice applications, or compresses may be appropriate.

WHEN TO DISCHARGE

When patient has reached maximum medical improvement or the need for referral is established.

REFERRAL

If fracture, dislocation, or neurologic complications are present. Daily treatment exceeding 2 weeks may signal the need for a second opinion or referral. Treatment exceeding 4 weeks or temporary disability for longer than 4 weeks with no objective signs of improvement, or worsening of the condition within the first 2 weeks, may signal the need for a second opinion or referral.

Suspected fracture, bone pathology, systemic disease, or infection signals the need for referral.[4]

REFERENCES

1. Clemente C: *Anatomy: a regional atlas of the human body,* ed 3, Baltimore, 1987, Urban & Schwarzenberg.
2. Gatterman M: *Chiropractic management of spine related disorders,* Baltimore, 1990, Williams & Wilkins.

3. Haldeman S, et al: Guidelines for chiropractic quality assurance & practice parameters, *The Proceedings of the Mercy Center Consensus Conference,* Gaithersburg, Md, 1993, Aspen Publishers.
4. Hansen DT: *Chiropractic standards of practice and utilization guidelines in the care and treatment of injured workers,* 1988, Washington State Department of Labor & Industries.
5. Lawrence D: *Fundamentals of chiropractic diagnosis and management,* Baltimore, 1991, Williams & Wilkins.
6. Schestack R: *Handbook of physical therapy,* ed 3, New York, 1977, Springer-Verlag.
7. Vear HJ: *Chiropractic standards of practice and quality of care,* Gaithersburg, Md, 1992, Aspen Publishers.

Ligamentous Injuries to the Knee

Lew Huff and David M. Brady

DEFINITION

A sprain or rupture of the anterior and/or posterior cruciates and/or lateral or medial collateral ligaments as they attach to the knee.

ETIOLOGY

May be due to muscular imbalance, athletic injuries, twisting injuries, rapid changes in direction, or trauma.

Lateral Collateral Ligament

Dashboard injury, blow to medial knee, or twisting injury.

Medial Collateral Ligament

Twisting injury with valgus strain (as in skiing injury), trauma, or repetitive stress.

Terrible Triad of O'Donohue

A torn medial capsule, torn medial collateral ligament, torn anterior cruciate ligament, and torn medial meniscus. Generally from blow to lateral knee.

SIGNS AND SYMPTOMS

Anterior Cruciate

1. Limb collapse
2. Decreased ranges of motion, locking
3. Instability
4. Patient walks in external rotation to stabilize knee
5. *70% of anterior cruciate rupture needs **immediate surgery***

Lateral Collateral Ligament

1. Walks with knee in slight flexion
2. Difficulty climbing or descending stairs
3. Difficulty with cutting moves in sports

Medial Collateral Ligament

1. Medial knee pain, above or below the joint
2. Palpable tenderness more proximal than distal
3. Acute edema

Posterior Cruciate

1. Tears are uncommon
2. Trouble ascending and descending stairs
3. Instability and difficulty performing cutting maneuvers in sports

ORTHOPEDIC TESTS

McIntosh's test
Lachman's test
McMurray's test

X-RAY EXAMINATION

Tunnel view and lateral view

TREATMENT GOALS

1. Promote soft tissue healing, protect while healing.
2. Relieve pain and prevent recurrence.
3. Increase pain-free ranges of motion.
4. Restore normal strength and stability to joint structure. Prevent degenerative changes to joint.
5. Quickly change to rehabilitation or restoration of function. Approximate previous performance levels.
6. Treatment conservatively is possible if:
   - Patient is willing to modify activities.
   - There is a low degree of instability and no rupture, fracture, or dislocation.
   - Patient has at least one normal meniscus and no other pathologic factors.

MANAGEMENT PROTOCOL (OPTIONS)

Acute Phase:
- Acute hyperemic phase: *PRICES*—*p*rotect, *r*est, *i*ce, *c*ompress, *e*levate, *s*tabilize.
- With moderate sprain, use crutches if needed for 5 days. From 7 to 10 days of bandaging may be adequate.
- Casting brace may be needed for the first 6 to 8 weeks in severe sprain.

Subacute Phase:
- Patient should be initially non-weight bearing. Gradually bear partial weight increasing to full weight bearing.
- Limit knee extension to 45 degrees for up to 6 months with anterior cruciate ligament sprain.
- No competitive sports for 1 to 3 weeks at a minimum.
- Rehabilitation: After 3 to 4 weeks, begin passive and active ROM exercises (or when pain permits). Move to gradual resumption of weight bearing.
- Special exercises:
  1. Range of motion: Start with passive, then active. Later move to active with resistance.
  2. Once painless knee extension is possible, use gentle ROM exercises, and isometric exercises may begin.
  3. The most important exercise should be resistance over the final 20% of extension to strengthen the vastus medialis along with resistive straight leg raising exercises.

4. Quad exercises should be limited to 45 degrees of extension. Exercise hamstrings as well.
5. Full extension exercises may begin when bracing is removed.
6. Bicycling is beneficial for strengthening phase.

Surgical Referral:

Refer to orthopedist if fracture, dislocation, ruptured ligaments or meniscus is present.

NUTRITIONAL MANAGEMENT PROTOCOL (OPTIONS)

Acute Pain and Inflammation:

- Proteolytic enzymes (trypsin, chymotrypsin, bromelin) (3-4 tablets qid in between meals). NOTE: Do not give to patients with ulcers!
- Bioflavonoids (quercetin, hesperidin, rutin, etc.) (200 mg mixed bioflavonoids q2h during acute phase).
- Herbals, such as boswellia, ginger, turmeric, cayenne (400 mg, 300 mg, 200 mg, 50 mg, respectively, q2h acute phase).

The above proteolytic enzymes can be obtained in Biozyme (Metagenics, Inc.) or Lyso-lymph Forte (Nutri-West, Inc.). Inflavonoid Intensive Care (Metagenics, Inc.) will provide the above bioflavonoids and herbals. Other manufacturers can provide quality proteolytic enzymes. Consult your product catalog.

Tissue Healing:

- Amino acids (glycine, L-cystine, L-proline, and L-lysine) (300-400 mg per day each in divided dosages). Supplies the amino acid pool necessary for the structural production of collagen.
- Vitamin C (3000-6000 mg per day in divided dosages).
- Iron (glycinate) (8-12 mg per day in divided dosages).
- Alpha-ketoglutaric acid (15 mg per day in divided dosages).

The above three nutrients are required for the hydroxylation of L-proline to L-hydroxyproline, which is needed for the production of quality collagen.

- Calcium (400 mg tid).
- Vitamin E (200 IU per day).
- Zinc (glycinate) (12-18 mg per day in divided dosages).
- Copper (glycinate) (600-900 μg per day in divided dosages).
- Manganese (glycinate) (4-6 mg per day in divided dosages).

The above provide antioxidant effects and serve as free radical scavengers to help remove cellular debris and promote healing. The zinc, copper, and manganese act as cofactors and catalysts for the potent antioxidant enzyme SOD and are therefore referred to as the *SOD induction complex*. Oral supplementation with SOD can be attempted; however, it has been reported that it is often destroyed in the stomach and intestinal tract before assimilation. SOD can be obtained in Cell Guard (Biotec Foods).

All the above tissue healing nutrients can be obtained in the formulary product Collagenics (Metagenics, Inc.). Other manufacturers make similar formulary products designed to aid in soft tissue repair, such as Rehab Plus (Professional Health Products). Consult the catalog of the reputable vendors you use for alternate products.

HOME CARE PROTOCOL (OPTIONS)

- Knee stretching and strengthening exercises.
- Brace for vigorous activities.

REFERENCES

1. Balch JF, Balch PA: *Prescription for natural healing,* Wayne, NJ, 1990, Avery Publishing.
2. Banks S, Willis J: Alar ligament injuries, *Spinal Manipulation* 3(2):1-3, 1987.
3. Bland JH, Cooper SM: Osteoarthritis: a review of the cell biology involved and evidence for reversibility, management rationally related to known genesis and pathophysiology, *Semin Arthritis Rheum* 14(2):106, 1984.
4. Brukner P: *Clinical sports medicine,* New York, 1993, McGraw-Hill.
5. Bucci LR: *Nutrition applied to injury rehabilitation and sports medicine,* Boca Raton, Fla, 1995, CRC Press.
6. Cichoke AJ, Marty L: The use of proteolytic enzymes with soft-tissue athletic injuries, *Am Chiropr,* October 1981, p 32.
7. Davis CD, Greger JL: Longitudinal changes of manganese-dependent superoxide dismutase and other indexes of manganese and iron status in women, *Am J Clin Nutr* 55:747, 1992.
8. D'Ambrosio E, et al: Glucosamine sulfate: a controlled clinical investigation in arthrosis, *Pharmatherapeutica* 2(8):504-508, 1981.
9. Drovanti A, et al: Oral glucosamine sulfate in osteoarthritis: a placebo controlled double-blind investigation, *Clin Ther* 3(4):260-272, 1980.

10. Fauci A, et al: *Harrison's principles of internal medicine,* ed 13, New York, 1994, McGraw-Hill.

11. Gatterman M: *Chiropractic management of spine related disorders,* Baltimore, 1990, Williams & Wilkins.

12. Grabowski RJ: *Current nutritional therapy,* San Antonio, Tex, 1993, Image Press.

13. Hammer W: *Functional soft tissue examination and treatment by manual methods,* Gaithersburg, Md, 1991, Aspen Publishers.

14. Havsteen B: Flavinoids, a class of natural products of high pharmacological potency, *Biochem Pharmacol* 33(24):3933-3939, 1984.

15. Lawrence D: *Fundamentals of chiropractic diagnosis and management,* Baltimore, 1991, Williams & Wilkins.

16. Liebenson C: *Rehabilitation of the spine,* Baltimore, 1996, Williams & Wilkins.

17. Lindahl O, Lindwall L: Double blind study of a *Valerian* preparation, *Pharmacol Biochem Behav* 32(4):10065-10066, 1989.

18. *Manual of medical therapeutics (the Washington manual),* ed 27, Boston, 1992, Little, Brown.

19. *The Merck manual,* ed 16, Rahway, NJ, 1992, Merck Co.

20. Niki E: Interaction of ascorbate and alpha-tocopherol, *Third Conference on Vitamin C* 498:187-189, 1987.

21. Rakel RE: *Conn's current therapy,* Philadelphia, 1996, WB Saunders.

22. Rakel RE: *Textbook of family practice,* ed 5, Philadelphia, 1995, WB Saunders.

23. Schwartz RI, et al: Ascorbate can act as an inducer of collagen pathway because most steps are tightly coupled, *Third Conference on Vitamin C* 498:172-184, 1987.

24. Scully RM, Barnes MR: *Physical therapy,* Philadelphia, 1990, JB Lippincott.

25. Souza T: Management of common knee disorders, *Topics Clin Chiropr* 1(2):24-33, 1994.

26. Speroni E, Minghetti A: Neuropharmacological activity of extracts from *Passiflora incarnata, Planta Med* 54(6):488-491, 1988.

27. Taraye JP, Lauressergues H: Advantages of combination of proteolytic enzymes, flavonoids and ascorbic acid in comparison with non-steroid inflammatory drugs, *Arzneimittelforschung* 27(1):1144-1149, 1977.

28. Tierney LM, McPhee SJ, Papadakis MA: *Current medical diagnosis and treatment,* ed 35, Norwalk, Conn, 1996, Appleton & Lange.

29. Werbach MR: *Nutritional influences on illness,* ed 2, Tarzana, Calif, 1996, Third Line Press.

30. Werbach MR, Murray MT: *Botanical influences on illness,* Tarzana, Calif, 1994, Third Line Press.

31. White AA, Panjabi MM: *Clinical biomechanics of the spine,* Philadelphia, 1990, JB Lippincott.

Meniscus Injuries to the Knee

LEW HUFF AND DAVID M. BRADY

DEFINITION

A medial or lateral meniscus tear; may be longitudinal tearing or more commonly a transverse or oblique tear. Meniscus tears are far more common on the medial side.

ETIOLOGY

Injury causing flexion or extension and rotation, possibly due to sports injuries, direct trauma, twisting injuries, and dashboard injuries. The meniscus is avascular and will not repair readily. A meniscus tear is usually caused by a rotatory stress on a weight-bearing joint.

SIGNS AND SYMPTOMS

Inspection

Locking of the knee joints and instability. Possible painful limp.

Palpation

Palpable tenderness over the medial joint space. May have generalized pain over knee joint as well.

Location

Patients with medial meniscus injury will point to the medial knee as site of pain. Lateral meniscus is less common; in this case, patient would point to lateral joint space.

Stressing the Joint

Pain with varus stress on the knee joint in medial meniscus, pain with valgus stress with lateral meniscus tear. McMurray's, Lachman's, and medial and lateral grinding tests may be positive.

DIFFERENTIAL DIAGNOSIS

Tumor
Lipoma
Xanthoma

ORTHOPEDIC TESTS

McMurray's
Medial, lateral grinding

X-RAY FINDINGS

Decreased joint space
Sclerosis
Osteophytes
May need CT scan or MRI

TREATMENT GOALS

1. Promote soft tissue healing.
2. Relieve pain and prevent recurrence.
3. Increase pain-free ranges of motion.
4. Restore normal strength and stability to joint structure.
5. Quickly change to rehabilitation and restoration of function.
6. Prevent degenerative changes to the joint.

MANAGEMENT PROTOCOL (OPTIONS)

Acute Phase:

- Ice packs to promote vasoconstriction to decrease inflammation, pain, edema, and muscle spasms. Ice packs over affected area for 20 minutes with dry towel between ice packs and subject. Interferential for pain and edema management.

Subacute or Chronic Phase:

- Short wave diathermy: Heat source is placed 18 inches from body part, treatment time is 20 minutes, use one towel between heat source and patient. Superficial heat, ultrasound, and transverse friction massage are beneficial.
- Transverse friction massage: A deep tissue massage at the site of involvement, stroking perpendicular to the fiber alignment to increase fiber mobility without longitudinal stress. This promotes orientation of fibers and induces hyperemia to hypovascular tissues. In addition, transverse friction massage has a mechanical influence on tissue maturation. Region may feel worse for the first few days, then improvement is noted.[12]
- Lawrence states that the treatment of choice is transverse friction massage over the painful lesion for 10 minutes daily. He advocates joint mobilization and manipulation/distraction of joint.[14]
- Hammer suggests cryotherapy and electrical stimulation along with diathermy, stretching, and strengthening exercises. He also advocates joint manipulation and distraction of the knee.[12]

NUTRITIONAL MANAGEMENT PROTOCOL (OPTIONS)

Acute Pain and Inflammation:

- Proteolytic enzymes (trypsin, chymotrypsin, bromelin) (3-4 tablets qid in between meals). NOTE: Do not give to patients with ulcers!
- Bioflavonoids (quercetin, hesperidin, rutin, etc.) (200 mg mixed bioflavonoids q2h during acute phase).
- Herbals, such as boswellia, ginger, turmeric, cayenne (400 mg, 300 mg, 200 mg, 50 mg, respectively, q2h acute phase).

The above proteolytic enzymes can be obtained in Biozyme (Metagenics, Inc.) or Lyso-lymph Forte (Nutri-West, Inc.). Inflavonoid Intensive Care (Metagenics, Inc.) will provide the above bioflavonoids and herbals. Other manufacturers can provide quality proteolytic enzymes. Consult your product catalog.

Tissue Healing:

- Amino acids (glycine, L-cystine, L-proline, and L-lysine) (300-400 mg per day each in divided dosages). Supplies the amino acid pool necessary for the structural production of collagen.

- Glucosamine sulfate (1500 mg per day in divided dosages). Supplies the needed nutrients for the production of healthy ground substance.
- Vitamin C (3000-6000 mg per day in divided dosages).
- Iron (glycinate) (8-12 mg per day in divided dosages).
- Alpha-ketoglutaric acid (15 mg per day in divided dosages).

The above three nutrients are required for the hydroxylation of L-proline to L-hydroxyproline, which is needed for the production of quality collagen.

- Calcium (400 mg tid).
- Vitamin E (200 IU per day).
- Zinc (glycinate) (12-18 mg per day in divided dosages).
- Copper (glycinate) (600-900 µg per day in divided dosages).
- Manganese (glycinate) (4-6 mg per day in divided dosages).

The above provide antioxidant effects and serve as free radical scavengers to help remove cellular debris and promote healing. The zinc, copper, and manganese act as cofactors and catalysts for the potent antioxidant enzyme SOD and are therefore referred to as the *SOD induction complex.* Oral supplementation with SOD can be attempted; however, it has been reported that it is often destroyed in the stomach and intestinal tract before assimilation. SOD can be obtained in Cell Guard (Biotec Foods).

All of the above tissue-healing nutrients can be obtained in the formulary product Collagenics (Metagenics, Inc.), with the exception of the Glucosamine Sulfate. For Glucosamine Sulfate, the sister product Collagenics Intensive Care must be used; however, this product does not contain the amino acid pool contained in the Collagenics. Other manufacturers make similar formulary products designed to aid in soft tissue repair, such as Rehab Plus (Professional Health Products). Consult the catalog of the reputable vendors you use for alternate products.

REFERENCES

1. Balch JF, Balch PA: *Prescription for natural healing,* Wayne, NJ, 1990, Avery Publishing.
2. Bland JH, Cooper SM: Osteoarthritis: a review of the cell biology involved and evidence for reversibility, management rationally related to known genesis and pathophysiology, *Semin Arthritis Rheum* 14(2):106, 1984.

3. Brukner P: *Clinical sports medicine,* New York, 1993, McGraw-Hill.

4. Bucci LR: *Nutrition applied to injury rehabilitation and sports medicine,* Boca Raton, Fla, 1995, CRC Press.

5. Cichoke AJ, Marty L: The use of proteolytic enzymes with soft-tissue athletic injuries, *Am Chiropr,* October 1981, p 32.

6. D'Ambrosio E, et al: Glucosamine sulfate: a controlled clinical investigation in arthrosis, *Pharmatherapeutica* 2(8):504-508, 1981.

7. Davis CD, Greger JL: Longitudinal changes of manganese-dependent superoxide dismutase and other indexes of manganese and iron status in women, *Am J Clin Nutr* 55:747, 1992.

8. Drovanti A, et al: Oral glucosamine sulfate in osteoarthritis: a placebo controlled double-blind investigation, *Clin Ther* 3(4):260-272, 1980.

9. Fauci A, et al: *Harrison's principles of internal medicine,* ed 13, New York, 1994, McGraw-Hill.

10. Gatterman M: *Chiropractic management of spine related disorders,* Baltimore, 1990, Williams & Wilkins.

11. Grabowski RJ: *Current nutritional therapy,* San Antonio, Tex, 1993, Image Press.

12. Hammer W: *Functional soft tissue examination and treatment by manual methods,* Gaithersburg, Md, 1991, Aspen Publishers.

13. Havsteen B: Flavinoids, a class of natural products of high pharmacological potency, *Biochem Pharmacol* 33(24):3933-3939, 1984.

14. Lawrence D: *Fundamentals of chiropractic diagnosis and management,* Baltimore, 1991, Williams & Wilkins.

15. Lindahl O, Lindwall L: Double blind study of a *Valerian* preparation, *Pharmacol Biochem Behav* 32(4):10065-10066, 1989.

16. *Manual of medical therapeutics (the Washington manual),* ed 27, Boston, 1992, Little, Brown.

17. *The Merck manual,* ed 16, Rahway, NJ, 1992, Merck Co.

18. Niki E: Interaction of ascorbate and alpha-tocopherol, *Third Conference on Vitamin C* 498:187-189, 1987.

19. Rakel RE: *Conn's current therapy,* Philadelphia, 1996, WB Saunders.

20. Rakel RE: *Textbook of family practice,* ed 5, Philadelphia, 1995, WB Saunders.

21. Schwartz RI, et al: Ascorbate can act as an inducer of collagen pathway because most steps are tightly coupled, *Third Conference on Vitamin C* 498:172-184, 1987.

22. Scully RM, Barnes MR: *Physical therapy,* Philadelphia, 1989, JB Lippincott.

23. Seplow W: Management of lateral meniscus injury, *J Sports Chiropr Rehab* 10(2):86-88, 1996.

24. Speroni E, Minghetti A: Neuropharmacological activity of extracts from *Passiflora incarnata, Planta Med* 54(6):488-491, 1988.

25. Taraye JP, Lauressergues H: Advantages of combination of proteo-lytic enzymes, flavonoids and ascorbic acid in comparison with non-steroid inflammatory drugs, *Arzneimittelforschung* 27(1):1144-1149, 1977.

26. Tierney LM, McPhee SJ, Papadakis MA: *Current medical diagnosis and treatment,* ed 35, Norwalk, Conn, 1996, Appleton & Lange.

27. Werbach MR: *Nutritional influences on illness,* ed 2, Tarzana, Calif, 1996, Third Line Press.

28. Werbach MR, Murray MT: *Botanical influences on illness,* Tarzana, Calif, 1994, Third Line Press.

Patellofemoral Pain Syndrome

KARLENE WISE, LEW HUFF, AND DAVID M. BRADY

DEFINITION

A syndrome of pain with or without the presence of pathologic changes of the articular cartilage of the patella. With cartilage degeneration, the diagnosis would be chondromalacia patella.

ETIOLOGY

May be due to trauma, recurrent subluxation, osteoarthritis, fracture, osteochondritis dessicans, twisting injuries, peripatellar tendinitis, overuse, valgus knee, external tibial torsion, increased Q angle, pronated feet, or short leg syndrome. Additional cause may be quad muscle imbalance. Patella alta may predispose to subluxation. Increased incidence in females 12 to 35 years of age.

SIGNS AND SYMPTOMS

Pain Pattern

Aching patellar pain; pain with running, weight bearing, or active motion. Stiffness relieved by activity, sensation of knee giving away or locking. Pain is aggravated by increased loads, ascending or descending stairs, skiing, or long-distance running.

Inspection

Possible valgus knee, swelling, increased Q angle, external tibial torsion, patella alta, or foot overpronation.

Palpation

Palpable tenderness over the anteromedial or anterolateral aspect of the knee. Tenderness over the joint line, crepitus during squatting, tight iliotibial band.

Muscle Testing

Quad weakness, general weakness about the knee. Patella seems to slide off to one side, usually laterally.

Other Manifestations

"Movie sign" or "cinema sign": increased achy pain when knees are flexed and unmoving for prolonged periods of time.

DIFFERENTIAL DIAGNOSIS

Osteoarthritis
Osteochondritis dessicans
Patella tendinitis
Overuse trauma

ORTHOPEDIC TESTS

Patellar grinding test (+)
Friction test (+)
Gait analysis
Apprehension test

X-RAY FINDINGS

Sclerosis
Spurring
Decreased joint space
(All are possible findings)

TREATMENT GOALS

1. Promote soft tissue and cartilage healing.
2. Relieve pain and prevent recurrence.

3. Increase pain-free ranges of motion.
4. Restore normal strength and stability to joint structure.
5. Quickly change to rehabilitation and restoration of function.
6. Prevent further degenerative changes in joint structure.

MANAGEMENT PROTOCOL (OPTIONS)

Acute Phase:

- Rest and avoidance of aggravating activities.
- Ice packs to promote vasoconstriction to decrease inflammation, pain, edema, and muscle spasms. Ice packs over affected area for 20 minutes with dry towel between ice packs and subject.
- Interferential for pain and edema management.

Subacute Phase:

- Electrical muscle stimulation with alternating, sinusoidal current. Frequency 80 to 150 Hz, continuous, 15 minutes with muscle contraction to reduce myospasms.[26]
- Short wave diathermy: Heat source is placed 18 inches from body part, treatment time is 20 minutes, use one towel between heat source and patient.
- Manipulation: Manipulate femur, tibia, and patella. General patella techniques, genu-stretch technique.
- ROM exercises followed by ice applications.
- Transverse friction massage: A deep tissue massage at the site of involvement, stroking perpendicular to the fiber alignment to increase fiber mobility without longitudinal stress.
- Detect and treat any myofascial trigger points in quads, hamstrings, and particularly vastus lateralis with ischemic compression held for 5 to 7 seconds and repeat 3 times each visit.
- Quad stretching with knee in extension and hip in external rotation to strengthen vastus medialis. Strengthening exercises of hamstrings.
- Strengthen vastus medialis muscle to improve patellar motion and decrease risk of lateral displacement.
- Isometric straight leg raising exercises along with low-load bicycling.
- Knee brace and heel lift may be beneficial.

NUTRITIONAL MANAGEMENT PROTOCOL (OPTIONS)

Acute Pain and Inflammation:

- Proteolytic enzymes (trypsin, chymotrypsin, bromelin) (3-4 tablets qid in between meals). NOTE: Do not give to patients with ulcers!
- Bioflavonoids (quercetin, hesperidin, rutin, etc.) (200 mg mixed bioflavonoids q2h during acute phase).
- Herbals, such as boswellia, ginger, turmeric, cayenne (400 mg, 300 mg, 200 mg, 50 mg, respectively, q2h acute phase).

The above proteolytic enzymes can be obtained in Biozyme (Metagenics, Inc.) or Lyso-lymph Forte (Nutri-West, Inc.). Inflavonoid Intensive Care (Metagenics, Inc.) will provide the above bioflavonoids and herbals. Other manufacturers can provide quality proteolytic enzymes. Consult your product catalog.

Tissue Healing:

- Amino acids (glycine, L-cystine, L-proline, and L-lysine) (300-400 mg per day each in divided dosages). Supplies the amino acid pool necessary for the structural production of collagen.
- Glucosamine sulfate (1500 mg per day in divided dosages). Supplies the needed nutrients for the production of healthy ground substance.
- Vitamin C (3000-6000 mg per day in divided dosages).
- Iron (glycinate) (8-12 mg per day in divided dosages).
- Alpha-ketoglutaric acid (15 mg per day in divided dosages).

The above three nutrients are required for the hydroxylation of L-proline to L-hydroxyproline, which is needed for the production of quality collagen.

- Calcium (400 mg tid)
- Vitamin E (200 IU per day)
- Zinc (glycinate) (12-18 mg per day in divided dosages)
- Copper (glycinate) (600-900 µg per day in divided dosages)
- Manganese (glycinate) (4-6 mg per day in divided dosages)

The above provide antioxidant effects and serve as free radical scavengers to help remove cellular debris and promote healing. The zinc, copper, and manganese act as cofactors and catalysts for the potent antioxidant enzyme SOD and are therefore referred to as the *SOD induction complex.* Oral supplementation with SOD can be attempted; however, it has been reported that it is often destroyed in the stomach and intestinal tract before assimilation. SOD can be obtained in Cell Guard (Biotec Foods).

All of the above tissue-healing nutrients can be obtained in the formulary product Collagenics (Metagenics, Inc.), with the exception of the Glucosamine Sulfate. For Glucosamine Sulfate, the sister product Collagenics Intensive Care must be used; however, this product does not contain the amino acid pool contained in the Collagenics. Other manufacturers make similar formulary products designed to aid in soft tissue repair, such as Rehab Plus (Professional Health Products). Consult the catalog of the reputable vendors you use for alternate products.

REFERENCES

1. Balch JF, Balch PA: *Prescription for natural healing,* Wayne, NJ, 1990, Avery Publishing.
2. Beneliyahu D: Conservative chiropractic management of patellofemoral pain syndrome: a case study, *Chiropr Sports Med* 6(2):57-63, 1992.
3. Bland JH, Cooper SM: Osteoarthritis: a review of the cell biology involved and evidence for reversibility, management rationally related to known genesis and pathophysiology, *Semin Arthritis Rheum* 14(2):106, 1984.
4. Boucher J, Hodgdon J: Anatomical, mechanical and functional factors in patellofemoral pain syndrome, *Chiropr Sports Med* 7(1):1-5, 1993.
5. Brukner P: *Clinical sports medicine,* New York, 1993, McGraw-Hill.
6. Bucci LR: *Nutrition applied to injury rehabilitation and sports medicine,* Boca Raton, Fla, 1995, CRC Press.
7. Cichoke AJ, Marty L: The use of proteolytic enzymes with soft-tissue athletic injuries, *Am Chiropr,* October 1981, p 32.
8. D'Ambrosio E, et al: Glucosamine sulfate: a controlled clinical investigation in arthrosis, *Pharmatherapeutica* 2(8):504-508, 1981.
9. Davis CD, Greger JL: Longitudinal changes of manganese-dependent superoxide dismutase and other indexes of manganese and iron status in women, *Am J Clin Nutr* 55:747, 1992.
10. Drovanti A, et al: Oral glucosamine sulfate in osteoarthritis: a placebo controlled double-blind investigation, *Clin Ther* 3(4):260-272, 1980.
11. Fauci A, et al: *Harrison's principles of internal medicine,* ed 13, New York, 1994, McGraw-Hill.
12. Grabowski RJ: *Current nutritional therapy,* San Antonio, Tex, 1993, Image Press.
13. Hammer W: *Functional soft tissue examination and treatment by manual methods,* Gaithersburg, Md, 1991, Aspen Publishers.

14. Havsteen B: Flavinoids, a class of natural products of high pharmacological potency, *Biochem Pharmacol* 33(24):3933-3939, 1984.

15. Lawrence D: *Fundamentals of chiropractic diagnosis and management,* Baltimore, 1991, Williams & Wilkins.

16. Lindahl O, Lindwall L: Double blind study of a *Valerian* preparation, *Pharmacol Biochem Behav* 32(4):10065-10066, 1989.

17. *Manual of medical therapeutics (the Washington manual),* ed 27, Boston, 1992, Little, Brown.

18. *The Merck manual,* ed 16, Rahway, NJ, 1992, Merck Co.

19. Meyer JJ, et al: Effectiveness of chiropractic management for patellofemoral pain syndrome's symptomatic control phase: a single subject experiment, *J Manipulative Physiol Ther* 13(9):539-549, 1990.

20. Niki E: Interaction of ascorbate and alpha-tocopherol, *Third Conference on Vitamin C* 498:187-189, 1987.

21. Nimmo R: Receptor, effecters and tonus: a new approach, *J Natl Chiropr Assoc,* November 1957.

22. Rakel RE: *Conn's current therapy,* Philadelphia, 1996, WB Saunders.

23. Rakel RE: *Textbook of family practice,* ed 5, Philadelphia, 1995, WB Saunders.

24. Schneider MJ: Chiropractic management of myofascial and muscular disorders. In Lawrence D, ed: *Advances in chiropractic,* vol 3, St Louis, 1996, Mosby.

25. Schwartz RI, et al: Ascorbate can act as an inducer of collagen pathway because most steps are tightly coupled, *Third Conference on Vitamin C* 498:172-184, 1987.

26. Scully RM, Barnes MR: *Physical therapy,* Philadelphia, 1989, JB Lippincott.

27. Speroni E, Minghetti A: Neuropharmacological activity of extracts from *Passiflora incarnata, Planta Med* 54(6):488-491, 1988.

28. Taraye JF, Lauressergues H: Advantages of combination of proteolytic enzymes, flavonoids and ascorbic acid in comparison with non-steroid inflammatory drugs, *Arzneimittelforschung* 27(1):1144-1149, 1977.

29. Tierney LM, McPhee SJ, Papadakis MA: *Current medical diagnosis and treatment,* ed 35, Norwalk, Conn, 1996, Appleton & Lange.

30. Travell JG, Simons DG: *Myofascial pain and dysfunction: the trigger point manual,* vol 2, Baltimore, 1992, Williams & Wilkins.

31. Werbach MR: *Nutritional influences on illness,* ed 2, Tarzana, Calif, 1996, Third Line Press.

32. Werbach MR, Murray MT: *Botanical influences on illness,* Tarzana, Calif, 1994, Third Line Press.

33. White AA, Panjabi MM: *Clinical biomechanics of the spine,* Philadelphia, 1990, JB Lippincott.

Anterior/Posterior Shin Splints

Lew Huff, David M. Brady, and Donald C. Stran

DEFINITION

A loosely defined condition that describes pain, aching, and tightness of the anterior or posterior muscle groups of the leg. It is a general term for pain below the knee joint. More specifically, it refers to an anatomic site of periostitis. It is also termed *tibial tendinitis, myositis, tendinoperiostitis,* or *tibial stress syndrome.*

ETIOLOGY

An overload phenomenon; may be due to overuse, running, or jumping on hard surfaces. The leg muscles are torn away from their bony insertions. May also be due to muscle imbalance or hard heel strike in the gait cycle. Hammer describes it as a periosteal inflammation associated with an overuse injury and pulling of the muscle from its myotendinous origin. Other causative factors may include overpronation during gait cycle, improper athletic shoes, and external femoral or tibial torsion.

SIGNS AND SYMPTOMS

Pain Pattern

Pain begins as a myositis or tendinitis left untreated. Pain onset begins after several minutes into athletic activity or immediately after cessation of activity. Pain described as a deep, dull ache, throbbing pain without radiation. Gradual onset, severity increases with continued stress.

Inspection

May reveal excessive pronation or excessive non-weight bearing plantar flexion.

Palpation

Extreme palpable tenderness over the medial tibia, anterolateral tibia, or posteromedial tibia. Palpable myospasms and hypertonicity of calf muscles, tibialis anterior, gastrocnemius, or soleus muscles.

Anterior Compartment

Frequently occurs in runners overtraining on hills and doing up-and-down running.

Symptoms become worse while running downhill.

Lateral Compartment

Frequently occurs in athletes with overpronation or excessive activity of peroneal muscle groups.

Medial Compartment

Posterior tibial shin splints are most common. Seen in runners and aerobic dancers.

DIFFERENTIAL DIAGNOSIS

Stress fracture
Trauma
Compartmental syndrome

ORTHOPEDIC EXAMINATION

Range of motion
Resisted muscle testing

X-RAY FINDINGS

Rule out stress fracture.
Reactive periostosis is possible.
Findings are usually negative.

TREATMENT GOALS

1. Promote soft tissue healing.
2. Relieve pain and prevent recurrence.
3. Increase pain-free ranges of motion.
4. Quickly change to rehabilitation and restoration of function.

MANAGEMENT PROTOCOL (OPTIONS)

- Rest area and cease aggravating activities. Decrease running time and style if an aggravating factor.

Acute Phase:

- Apply ice packs for 15 to 20 minutes with dry towel between the patient and the ice packs. Use every 2 hours for reduction of pain and edema.
- Ice massage: Freeze ¾ cup water in Styrofoam cup; break off bottom of cup, exposing about ¼ inch of frozen ice; and slowly in a circular pattern massage the involved painful area for about 3 minutes.
- Ultrasound (pulsed) at 0.5 W/cm^2 over area for 5 minutes. Ultrasound causes the resolution of inflammatory exudates and increases blood flow.

Subacute Phase:

- Transverse friction massage: A deep tissue massage at the site of involvement, stroking perpendicular to the fiber alignment to increase fiber mobility without longitudinal stress. This promotes orientation of fibers and induces hyperemia to hypovascular tissues. In addition, transverse friction massage has a mechanical influence on tissue maturation.[24]
- Muscle stretching techniques and reduction of ankle equinus.[24]
- Stretch quads, hamstrings, tibialis anterior, gastrocnemius, and soleus.

- Reduction of any myofascial trigger points in gastrocnemius, soleus, anterior and posterior tibialis, peroneal, and popliteus muscles using ischemic compression techniques held 5 to 7 seconds, repeat 3 times each visit.
- Avoid overpronation, acquire suitable running shoes, and use semiflexible orthotic devices.[24]
- Manipulation: Check tarsals, metatarsal, and subtalar joint. Reduce subluxations of the lumbar spine and pelvis.

NUTRITIONAL MANAGEMENT PROTOCOL (OPTIONS)

Acute Pain and Inflammation:

- Proteolytic enzymes (trypsin, chymotrypsin, bromelin) (3-4 tablets qid in between meals). NOTE: Do not give to patients with ulcers!
- Bioflavonoids (quercetin, hesperidin, rutin, etc.) (200 mg mixed bioflavonoids every q2h during acute phase).
- Herbals, such as boswellia, ginger, turmeric, cayenne (400 mg, 300 mg, 200 mg, 50 mg, respectively, q2h acute phase).

The above proteolytic enzymes can be obtained in Biozyme (Metagenics, Inc.) or Lyso-lymph Forte (Nutri-West, Inc.). Inflavonoid Intensive Care (Metagenics, Inc.) will provide the above bioflavonoids and herbals. Other manufacturers can provide quality proteolytic enzymes. Consult your product catalog.

Tissue Healing:

- Amino acids (glycine, L-cystine, L-proline, and L-lysine) (300-400 mg per day each in divided dosages). Supplies the amino acid pool necessary for the structural production of collagen.
- Vitamin C (3000-6000 mg per day in divided dosages).
- Iron (glycinate) (8-12 mg per day in divided dosages).
- Alpha-ketoglutaric acid (15 mg per day in divided dosages).

The above three nutrients are required for the hydroxylation of L-proline to L-hydroxyproline, which is needed for the production of quality collagen.

- Calcium (400 mg tid)
- Vitamin E (200 IU per day)
- Zinc (glycinate) (12-18 mg per day in divided dosages)
- Copper (glycinate) (600-900 µg per day in divided dosages)
- Manganese (glycinate) (4-6 mg per day in divided dosages)

The above provide antioxidant effects and serve as free radical scavengers to help remove cellular debris and promote healing. The zinc, copper, and manganese act as cofactors and catalysts for the potent antioxidant enzyme SOD and are therefore referred to as the *SOD induction complex*. Oral supplementation with SOD can be attempted; however, it has been reported that it is often destroyed in the stomach and intestinal tract before assimilation. SOD can be obtained in Cell Guard (Biotec Foods).

All of the above tissue-healing nutrients can be obtained in the formulary product Collagenics (Metagenics, Inc.). Other manufacturers make similar formulary products designed to aid in soft tissue repair, such as Rehab Plus (Professional Health Products). Consult the catalog of the reputable vendors you use for alternate products.

HOME CARE PROTOCOL (OPTIONS)

- Use shock-absorbing running shoes.[28] Orthotic shoe inserts are most effective in treatment of symptoms arising from biomechanical abnormalities, such as excessive pronation or leg length discrepancy
- Rest and avoid aggravating activities.
- Gradually work up to prior training levels.
- Stretching may help prevent injury.
- Consider changing running style.

REFERENCES

1. Austin WM: Shin splints with underlying posterior tibial tendinitis: a case report, *J Sports Chiropr Rehab* 10(4):163-168, 1994.
2. Balch JF, Balch PA: *Prescription for natural healing,* Wayne, NJ, 1990, Avery Publishing.
3. Batt ME: Shin-splints: a review of terminology, *Clin J Sport Med* 5(1):153-157, 1995.
4. Bland JH, Cooper SM: Osteoarthritis: a review of the cell biology involved and evidence for reversibility, management rationally related to known genesis and pathophysiology, *Semin Arthritis Rheum* 14(2):106, 1984.
5. Brukner P: *Clinical sports medicine,* New York, 1993, McGraw-Hill.
6. Bucci LR: *Nutrition applied to injury rehabilitation and sports medicine,* Boca Raton, Fla, 1995, CRC Press.
7. Cibulka MT, et al: Shin-splints and forefoot contact running: a case report, *J Orthop Sports Phys Ther* 20(2):98-102, 1994.

8. Cichoke AJ, Marty L: The use of proteolytic enzymes with soft-tissue athletic injuries, *Am Chiropr,* October 1981, p 32.

9. D'Ambrosio E, et al: Glucosamine sulfate: a controlled clinical investigation in arthrosis, *Pharmatherapeutica* 2(8):504-508, 1981.

10. Davis CD, Greger JL: Longitudinal changes of manganese-dependent superoxide dismutase and other indexes of manganese and iron status in women, *Am J Clin Nutr* 55:747, 1992.

11. Drovanti A, et al: Oral glucosamine sulfate in osteoarthritis: a placebo controlled double-blind investigation, *Clin Ther* 3(4):260-272, 1980.

12. Fauci A, et al: *Harrison's principles of internal medicine,* ed 13, New York, 1994, McGraw-Hill.

13. Gatterman M: *Chiropractic management of spine related disorders,* Baltimore, 1990, Williams & Wilkins.

14. Gerow G, et al: Compartment syndrome and shin splints of the lower leg, *J Manipulative Physiol Ther* 16(4):245-252, 1993.

15. Grabowski RJ: *Current nutritional therapy,* San Antonio, Tex, 1993, Image Press.

16. Gross ML, et al: Effectiveness of orthotic shoe inserts in the long distance runner, *Am J Sports Med* 19(4):409-412, 1991.

17. Hammer W: *Functional soft tissue examination and treatment by manual methods,* Gaithersburg, Md, 1991, Aspen Publishers.

18. Havsteen B: Flavinoids, a class of natural products of high pharmacological potency, *Biochem Pharmacol* 33 (24):3933-3939, 1984.

19. Lawrence D: *Fundamentals of chiropractic diagnosis and management,* Baltimore, 1991, Williams & Wilkins.

20. Liebenson C: *Rehabilitation of the spine,* Baltimore, 1996, Williams & Wilkins.

21. Lindahl O, Lindwall L: Double blind study of a *Valerian* preparation, *Pharmacol Biochem Behav* 32(4):10065-10066, 1989.

22. *Manual of medical therapeutics (the Washington manual),* ed 27, Boston, 1992, Little, Brown.

23. *The Merck manual,* ed 16, Rahway, NJ, 1992, Merck Co.

24. Morris R: Medial tibial syndrome: a treatment protocol using electrical current, *Chiropr Sports Med* 5(1):5-8, 1991.

25. Niki E: Interaction of ascorbate and alpha-tocopherol, *Third Conference on Vitamin C* 498:187-189, 1987.

26. Nimmo R: Receptor, effecters and tonus: a new approach, *J Natl Chiropr Assoc,* November 1957.

27. Rakel RE: *Conn's current therapy,* Philadelphia, 1996, WB Saunders.

28. Rakel RE: *Saunders manual of medical practice,* Philadelphia, 1996, WB Saunders.

29. Rakel RE: *Textbook of family practice,* ed 5, Philadelphia, 1995, WB Saunders.

30. Schneider MJ: Chiropractic management of myofascial and muscular disorders. In Lawrence D, ed: *Advances in chiropractic,* vol 3, St Louis, 1996, Mosby.

31. Schwartz RI, et al: Ascorbate can act as an inducer of collagen pathway because most steps are tightly coupled, *Third Conference on Vitamin C* 498:172-184, 1987.

32. Scully RM, Barnes MR: *Physical therapy,* Philadelphia, 1989, JB Lippincott.

33. Speroni E, Minghetti A: Neuropharmacological activity of extracts from *Passiflora incarnata, Planta Med* 54(6):488-491, 1988.

34. Taraye JP, Lauressergues H: Advantages of combination of proteo-lytic enzymes, flavonoids and ascorbic acid in comparison with non-steroid inflammatory drugs, *Arzneimittelforschung* 27(1):1144-1149, 1977.

35. Tierney LM, McPhee SJ, Papadakis MA: *Current medical diagnosis and treatment,* ed 35, Norwalk, Conn, 1996, Appleton & Lange.

36. Travell JG, Simons DG: *Myofascial pain and dysfunction: the trigger point manual,* vol 2, Baltimore, 1992, Williams & Wilkins.

37. Werbach MR: *Nutritional influences on illness,* ed 2, Tarzana, Calif, 1996, Third Line Press.

38. Werbach MR, Murray MT: *Botanical influences on illness,* Tarzana, Calif, 1994, Third Line Press.

39. White AA, Panjabi MM: *Clinical biomechanics of the spine,* Philadelphia, 1990, JB Lippincott.

Compartment Syndrome

LEW HUFF, DAVID M. BRADY, AND DONALD C. STRAN

DEFINITION

A condition of increased pressure within one of the four compartments of the lower leg, leading to motor and sensory disturbances. The four compartments are defined as the anterior, deep posterior, peroneal, and superficial posterior.

ETIOLOGY

Increased pressure within a closed osteofascial space or lack of fascia laxity, which would prevent increased blood flow during exercise. Decreased blood flow to tissues during periods in which the pressure is high within the compartment results in insufficient metabolic flow to muscle and nerves, leading to muscle necrosis.[2] Other causes include soft tissue swelling, calcified hematoma, deep venous thrombosis, and healing fracture. This disorder is generally associated with runners, sprinters, track and field athletes, skiers, dancers, and boxers.[6]

SIGNS AND SYMPTOMS

Inspection

Edema may be present. Patient is often left with a fixed inverted deformity of the ankle with a painful high arch and claw toes if severe and untreated.

Palpation

Not an arterial injury, so distal pulses may be palpable. Extreme tenderness within the compartment is present.

Quality

Painful tight sensation in the calf. Extreme pain on passive stretch of the involved muscles.

Differential Diagnosis

Peripheral vascular disease, tendinitis, claudication, fatigue fractures, shin splints

Anterior Compartment Syndrome

Transient or persistent footdrop with possible paresthesia. Paresthesia is often felt over dorsum of the foot.

Deep Posterior Compartment

Paresthesias of the instep of the foot
    CAUTION: Compartment pressures over 30 to 40 mm Hg for 4 to 12 hours are associated with ischemia and permanent neuromuscular damage if not relieved.[2,6]

Clinical Note

The pathogenesis of acute compartment syndrome is associated with external pressure or hemorrhage. If the tissue pressure were to rise above 30 to 40 mm Hg for 4 to 12 hours, irreversible muscular damage would result. Emergency intervention is the only appropriate treatment of severe acute compartment syndrome.

TREATMENT GOALS

1. Decrease pain and pressure within the compartment.
2. Restore normal function of the muscle groups.
3. Gradually resume preinjury activities.

MANAGEMENT PROTOCOL (OPTIONS)

- *Surgery* may be necessary for patients who have compartment pressures greater than 30 to 35 mm Hg.[6]

- Compartment syndrome can develop 2 hours to 7 days after injury. Monitor for swelling. An ischemic event of 6 hours is sufficient to produce permanent muscle and nerve damage. Be prepared to refer for fasciotomy.[2]
- For chronic compartment syndrome, orthotics may be helpful.[6] For chronic compartment syndrome with elevated pressures on a transient basis and influenced by activity, conservative management is felt to be effective.[9]

NUTRITIONAL MANAGEMENT PROTOCOL (OPTIONS)

Acute Pain and Inflammation:
- Proteolytic enzymes (trypsin, chymotrypsin, bromelin) (3-4 tablets qid in between meals). NOTE: Do not give to patients with ulcers!
- Bioflavonoids (quercetin, hesperidin, rutin, etc.) (200 mg mixed bioflavonoids q2h during acute phase).
- Herbals, such as boswellia, ginger, turmeric, cayenne (400 mg, 300 mg, 200 mg, 50 mg, respectively, q2h acute phase).

The above proteolytic enzymes can be obtained in Biozyme (Metagenics, Inc.) or Lyso-lymph Forte (Nutri-West, Inc.). Inflavonoid Intensive Care (Metagenics, Inc.) will provide the above bioflavonoids and herbals. Other manufacturers can provide quality proteolytic enzymes. Consult your product catalog.

REFERENCES

1. Balch JF, Balch PA: *Prescription for natural healing,* Wayne, NJ, 1990, Avery Publishing.
2. Beneliyahu D: Dynamic electrodiagnostic evaluation and conservative management of chronic exertional compartment syndrome of the leg: a case report, *Chiropr Sports Med* 9(2):39-43, 1995.
3. Brukner P: *Clinical sports medicine,* New York, 1993, McGraw-Hill.
4. Cichoke AJ, Marty L: The use of proteolytic enzymes with soft-tissue athletic injuries, *Am Chiropr,* October 1981, p 32.
5. Fauci A, et al: *Harrison's principles of internal medicine,* ed 13, New York, 1994, McGraw-Hill.
6. Gerow G, et al: Compartment syndrome and shin splints of the lower leg, *J Manipulative Physiol Ther* 16(4):245, 1993.
7. Grabowski RJ: *Current nutritional therapy,* San Antonio, Tex, 1993, Image Press.

8. Gross ML, et al: Effectiveness of orthotic shoe inserts in the long distance runner, *Am J Sports Med* 19(4):409-412, 1991.

9. Hammer W: *Functional soft tissue examination and treatment by manual methods*, Gaithersburg, Md, 1991, Aspen Publishers.

10. Havsteen B: Flavinoids, a class of natural products of high pharmacological potency, *Biochem Pharmacol* 33(24):3933-3939, 1984.

11. Lawrence D: *Fundamentals of chiropractic diagnosis and management*, Baltimore, 1991, Williams & Wilkins.

12. *Manual of medical therapeutics (the Washington manual)*, ed 27, Boston, 1992, Little, Brown.

13. Niki E: Interaction of ascorbate and alpha-tocopherol, *Third Conference on Vitamin C* 498:187-189, 1987.

14. Nimmo R: Receptor, effecters and tonus: a new approach, *J Natl Chiropr Assoc*, November 1957.

15. Rakel RE: *Conn's current therapy*, Philadelphia, 1996, WB Saunders.

16. Rakel RE: *Saunders manual of medical practice*, Philadelphia, 1996, WB Saunders.

17. Rakel RE: *Textbook of family practice*, ed 5, Philadelphia, 1995, WB Saunders.

18. Schneider MJ: Chiropractic management of myofascial and muscular disorders. In Lawrence D, ed: *Advances in chiropractic*, vol 3, St Louis, 1996, Mosby.

19. Scully RM, Barnes MR: *Physical therapy*, Philadelphia, 1989, JB Lippincott.

20. Tierney LM, McPhee SJ, Papadakis MA: *Current medical diagnosis and treatment*, ed 35, Norwalk, Conn, 1996, Appleton & Lange.

21. Travell JG, Simons DG: *Myofascial pain and dysfunction: the trigger point manual*, vol 2, Baltimore, 1992, Williams & Wilkins.

22. Werbach MR: *Nutritional influences on illness*, ed 2, Tarzana, Calif, 1996, Third Line Press.

23. Werbach MR, Murray MT: *Botanical influences on illness*, Tarzana, Calif, 1994, Third Line Press.

Injuries to the Foot and Ankle: General Overview

Lew Huff

ANKLE INJURIES

The ankle is prone to injuries resulting from sports, occupational, and daily activities. Weight-bearing forces of the entire body are transmitted to the ankle via the knee. The commonly injured ligaments are the calcaneofibular, anterior talofibular, dorsal calcaneo, cuboid, and deltoid ligaments. Anterior talofibular ligament is the most common ligament injury.

PLANTAR FASCIITIS

An overuse syndrome causing a strain or tear of the plantar fascia characterized by pain primarily at the plantar medial calcaneal area, or the origin of the plantar fascia.

TARSAL TUNNEL

An entrapment neuropathy involving the tarsal tunnel of the foot caused by ill-fitting shoes, chronic foot strain, bone spurs, repetitive stress, abnormal calcaneal eversion, and foot pronation.

SITE OF PAIN

Ankle Sprain

Pain from a ligament sprain is superficial and well localized. Approximately 90% of ankle sprains are inversion sprains with no fractures. Commonly seen with ankle sprains are diffuse swelling, ecchymosis, and skin temperature elevation. The mechanism of injury is most often plantar flexion and inversion. The site of pain is localized to the area of injury.

Plantar Fasciitis

Palpable tenderness and crepitus noted over the plantar calcaneal aspect of the foot and calcaneal tuberosity. Medial heel pad may be callused. Plantar pain increases with running or toe rises. Site of pain is the anteromedial plantar calcaneal area.

Tarsal Tunnel

Burning pain under the ball and sole of the foot and burning and paresthesia of the toes and soles occur. Pain is aggravated by valgus pressure and may radiate to the calf or toes.

EXAMINATION
Ankle Sprain

Examine the quads, hamstrings, anterior and posterior tibialis, gastrocnemius, and soleus for injury. Examine gait patterns and ranges of motion in all planes. A person with complete rupture of a ligament may have no pain because a complete rupture causes loss of continuity of fibers, which are unable to be stressed, producing no pain. Painless hypermobility is seen in chronic ligamentous rupture. Examine the entire fibula for fracture.

Eversion sprains may cause avulsion of the medial malleolus rather than ligamentous damage. Tenderness along the anterior talofibular ligament suggests sprain (drawer sign). Gross lateral instability is noted with a tear of the anterior talofibular and calcaneofibular ligament. Medial instability is common with a deltoid ligament tear.

Plantar Fasciitis

Examine the gastrocnemius, soleus, anterior and posterior tibialis, and intrinsic muscles of the foot. With patient supine, extend knee and dorsiflex the ankle and digits (especially the hallux) to the maximum dorsiflexion possible. Symptoms should appear. Blood work, including human leukocyte antigen (HLA-B27), complete blood count (CBC), uric acid, rheumatoid arthritis factor (RA factor), ESR, C-reactive protein, and a multichannel 24, should be included to rule out systemic inflammatory arthritis.

Tarsal Tunnel

Examine the gastrocnemius, soleus, anterior and posterior tibialis, and intrinsic muscles of the foot. Examine for overpronation, varus heel, or valgus heel. Note tenderness on palpation or mass at the tunnel region. Tinel's sign many be present. Examine the strength of the foot flexors and extensors. Tourniquet applied above the ankle may reproduce symptoms.

RADIATION, REFERRED PAIN

Ankle Sprain

Referred pain is common to the knee, lower leg, or foot.

Tarsal Tunnel

Pain may radiate to the calf area or toward the toes.

ACTIVITIES OF DAILY LIVING

A patient with a ankle injury will have difficulty walking, turning, running, or weight bearing. A crutch or casting may be needed.

UNINJURED AREA

Examination and radiographic examination for bilateral comparison if necessary.

REINJURY/FLARE-UP

Restrict aggravating activities, continue care, and start low-impact rehabilitative exercises.

HOME CARE

ROM exercises, passive stretching, surgical tubing exercises, ice applications, or compresses may be appropriate.

WHEN TO DISCHARGE

When patient has reached maximum medical improvement or the need for referral is established.

REFERRAL

If fracture, dislocation, or neurologic complications are present. Daily treatment exceeding 2 weeks may signal the need for a second opinion or referral. Treatment exceeding 4 weeks, temporary disability for longer than 4 weeks with no objective signs of improvement, or worsening of the condition within the first 2 weeks may signal the need for a second opinion or referral.[4]

REFERENCES

1. Clemente C: *Anatomy: a regional atlas of the human body,* ed 3, Baltimore, 1987, Urban & Schwarzenberg.
2. Gatterman M: *Chiropractic management of spine related disorders,* Baltimore, 1990, Williams & Wilkins.
3. Haldeman S, et al: Guidelines for chiropractic quality assurance & practice parameters, *The Proceedings of the Mercy Center Consensus Conference,* Gaithersburg, Md, 1993, Aspen Publishers.
4. Hansen DT: *Chiropractic standards of practice and utilization guidelines in the care and treatment of injured workers,* 1988, Washington State Department of Labor & Industries.
5. Lawrence D: *Fundamentals of chiropractic diagnosis and management,* Baltimore, 1991, Williams & Wilkins.
6. Schestack R: *Handbook of physical therapy,* ed 3, New York, 1977, Springer-Verlag.
7. Vear HJ: *Chiropractic standards of practice and quality of care,* Gaithersburg, Md, 1992, Aspen Publishers.

Ankle Sprain

LEW HUFF, DAVID M. BRADY, AND DONALD C. STRAN

DEFINITION

A tearing or rupture of the tendons and ligaments of the ankle mortise.

Grade 1: Mild or moderate sprain without tearing of ligaments but some swelling. Anterior talofibular (ATF) ligament.

Grade 2: Moderate sprain, partial rupture of ligaments, swelling, and ecchymosis. ATF, calcaneofibular (CF) ligaments.

Grade 3: Complete ligamentous tearing, swelling, hemorrhage, and instability. ATF, CF, and posterior talofibular (PTF) ligaments.

ETIOLOGY

Predisposed to ankle sprain with ligamentous laxity, a vast range of motion of the joint, and/or weakness of the peroneal muscles. Approximately 80% of ankle sprains are caused by inversion with injury to the lateral ligaments. ATF ligament is the most common to tear.

SIGNS AND SYMPTOMS

History

Ask questions regarding mechanism of injury, prior injury, disability, treatment, and pain.[16]

Inspection

Abnormal gait, decreased range of motion, rapid swelling and ecchymosis, weight-bearing instability.

Palpation

Exquisite pain or localized tenderness of ankle mortise. Point tenderness over ligament or insertion point. Pain over sinus tarsi area suggests tear of ATF ligament.

Examination

Examination for ecchymosis, edema, areas of tenderness and laxity.[16]

Other Manifestations

Inability to continue activity after injury. Ligamentous laxity when stressed.

ORTHOPEDIC EXAMINATION

Drawer sign (+)
Range of motion
Palpation of joint spaces
Syndesmotic sprain test
Talar tilt test

X-RAY FINDINGS

Stress view, mortise view may be needed.
  Rule out fracture of fibula and widening of mortise.
  Rule out avulsion of bone or fifth metatarsal fracture.
  Criteria for radiographic examination. Inability to bear weight initially or when examined and tenderness over the medial or lateral malleolus.[15]
  NOTE: Need MRI if pain continues to rule out talar bone lesion which is very often missed. Stress views should be done under anesthesia.

TREATMENT GOALS

1. Promote soft tissue healing.
2. Relieve pain and prevent recurrence.
3. Increase pain-free ranges of motion.
4. Restore normal strength and stability to joint structure

5. Quickly change to rehabilitation for restoration of function.

MANAGEMENT PROTOCOL (OPTIONS)

- **Rule out** fracture and ruptured syndesmosis for immediate surgical referral.

Acute Phase:

- Immobilize to allow ligament ends to heal to prevent necrosis. Later, weight bearing and functional therapy is treatment of choice for Grade 1 and Grade 2 sprains. Ace wrap for Grade 1, soft brace or posterior splint for Grade 2.
- PRICES, *p*rotect, *r*est, *i*ce, *c*ompress, *e*levate, and *s*tabilize, for early acute intervention. If possible, use immediate ice pack and elastic wrapping.
- Ice packs or frozen bag of peas applied for 20 to 30 minutes every 3 to 4 hours day and night for 48 hours.[1]
- Continuous compression for the first 48 hours. Elevate above the heart for the first 48 hours.

Subacute Phase:

- 48 hours to several days: PRICES therapy before each exercise session. Patient stands in moderately hot water in tub, followed by slow stretching in plantar and dorsiflexion. Later, follow with ergometric cycling with light resistance.
- Several days to 10 weeks: Linear movement exercises with increasing load and speed, toe rises, jogging, squats, jumping in place.
- Resistance exercises should include movement in all planes, emphasizing resistance to eversion and dorsiflexion. This should not elicit pain.
- Strengthening of weak lateral musculature (i.e., peroneal muscles) is essential to avoid repeated inversion sprain/ strains. Manual "resetting" of muscle spindle gain may be necessary, along with eliminating any trigger points with ischemic compression and strengthening exercises for full functionality of muscles to return.
- Taping or bracing should be used with vigorous activity or walking on uneven surfaces.
- Rehabilitation program should include at least 10 weeks of proprioception training on a balance board in severe cases.

Proprioception training with balance board can begin from 1 to 3 weeks after injury.[1]
- Manipulation: Adjust any lateral talus or anterior talus malpositions, fixated mortise joint, or any other foot or ankle articular segmental dysfunctions.

NUTRITIONAL MANAGEMENT PROTOCOL (OPTIONS)

Acute Pain and Inflammation:
- Proteolytic enzymes (trypsin, chymotrypsin, bromelin) (3-4 tablets qid in between meals). NOTE: Do not give to patients with ulcers!
- Bioflavonoids (quercetin, hesperidin, rutin, etc.) (200 mg mixed bioflavonoids q2h during acute phase).
- Herbals, such as boswellia, ginger, turmeric, cayenne (400 mg, 300 mg, 200 mg, 50 mg, respectively, q2h acute phase).

The above proteolytic enzymes can be obtained in Biozyme (Metagenics, Inc.) or Lyso-lymph Forte (Nutri-West, Inc.). Inflavonoid Intensive Care (Metagenics, Inc.) will provide the above bioflavonoids and herbals. Other manufactures can provide quality proteolytic enzymes. Consult your product catalog.

Tissue Healing:
- Amino acids (glycine, L-cystine, L-proline, and L-lysine) (300-400 mg per day each in divided dosages). Supplies the amino acid pool necessary for the structural production of collagen.
- Vitamin C (3000-6000 mg per day in divided dosages).
- Iron (glycinate) (8-12 mg per day in divided dosages).
- Alpha-ketoglutaric acid (15 mg per day in divided dosages).

The above three nutrients are required for the hydroxylation of L-proline to L-hydroxyproline, which is needed for the production of quality collagen.
- Calcium (400 mg tid)
- Vitamin E (200 IU per day)
- Zinc (glycinate) (12-18 mg per day in divided dosages)
- Copper (glycinate) (600-900 µg per day in divided dosages)
- Manganese (glycinate) (4-6 mg per day in divided dosages)

The above provide antioxidant effects and serve as free radical scavengers to help remove cellular debris and promote healing. The zinc, copper, and manganese act as cofactors and catalysts for the potent antioxidant enzyme SOD and are therefore referred to as the *SOD induction complex*. Oral supplementation with SOD can be attempted; however, it has been reported that it is often destroyed in the stomach and intestinal tract before assimilation. SOD can be obtained in Cell Guard (Biotec Foods).

All of the above tissue-healing agents can be obtained in the formulary product Collagenics (Metagenics, Inc.). Other manufacturers make similar formulary products designed to aid in soft tissue repair, such as Rehab Plus (Professional Health Products). Consult the catalog of the reputable vendors you use for alternate products.

HOME CARE PROTOCOL (OPTIONS)

- Acute: PRICES at home.
- Subacute/chronic: Taping before vigorous activity.
- Avoid aggravating activities.
- Wear good supportive shoes.
- Walking on sand is good rehabilitation when tolerated.
- Prevention:
  1. Use of external ankle support.
  2. Slow static stretching of calf muscles reduces severity of injury.[1]

REFERENCES

1. Bahr R: Acute ankle sprains: a functional treatment plan for injured athletes, *Consultant*, April 1996.
2. Balch JF, Balch PA: *Prescription for natural healing*, Wayne, NJ, 1990, Avery Publishing.
3. Brukner P: *Clinical sports medicine*, New York, 1993, McGraw-Hill.
4. Bucci LR: *Nutrition applied to injury rehabilitation and sports medicine*, Boca Raton, Fla, 1995, CRC Press.
5. Charrette M: Ankle sprain, *Digest of Chiropractic Economics* 36(3):36-38, 40-41, 1993.
6. Cichoke AJ, Marty L: The use of proteolytic enzymes with soft-tissue athletic injuries, *Am Chiropr*, October 1981, p 32.
7. Davis CD, Greger JL: Longitudinal changes of manganese-dependent superoxide dismutase and other indexes of manganese and iron status in women, *Am J Clin Nutr* 55:747, 1992.
8. Grabowski RJ: *Current nutritional therapy*, San Antonio, Tex, 1993, Image Press.

9. Hammer W: *Functional soft tissue examination and treatment by manual methods,* Gaithersburg, Md, 1991, Aspen Publishers.

10. Havsteen B: Flavinoids, a class of natural products of high pharmacological potency, *Biochem Pharmacol* 33(24):3933-3939, 1984.

11. Lawrence D: *Fundamentals of chiropractic diagnosis and management,* Baltimore, 1991, Williams & Wilkins.

12. *Manual of medical therapeutics (the Washington manual),* ed 27, Boston, 1992, Little, Brown.

13. Murtagh J: *General practice,* New York, 1994, McGraw-Hill.

14. Niki E: Interaction of ascorbate and alpha-tocopherol, *Third Conference on Vitamin C* 498:187-189, 1987.

15. Picone J: Acute/chronic ankle sprain: a case study, *Chiropr Sports Med* 3(3):74-80, 1989.

16. Rakel RE: *Saunders manual of medical practice,* Philadelphia, 1996, WB Saunders.

17. Rakel RE: *Textbook of family practice,* ed 5, Philadelphia, 1995, WB Saunders.

18. Rifat SF, McKeag DB: Practical methods of preventing ankle injuries, *Am Fam Physician* 53(8):2491-2498, 1996.

19. Rubin A, Sallis R: Evaluation and diagnosis of ankle injuries, *Am Fam Physician* 54(5):1609-1618, 1996.

20. Schneider MJ: Chiropractic management of myofascial and muscular disorders. In Lawrence D, ed: *Advances in chiropractic,* vol 3, St Louis, 1996, Mosby.

21. Schwartz RI, et al: Ascorbate can act as an inducer of collagen pathway because most steps are tightly coupled, *Third Conference on Vitamin C* 498:172-184, 1987.

22. Scully RM, Barnes MR: *Physical therapy,* Philadelphia, 1989, JB Lippincott.

23. Tierney LM, McPhee SJ, Papadakis MA: *Current medical diagnosis and treatment,* ed 35, Norwalk, Conn, 1996, Appleton & Lange.

24. Ward D: Syndesmotic ankle sprain in a recreational hockey player, *J Chiropr* 17(6):385-394, 1994.

25. Werbach MR: *Nutritional influences on illness,* ed 2, Tarzana, Calif, 1996, Third Line Press.

26. Werbach MR, Murray MT: *Botanical influences on illness,* Tarzana, Calif, 1994, Third Line Press.

Achilles Tendinitis (Achillobursitis)

Lew Huff, David M. Brady, and Donald C. Stran

DEFINITION

An inflammation of the anterior Achilles bursa and tendon. Achillobursitis is also known as *Albert's disease* or *retrocalcaneal bursitis*. Tendinitis may precede the development of bursitis.

ETIOLOGY

Achilles tendinitis is classified as a fatigue disorder and may be due to overuse, trauma, repetitive stress, sudden or excessive stretching of the tendon, or shock forces from running on hard surfaces. Achilles bursitis may be due to tendon damage, excessive pressure on the heels, or oversized or tight shoes. Rapid onset is due to trauma, whereas gradual onset may be due to rheumatoid arthritis. Other causes may include rear foot pronation, exostosis, or calcification of the tendon.

SIGNS AND SYMPTOMS

Pain Pattern

Pain, heat, and edema of distal Achilles tendon. Heel pain on running heel strike. Pain may be constant or just with movement.

Inspection

Localized swelling anterior to Achilles tendon. Difficulty with walking, running. Erythema may be seen. Limited ranges of motion of the ankle and foot. Enlargement of posterior-superior calcaneus—usually lateral. Discomfort wearing shoes.

Palpation

Heat felt over retrocalcaneal surface. Palpable tenderness over tendon and soft tissue. Crepitus on movement of the tendon.

Other

Painful passive dorsiflexion of the foot. Difficulty climbing stairs, walking on sand, or jogging. Weakness of the calf muscle secondary to tendon pain.

DIFFERENTIAL DIAGNOSIS

Rheumatoid arthritis
Retrocalcaneal heel spur
Cellulitis
Tendinitis

X-RAY FINDINGS

Rule out fracture, rheumatoid arthritis, and erosive changes of the calcaneus

TREATMENT GOALS

1. Decrease pain of heel.
2. Increase pain-free mobility.
3. Gradually return to preinjury status.

MANAGEMENT PROTOCOL (OPTIONS)

Acute Phase:
- Ice massage to painful area for 15 minutes every 2 hours.
- Avoid aggravating activities and limit movements to allow inflammation to subside. Stop running for 1 to 2 weeks.
- Ultrasound (pulsed) over related muscle tissues. Pulsed at 0.5 W/cm² at 5 to 8 minutes followed by stretching exercises and ice applications.
- High-volt galvanism or interferential to decrease pain.

Subacute Phase:
- Transverse friction massage: A deep tissue massage at the site of involvement, stroking perpendicular to the fiber alignment to increase fiber mobility without longitudinal stress. Longitudinal friction massage is beneficial.
- Correct talus and calcaneal subluxations.
- When pain and inflammation subside, graded strengthening exercises should begin.
  1. Surgical tubing exercises
  2. Stretching, flexibility exercises
  3. Muscle strengthening of gastrocnemius, soleus, and tibialis anterior
- Assess need for new shoes or orthotics. Change to strapless shoes, latex shields, or heel lift to raise calcaneus. Foot strapping to prevent overpronation. Consider temporary heel lift to decrease tension on the Achilles tendon.

NUTRITIONAL MANAGEMENT PROTOCOL (OPTIONS)

Acute Pain and Inflammation:
- Proteolytic enzymes (trypsin, chymotrypsin, bromelin) (3-4 tablets qid in between meals). NOTE: Do not give to patients with ulcers!
- Bioflavonoids (quercetin, hesperidin, rutin, etc.) (200 mg mixed bioflavonoids q2h during acute phase).
- Herbals, such as boswellia, ginger, turmeric, cayenne (400 mg, 300 mg, 200 mg, 50 mg, respectively, q2h acute phase).

The above proteolytic enzymes can be obtained in Biozyme (Metagenics, Inc.) or Lyso-lymph Forte (Nutri-West, Inc.). Inflavonoid Intensive Care (Metagenics, Inc.) will provide the above bioflavonoids and herbals. Other manufacturers can provide quality proteolytic enzymes. Consult your product catalog.

HOME CARE PROTOCOL (OPTIONS)

- Do not run too many miles per week or increase mileage too quickly.
- Do not increase running intensity too quickly.
- Invest in good running shoes, and avoid worn-out shoes or poor heel counters.
- Use ankle brace for vigorous activities.

REFERENCES

1. Balch JF, Balch PA: *Prescription for natural healing,* Wayne, NJ, 1990, Avery Publishing.
2. Brukner P: *Clinical sports medicine,* New York, 1993, McGraw-Hill.
3. Cichoke AJ, Marty L: The use of proteolytic enzymes with soft-tissue athletic injuries, *Am Chiropr,* October 1981, p 32.
4. Fauci A, et al: *Harrison's principles of internal medicine,* ed 13, New York, 1994, McGraw-Hill.
5. Grabowski RJ: *Current nutritional therapy,* San Antonio, Tex, 1993, Image Press.
6. Hammer W: *Functional soft tissue examination and treatment by manual methods,* Gaithersburg, Md, 1991, Aspen Publishers.
7. Havsteen B: Flavinoids, a class of natural products of high pharmacological potency, *Biochem Pharmacol* 33(24):3933-3939, 1984.
8. Lawrence D: *Fundamentals of chiropractic diagnosis and management,* Baltimore, 1991, Williams & Wilkins.
9. *Manual of medical therapeutics (the Washington manual),* ed 27, Boston, 1992, Little, Brown.
10. *The Merck manual,* ed 16, Rahway, NJ, 1992, Merck Co.
11. Niki E: Interaction of ascorbate and alpha-tocopherol, *Third Conference on Vitamin C* 498:187-189, 1987.
12. Rakel RE: *Conn's current therapy,* Philadelphia, 1996, WB Saunders.
13. Rakel RE: *Saunders manual of medical practice,* Philadelphia, 1996, WB Saunders.
14. Rakel RE: *Textbook of family practice,* ed 5, Philadelphia, 1995, WB Saunders.
15. Scully RM, Barnes MR: *Physical therapy,* Philadelphia, 1989, JB Lippincott.
16. Tierney LM, McPhee SJ, Papadakis MA: *Current medical diagnosis and treatment,* Norwalk, Conn, 1996, Appleton & Lange.
17. Werbach MR: *Nutritional influences on illness,* ed 2, Tarzana, Calif, 1996, Third Line Press.
18. Werbach MR, Murray MT: *Botanical influences on illness,* Tarzana, Calif, 1994, Third Line Press.
19. White AA, Panjabi MM: *Clinical biomechanics of the spine,* Philadelphia, 1990, JB Lippincott.

Plantar Fasciitis

Lew Huff, David M. Brady, and Donald C. Stran

DEFINITION

A strain or tear of the plantar fascia characterized by pain primarily at the plantar medial calcaneal area or the origin of the plantar fascia. An overuse syndrome causing microtears of the plantar fascia. Also known as *heel spur syndrome,* although a heel spur is not always present.

ETIOLOGY

May be due to abnormal heel impact in the gait cycle, rapid acceleration or deceleration, pes planus, pes cavus, ill-fitting shoes, or leg length discrepancy. Excess subtalar joint pronation may lower the arch, placing a traction force on the plantar fascia and often leading to the development of heel spurs. Often associated with walking, running, tennis, gymnastics, and basketball. May be due to new or unusual activity, such as a walking program or shopping spree.

SIGNS OR SYMPTOMS

Inspection

Overpronation of the foot
Increased pain with weight bearing
Shoe may poorly control the ankle area
Medial heel pad may be callused

Palpation

Palpable tenderness and crepitus noted over the plantar calcaneal aspect of the foot and the calcaneal tuberosity.

Pain Pattern

Pain is originally worse upon rising out of bed or after long rest periods because ligaments get cold and shortened. Plantar pain increases with running or toe rises. Pain increases toward end of day or while running on hard surfaces.

Quality

Pain ranges from dull to sharp over the anteromedial plantar calcaneal area, especially when rising from rest and during initial periods of weight bearing.

EXAMINATION

With patient supine, extend knee and dorsiflex the ankle and digits (especially the hallux) to the maximum dorsiflexion possible. Symptoms should appear. Take an x-ray of the lateral foot weight bearing.

DIFFERENTIAL DIAGNOSIS

Tenosynovitis
Ruptured plantar fascia
Reiter's syndrome
Ankylosing spondylitis
Tarsal tunnel syndrome
Gouty arthritis
Rheumatoid arthritis

X-RAY FINDINGS

Possible calcific calcaneal spur
Possible neoplasm

LABORATORY WORK

Blood work, including HLA-B27, CBC, uric acid, RA factor, ESR, C-reactive protein, and a multichannel 24, should be included to rule out systemic inflammatory arthritis.

TREATMENT GOALS

1. Promote soft tissue healing.
2. Relieve pain and prevent recurrence.
3. Increase pain-free ranges of motion.
4. Restore normal strength and stability to joint structure.
5. Quickly change to rehabilitation or restoration of function.

MANAGEMENT PROTOCOL (OPTIONS)

Acute Phase:

- Ultrasound (pulsed) underwater: Use 1.0 W/cm^2 at 5 to 8 minutes followed by stretching exercises and ice applications. Ultrasound as a micromassage is beneficial.
- Ice massage: Freeze a Styrofoam cup full of water; remove the cup and break off the bottom, exposing the ice; and massage in a small circular pattern for about 3 minutes over the involved area. Ice massage to tolerance for 20 minutes a day is beneficial.[15]

Subacute Phase:

- Transverse friction massage and longitudinal friction massage are beneficial.[17]
- Reduction of myofascial trigger points in all plantar musculature using ischemic compression techniques (5 to 7 seconds), repeat 3 times.
- Correct subluxations of calcaneus, cuboids, navicular, and metatarsals. Active stretching of gastrocnemius and soleus and the Achilles tendon is the cornerstone of the rehabilitation program.[23] Strengthen all antipronator muscles of the ankle with elastic tubing exercises.
- Isometric training should begin almost immediately in the rehabilitation process. Progress to isotonic training as soon as possible.
- Balance boards are used to improve proprioception and balance.[22]
- In runners, a return to running should begin as soon as symptoms allow. Distance should be increased gradually and in small increments. Ice after workout.
- Use Sorbothane or other shock-absorbing heel pads. Orthotics for long-term care are beneficial.

NUTRITIONAL MANAGEMENT PROTOCOL (OPTIONS)

Acute Pain and Inflammation:

- Proteolytic enzymes (trypsin, chymotrypsin, bromelin) (3-4 tablets qid in between meals). NOTE: Do not give to patients with ulcers!
- Bioflavonoids (quercetin, hesperidin, rutin, etc.) (200 mg mixed bioflavonoids q2h during acute phase).
- Herbals, such as boswellia, ginger, turmeric, cayenne (400 mg, 300 mg, 200 mg, 50 mg, respectively, q2h acute phase).

The above proteolytic enzymes can be obtained in Biozyme (Metagenics, Inc.) or Lyso-lymph Forte (Nutri-West, Inc.). Inflavonoid Intensive Care (Metagenics, Inc.) will provide the above bioflavonoids and herbals. Other manufacturers can provide quality proteolytic enzymes. Consult your product catalog.

HOME CARE PROTOCOL (OPTIONS)

- Avoid sprinting or running on uneven surfaces or running uphill.
- Decrease running mileage when reconditioning.
- Look for shoes with a close-fitting heel counter and adequate medial arch.

REFERENCES

1. Balch JF, Balch PA: *Prescription for natural healing,* Wayne, NJ, 1990, Avery Publishing.
2. Batt M, Tanji J: Management options for plantar fasciitis, *Physician Sports Med* 23(6):77-80, 83-86, 1995.
3. Brukner P: *Clinical sports medicine,* New York, 1993, McGraw-Hill.
4. Cichoke AJ, Marty L: The use of proteolytic enzymes with soft-tissue athletic injuries, *Am Chiropr,* October 1981, p 32.
5. Fauci A, et al: *Harrison's principles of internal medicine,* ed 13, New York, 1994, McGraw-Hill.
6. Grabowski RJ: *Current nutritional therapy,* San Antonio, Tex, 1993, Image Press.
7. Hammer W: *Functional soft tissue examination and treatment by manual methods,* Gaithersburg, Md, 1991, Aspen Publishers.
8. Havsteen B: Flavinoids, a class of natural products of high pharmacological potency, *Biochem Pharmacol* 33(24):3933-3939, 1984.
9. Lawrence D: *Fundamentals of chiropractic diagnosis and management,* Baltimore, 1991, Williams & Wilkins.

10. *Manual of medical therapeutics (the Washington manual),* ed 27, Boston, 1992, Little, Brown.

11. Michelson JD: Heel pain: when is it plantar fasciitis? *J Musculo Med* 12(3):22-29, 1995.

12. Murtagh J: *General practice,* New York, 1994, McGraw-Hill.

13. Niki E: Interaction of ascorbate and alpha-tocopherol, *Third Conference on Vitamin C* 498:187-189, 1987.

14. Nimmo R: Receptor, effecters and tonus: a new approach, *J Natl Chiropr Assoc,* November 1957.

15. Polkinghorn B: Posterior calcaneal subluxation: an important consideration in chiropractic treatment of plantar fasciitis (heel spur syndrome), *Chiropr Sports Med* 9(2):44-51, 1995.

16. Rakel RE: *Textbook of family practice,* ed 5, Philadelphia, 1995, WB Saunders.

17. Ryan J: Use of posterior night splints in the treatment of plantar fasciitis, *Am Fam Physician* 52(3):891-898, 1995.

18. Scully RM, Barnes MR: *Physical therapy,* Philadelphia, 1989, JB Lippincott.

19. Schneider MJ: Chiropractic management of myofascial and muscular disorders. In Lawrence D, ed: *Advances in chiropractic,* vol 3, St Louis, 1996, Mosby.

20. Tierney LM, McPhee SJ, Papadakis MA: *Current medical diagnosis and treatment,* Norwalk, Conn, 1996, Appleton & Lange.

21. Travell JG, Simons DG: *Myofascial pain and dysfunction: the trigger point manual,* vol 2, Baltimore, 1992, Williams & Wilkins.

22. Wapner KL, Sharkey PF: The use of night splints for treatment of recalcitrant plantar fasciitis, *Foot Ankle Int* 12(3):135-137, 1991.

23. Werbach MR: *Nutritional influences on illness,* ed 2, Tarzana, Calif, 1996, Third Line Press.

24. Werbach MR, Murray MT: *Botanical influences on illness,* Tarzana, Calif, 1994, Third Line Press.

25. White AA, Panjabi MM: *Clinical biomechanics of the spine,* Philadelphia, 1990, JB Lippincott.

Tarsal Tunnel Syndrome

Lew Huff, David M. Brady, and Donald C. Stran

DEFINITION

An entrapment neuropathy involving the posterior tibial nerve in the tarsal tunnel beneath the flexor retinaculum on the medial side of the ankle.

ETIOLOGY

Causes may include ill-fitting shoes, tenosynovitis, chronic foot strain, chronic thrombophlebitis, gouty arthritis, hypertrophy of the abductor hallucis muscle, bone spurs, repetitive stress, abnormal calcaneal eversion, and foot pronation. Overpronation is the most common cause. Lorei and Hershman state that in 3 out of 4 cases, it is a late consequence of twisting injury or fracture of the ankle.[11]

SIGNS AND SYMPTOMS

Inspection

Overpronation, varus heel, or valgus heel may be noted.

Palpation

Tenderness on digital palpation, pressure, or percussion. Palpable mass at tunnel region.

Pain Pattern

Burning pain under the ball and sole of the foot. Burning and paresthesia of the toes and soles of the feet. Pain aggravated by valgus pressure. Local pain decreased by walking.[11]

Radiation

Pain may radiate to the calf area or toward the toes.

Neurological Manifestations

(+) Tinel's sign. Numbness of the feet and legs. Sensory deficits over the medial and lateral plantar and calcaneal distribution. Weakness of the foot flexors.

Quality

Symptoms may be vague. Aching, burning, and numbness are common.

Other

Nocturnal exacerbations are common. Tourniquet applied above the ankle may reproduce symptoms.

DIFFERENTIAL DIAGNOSIS

Interdigital neuroma (Morton's)
Peripheral neuritis
Tenosynovitis
Plantar fasciitis
Gouty arthritis

SPECIAL TESTS

To confirm neurologic manifestations
NCV, EMG (+/−)

TREATMENT GOALS

1. Promote soft tissue healing.
2. Relieve pain and prevent recurrence.
3. Increase pain-free ranges of motion.
4. Restore normal strength and stability to joint structure.
5. Quickly change to rehabilitation or restoration of function.

MANAGEMENT PROTOCOL (OPTIONS)

Acute Phase:
- Rest the area and avoid aggravating activities.
- Ice massage: Freeze a Styrofoam cup full of water; remove the cup and break off the bottom, exposing the ice; and massage in a small circular pattern for about 3 minutes over the involved area. Ice massage to tolerance for 20 minutes a day is beneficial.
- Ultrasound (pulsed) underwater: Use 1.0 W/cm^2 at 5 to 8 minutes followed by stretching exercises and ice applications. Ultrasound as a micromassage is beneficial.
- High-volt galvanic and interferential are beneficial.

Subacute Phase:
- Adjustment of the calcaneus, distal tibia, and talus helps mobilize the area, break adhesions, and promote circulation.[13]
- Use of medial or lateral heel wedge is beneficial along with semirigid or rigid orthotics to prevent overpronation. Treatment with foot orthotics and cessation of running activities will decrease signs and symptoms.[15] Use orthotics for long-term pronator control.

NUTRITIONAL MANAGEMENT PROTOCOL (OPTIONS)

Acute Pain and Inflammation:
- Proteolytic enzymes (trypsin, chymotrypsin, bromelin) (3-4 tablets qid in between meals). NOTE: Do not give to patients with ulcers!
- Bioflavonoids (quercetin, hesperidin, rutin, etc.) (200 mg mixed bioflavonoids q2h during acute phase).
- Herbals, such as boswellia, ginger, turmeric, cayenne (400 mg, 300 mg, 200 mg, 50 mg, respectively, q2h acute phase).

The above proteolytic enzymes can be obtained in Biozyme (Metagenics, Inc.) or Lyso-lymph Forte (Nutri-West, Inc.). Inflavonoid Intensive Care (Metagenics, Inc.) will provide the above bioflavonoids and herbals. Other manufacturers can provide quality proteolytic enzymes. Consult your product catalog.

HOME CARE PROTOCOL (OPTIONS)

Avoid jogging, hiking, or walking on uneven surfaces.

REFERENCES

1. Balch JF, Balch PA: *Prescription for natural healing,* Wayne, NJ, 1990, Avery Publishing.
2. Brukner P: *Clinical sports medicine,* New York, 1993, McGraw-Hill.
3. Bucci LR: *Nutrition applied to injury rehabilitation and sports medicine,* Boca Raton, Fla, 1995.
4. Cichoke AJ, Marty L: The use of proteolytic enzymes with soft-tissue athletic injuries, *Am Chiropr,* October 1981, p 32.
5. Fauci A, et al: *Harrison's principles of internal medicine,* ed 13, New York, 1994, McGraw-Hill.
6. Goodheart G: The tarsal tunnel syndrome, *Digest of Chiropractic Economics* 13(5):6-7, 1971.
7. Grabowski RJ: *Current nutritional therapy,* San Antonio, Tex, 1993, Image Press.
8. Hammer W: *Functional soft tissue examination and treatment by manual methods,* Gaithersburg, Md, 1991, Aspen Publishers.
9. Havsteen B: Flavinoids, a class of natural products of high pharmacological potency, *Biochem Pharmacol* 33(24):3933-3939, 1984.
10. Lawrence D: *Fundamentals of chiropractic diagnosis and management,* Baltimore, 1991, Williams & Wilkins.
11. Lorei MP, Hershman EB: Peripheral nerve injury in athletes: treatment and prevention, *Sports Med* 16(2):130-147, 1993.
12. *Manual of medical therapeutics (the Washington manual),* ed 27, Boston, 1992, Little, Brown.
13. Mavissakalian S, et al: Tarsal tunnel syndrome and the chiropractic adjustment: a case report, *J Am Chiropr Assoc* 32(2):77-78, 1995.
14. *The Merck manual,* ed 16, Rahway, NJ, 1992, Merck Co.
15. Mumenthaler M: Tarsal tunnel syndrome: diagnosis and differential diagnosis, *Wien Klin Wochenschr* 105(16):459-461, 1993.
16. Murtagh J: *General practice,* New York, 1994, McGraw-Hill.
17. Niki E: Interaction of ascorbate and alpha-tocopherol, *Third Conference on Vitamin C* 498:187-189, 1987.
18. Pla ME, et al: Painful legs and moving toes associated with tarsal tunnel syndrome and accessory soleus muscle, *Mov Disord* 119(1):82-86, 1996.
19. Rakel RE: *Conn's current therapy,* Philadelphia, 1996, WB Saunders.
20. Rakel RE: *Saunders manual of medical practice,* Philadelphia, 1996, WB Saunders.
21. Rakel RE: *Textbook of family practice,* ed 5, Philadelphia, 1995, WB Saunders.
22. Scully RM, Barnes MR: *Physical therapy,* Philadelphia, 1989, JB Lippincott.
23. Tierney LM, McPhee SJ, Papadakis MA: *Current medical diagnosis and treatment,* Norwalk, Conn, 1996, Appleton & Lange.

24. Werbach MR: *Nutritional influences on illness,* ed 2, Tarzana, Calif, 1996, Third Line Press.
25. Werbach MR, Murray MT: *Botanical influences on illness,* Tarzana, Calif, 1994, Third Line Press.
26. White AA, Panjabi MM: *Clinical biomechanics of the spine,* Philadelphia, 1990, JB Lippincott.

SECTION X

Related Disorders

Ankylosing Spondylitis

Rheumatoid Arthritis

Degenerative Joint Disease (Osteoarthritis)

Diabetes Mellitus

Fibromyalgia

Hypertension

Osteoporosis

Ankylosing Spondylitis

BRIAN BATENCHUK, LEW HUFF, AND DAVID M. BRADY

DEFINITION

Ankylosing spondylitis (AS) is a chronic progressive inflammatory disease characterized by pain, inflammation, and progressive stiffening of the spine and bilateral sacroiliitis.

ETIOLOGY

Etiology unknown. Approximately 90% of cases are men, usually under age 30 years when symptoms first appear. Primarily affects young males, commencing in the late teens or early 20s. There appears to be a strong genetic component.

SIGNS AND SYMPTOMS

Onset

First sign is low back pain localized to SI joints and/or lumbar spine; low back pain is insidious and nontraumatic.

Location

Localized pain of SI joints and lumbar spine.

Inspection

Increased thoracic kyphosis, painful gait and posture. Stooped "question mark" posture.

Palpation

SI joints are tender upon percussion and springing of pelvis.

Pain Pattern

Pain worse at rest, often felt over buttocks. Pain may awaken the patient at night. Morning stiffness improves during exercise. Pain is characterized by exacerbations and remissions.

Aggravating Factors

Pain may increase with walking.

Ranges of Motion

Decreased ranges of motion and joint play of spine. Decreased chest expansion in later stages. Loss of lateral flexion.

Systemic Manifestations

May include anemia, myalgia, fatigue, weight loss, vague chest pain, iritis in 25%, heart involvement in 5%, and low-grade fever.

Radiation of Pain

Asymmetrical SI pain with radiation to buttock and thigh is not unusual. Radicular symptoms may occur years later as a result of cauda equina fibrosis.

Arthritic Changes

Transient acute arthritis is seen in peripheral joints (especially the larger joints) in 50% of cases. Permanent arthritic changes are seen, especially in hips, shoulders, and knees, in 25% of cases.

Complications

Aortic aneurysm, aortic insufficiency, conjunctivitis, cardiac conduction defects, pulmonary fibrosis, asymmetrical oligoarthritis, urethritis, and mucocutaneous lesions. Arthritis of costotransverse, costosternal, manubriosternal, sternoclavicular, and AC joints is common.[10,28]

DIFFERENTIAL DIAGNOSIS

The history and physical findings distinguish AS from back pain caused by disk disease, osteoporosis, soft tissue trauma, and tumors. The appearance in the SI joints is the most distinguishing radiographic sign of AS that helps differentiate it from other inflammatory arthropathies. Differentiate from osteitis ilii. Testing for HLA-B27 should not be considered an absolute diagnostic criteria.[27] (See Fig. 3.)

IMAGING FINDINGS

Major signs include osteoporosis, erosions with sclerosis, and bony ankylosis. First changes are seen in the SI joints, then the thoracolumbar and lumbosacral junction. Enthesopathy is usually associated with SI changes. SI changes are frequently bilateral and symmetrical. In the spine the discovertebral junctions and zygapophyseal and costovertebral articulations are involved.

NOTE: **Atlantoaxial instability may be present due to odontoid erosions and transverse ligament involvement, manipulation would be a contraindication.**

LABORATORY FINDINGS

ESR elevated in 85% of cases. Serological tests for RA factor are negative. Anemia may be present but is usually mild. HLA-B27 is found in 90% of cases compared with 8% of normal population.

MANAGEMENT PROTOCOL (OPTIONS)

- *Manipulation is contraindicated in the inflammatory stage.*[8,27] Manipulation may be tolerated after acute phase with no excessive force.[8]
- Gentle manipulation of the costovertebral joints may be beneficial to normal respiratory movements.[8] ***Beware of osteopenia, aortic aneurysm, and dens erosion.***
- Swimming exercises, stretching, and hyperflexion/hyperextension exercises may prevent flexion deformities.
- Physical medicine modalities may be beneficial for pain relief.

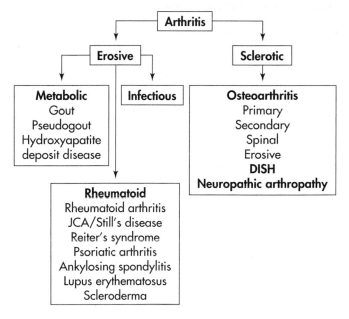

FIG. 3. Arthritis classification diagram.

NUTRITIONAL MANAGEMENT PROTOCOL (OPTIONS)

Acute Pain and Inflammation:

- Proteolytic enzymes (trypsin, chymotrypsin, bromelin) (3-4 tablets qid in between meals). NOTE: Do not give to patients with ulcers!
- Bioflavonoids (quercetin, hesperidin, rutin, etc.) (200 mg mixed bioflavonoids q2h during acute phase).
- Herbals, such as boswellia, ginger, turmeric, cayenne (400 mg, 300 mg, 200 mg, 50 mg, respectively, q2h acute phase).

The above proteolytic enzymes can be obtained in Biozyme (Metagenics, Inc.) or Lyso-lymph Forte (Nutri-West, Inc.). Inflavonoid Intensive Care (Metagenics, Inc.) will provide the above bioflavonoids and herbals. Other manufacturers can provide quality proteolytic enzymes. Consult your product catalog.

HOME CARE PROTOCOL (OPTIONS)

- Perform ROM, posture, and breathing exercises.
- Sleep supine on a firm mattress without a pillow.
- Take daily warm baths for stiffness.
- Avoid heavy lifting.
- Practice standing and sitting up straight.

REFERENCES

1. Balch JF, Balch PA: *Prescription for natural healing,* Wayne, NJ, 1990, Avery Publishing.
2. Bose R: Ankylosing spondylitis: treatment, *Am Chiropr,* June 1982, p 50.
3. Brukner P: Clinical sports medicine, *New York,* 1993, McGraw-Hill.
4. Bucci LR: *Nutrition applied to injury rehabilitation and sports medicine,* Boca Raton, Fla, 1995, CRC Press.
5. Cichoke AJ, Marty L: The use of proteolytic enzymes with soft-tissue athletic injuries, *Am Chiropr,* October 1981, p 32.
6. Fauci A, et al: *Harrison's principles of internal medicine,* ed 13, New York, 1994, McGraw-Hill.
7. Forbes CD, Jackson WF: *Color atlas and text of clinical medicine,* St Louis, 1993, Mosby.
8. Gatterman M: *Chiropractic management of spine related disorders,* Baltimore, 1990, Williams & Wilkins.
9. Grabowski RJ: *Current nutritional therapy,* San Antonio, Tex, 1993, Image Press.
10. Haldeman S: *Principles and practice of chiropractic,* ed 2, Norwalk, Conn, 1992, Appleton & Lange.
11. Hammer W: *Functional soft tissue examination and treatment by manual methods,* Gaithersburg, Md, 1991, Aspen Publishers.
12. Havsteen B: Flavinoids, a class of natural products of high pharmacological potency, *Biochem Pharmacol* 33(24):3933-3939, 1984.
13. Kelley WN: *Essentials of internal medicine,* Philadelphia, 1994, JB Lippincott.
14. Kirkaldy-Willis WH: *Managing low back pain,* ed 2, Edinburgh, 1989, Churchill Livingston.
15. *Manual of medical therapeutics (the Washington manual),* ed 27, Boston, 1992, Little, Brown.
16. *The Merck manual,* ed 16, Rahway, NJ, 1992, Merck Co.
17. Rakel RE: *Conn's current therapy,* Philadelphia, 1996, WB Saunders.
18. Rakel RE: *Textbook of family practice,* ed 5, Philadelphia, 1995, WB Saunders.
19. Sandman KB: Ankylosing spondylitis: a review and clinical update, *J Manipulative Physiol Ther* 5(4):183-185, 1982.

20. Taraye JP, Lauressergues H: Advantages of combination of proteolytic enzymes, flavonoids and ascorbic acid in comparison with non-steroid inflammatory drugs, *Arzneimittelforschung* 27(1):1144-1149, 1977.

21. Tierney LM, McPhee SJ, Papadakis MA: *Current medical diagnosis and treatment,* ed 35, Norwalk, Conn, 1996, Appleton & Lange.

22. Underwood M, Dawes P: Inflammatory back pain in primary care, *Br J Rheumatol* 34(11):1074-1077, 1995.

23. Werbach MR: *Nutritional influences on illness,* ed 2, Tarzana, Calif, 1996, Third Line Press.

24. Werbach MR, Murray MT: *Botanical influences on illness,* Tarzana, Calif, 1994, Third Line Press.

25. White AH, Schofferman JA: *Spine care,* vol 1, St Louis, 1995, Mosby.

26. White AA, Panjabi MM: *Clinical biomechanics of the spine,* Philadelphia, 1990, JB Lippincott.

27. Yochum T: Ankylosing spondylitis, *Eur J Chiropr* 30(4):221-226, 1982.

28. Yochum TR, Rowe LJ: *Essentials of skeletal radiology,* ed 2, Baltimore, 1995, Williams & Wilkins.

Rheumatoid Arthritis

BRIAN BATENCHUK, LEW HUFF, AND DAVID M. BRADY

DEFINITION

Rheumatoid arthritis (RA) is a connective tissue disorder that targets synovial joints, especially of the hands, feet, larger joints, and the cervical spine. Other body systems may be involved, including the heart, lungs, small blood vessels, nervous system, eyes, and reticuloendothelial system. In Western populations the prevalence is approximately 3%, with women more commonly affected than men, and a peak age of onset of 30 to 50 years.

ETIOLOGY

The etiology is unknown but is most likely multifactorial. The high risk conferred by HLA-D4 and common family history suggest a genetic component. Environmental factors such as viral infections, toxicity, and food allergies have been suggested. RA may be triggered by infection, surgery, trauma, emotional stress, and increased intestinal permeability resulting in modified food allergics.[31]

SIGNS AND SYMPTOMS

Pain Pattern

Joint pain, stiffness, and swelling (worse in early morning). Pain on motion or tenderness of at least one joint.

Location

Bilateral and symmetrical polyarthritis, usually of insidious onset. (70% of patients).

Inspection

Soft tissue swelling or joint effusion of at least one joint. Swelling of at least one other joint (within 3 months). Bilateral, symmetrical, and simultaneous joint swelling (except distal interphalangeal [DIP] joints). Subcutaneous nodules (bony protuberances) of extensor surfaces.

Joint Deformities

In the hands, there is subluxation and ulnar deviation at the metacarpophalangeal joints in advanced cases. Swan-neck and boutonniere deformities can occur at the interphalangeal joints. Dorsal subluxation of the ulnar styloid at the wrist is common and may contribute to rupture of the fourth and fifth extensor tendons when there is also inflammation within the extensor tendon sheaths. In the forefoot, the metatarsophalangeal joints become dislocated. There is sometimes reported a clawing of the toes, and patients complain of painful sensation like "walking on pebbles." Varus and fixed flexion deformities of the knees are common, and popliteal (Baker's) cysts are sometimes felt. Rupture of these cysts causes sudden calf pain with swelling, which can mimic deep venous thrombosis.

Systemic Manifestations

Skin manifestations include subcutaneous nodules. Vasculitic skin rashes and nail fold and finger pulp infarcts are common. Patients may also complain of Raynaud's phenomenon. Keratoconjunctivitis sicca (dry eyes) and episcleritis are common ocular manifestations. Scleritis and scleromalacia are rare complications. Cardiac and pulmonary complications are usually limited to pericardial and pleural involvement. Neurological manifestations include mononeuritis, carpal tunnel syndrome, and cervical myelopathy. Amyloid may deposit in the kidneys. Other systemic manifestations include fever, weight loss, malaise, paresthesias, low-grade fever, anorexia, fatigue, weakness, and pulmonary complications.

DIAGNOSTIC CRITERIA

Physical

1. Morning stiffness
2. Pain on motion or tenderness in at least one joint
3. Soft tissue swelling or joint effusion in at least one joint
4. Swelling of at least one other joint (within 3 months)
5. Bilateral, symmetrical, and simultaneous joint swelling (except DIP joints)
6. Juxtaarticular, subcutaneous nodules (bony protuberances) over extensor surfaces

Objective Indicators

1. Positive sheep agglutination test (rheumatoid factor)
2. Poor mucin precipitate from synovial fluid
3. Synovium—at least three of:
   a. Marked villous hypertrophy
   b. Superficial synovial cell proliferation
   c. Marked inflammatory cell infiltrate fibrin deposition
   d. Foci of cell necrosis
4. Nodule-granulomas with central necrosis, proliferated fixed cells, peripheral fibrosis, and chronic inflammatory cell infiltrate
5. Typical changes—uniform joint space loss, marginal erosions, etc.
6. Increased serum ANA latex, ESR, and C-reactive protein

LABORATORY FINDINGS

1. Positive rheumatoid factor (80% of patients).
2. The most common hematological manifestation is a normochromic, normocytic anemia, but hypochromic anemia may occur, especially where nonsteroidal antiinflammatory drug (NSAID) therapy has caused GI blood loss.
3. Platelet and white cell count may be high, and the ESR, antinuclear antibody (ANA) latex, and C-reactive protein may be elevated.

CLASSIFICATION

Classic: More than six criteria (with swelling for >6 months)

Definite: More than five criteria (with continuous joint symptoms >6 weeks)

Probable: More than three criteria (with continuous joint symptoms >4-6 weeks)

Possible: At least two of stiffness, pain, swelling, nodules, elevated ESR or C-reactive protein, or iritis, with joint symptoms of at least 3 weeks.

IMAGING FINDINGS

1. Bilateral symmetrical joint changes
2. Periarticular soft tissue swelling
3. Juxtaarticular osteoporosis
4. Uniform loss of joint space
5. Marginal bony erosion ("rat bite" erosions)
6. Juxtaarticular periostitis (rare)
7. Large pseudocysts in bone
8. Deformity

DIFFERENTIAL DIAGNOSIS

Differentiate RA from other inflammatory spondyloarthropathies such as AS, psoriatic arthritis, or Reiter's syndrome, as well as systemic lupus erythematosus.

TREATMENT GOALS

1. Promote soft tissue healing.
2. Relieve pain.
3. Increase pain-free ranges of motion.
4. Eliminate allergenic triggers.

Clinical Notes

Peer-reviewed refereed journals suggest that there is strong evidence that RA patients on appropriate nutritional supplementation may reduce their intake of antirheumatoid drugs without suffering deterioration in their arthritis.[4]

RA patients may initially complain of systemic manifestations, such as weight loss, fatigue, or anorexia, and generalized aching or stiffness. The diagnosis of RA depends on a pattern of clinical symptoms and signs that must be present for at least 6 weeks. The Mercy Center Consensus Conference document has assigned *cervical manipulation as an absolute contraindication* in a patient with RA.[5]

MANAGEMENT PROTOCOL (OPTIONS)

- Osteoarthrosis and instability caused by RA of the upper cervical spine are contraindications to rotary high velocity thrust techniques.[24] Manipulation is an absolute contraindication in the acute phase.
- *Forceful manipulation is contraindicated;* use gentle manipulation only.[25] Rule out *cervical instability* resulting from inflammation of transverse ligament.
- Appropriate chiropractic and physiotherapeutic treatment to maintain full joint movement and strengthen weak muscles.
- Treat with rest and relieve joint symptoms using wax baths, ice packs, ultrasound, and weak electrical current stimulation (interferential therapy).
- Lightweight splints may be used, especially at night.

NUTRITIONAL MANAGEMENT PROTOCOL (OPTIONS)

Acute:
- Copper salicylate: 60-120 mg/day with meals for 10 days during acute periods. NOTE: Local application of elemental copper, such as wearing a copper bracelet, may have some therapeutic value.
- Proteolytic enzymes (trypsin, chymotrypsin, bromelin) (3-4 tablets qid in between meals). NOTE: Do not give to patients with ulcers!
- Bioflavonoids (quercetin, hesperidin, rutin, etc.) (200 mg mixed bioflavonoids q2h during acute phase).
- Herbals, such as boswellia, ginger, turmeric, cayenne (400 mg, 300 mg, 200 mg, 50 mg, respectively, q2h acute phase).

The above proteolytic enzymes can be obtained in Biozyme

(Metagenics, Inc.) or Lyso-lymph Forte (Nutri-West, Inc.). Inflavonoid Intensive Care (Metagenics, Inc.) will provide the above bioflavonoids and herbals. Other manufacturers can provide quality proteolytic enzymes. Consult your product catalog.
Chronic:

- Pantothenic acid (calcium pantothenate) (2 g daily)
- Vitamin C (1 g 3 to 5 times daily)
- Vitamin E (400 IU daily)
- Zinc (50 mg three 3 daily)
- Omega-3 fatty acids (EPA-DHA) (1-2 g 3 times daily)

NOTE: Many patients with RA show signs of microcytic anemia (i.e., low RBC, mean corpuscular volume [MCV], hemoglobin [Hgb]). However, iron supplementation should be used with caution. Iron supplementation should only be considered when serum ferritin levels fall below 60 μg/L. Iron deficiency may not be the cause of the anemia and supplementation with iron may result in hydroxyl radicals, which can be highly irritating to the synovial joint linings. Consider trying to correct the anemia with folic acid, vitamin B_{12}, and copper supplementation and adequate dietary iron alone.

Clinical Notes

Screen for increased *intestinal permeability ("leaky gut syndrome")* and *hepatic toxicity.* Increased toxic load and large food proteins entering the bloodstream through a hyperpermeable gut, or an inability of the liver to adequately detoxify, can be the possible trigger of the hyperimmune response that leads to RA. Functional tests for these disorders are available through Great Smokies Diagnostic Labs, including intestinal permeability and functional liver detoxification panels. We prefer the use of Ultra Clear Sustain and Ultra Clear products (Health Comm, Inc.) for treating increased intestinal permeability and hepatic dysfunction, respectively. Refraining from using NSAIDS is essential to avoid increased intestinal permeability. A complete discussion of these techniques is beyond the scope of this book; however, research into the work of Jeffrey Bland, PhD, will provide detailed techniques in handling these difficult problems.

A diet based on low-fat fresh (whole) food is recommended. Foods of convenience, such as prepackaged, pre-prepared "high-tech" foods, should be eliminated. Hydrogenated and partially hydrogenated oils and spreads should be avoided. (Yes, use butter instead of margarine!) Coffee, tea, alcohol, fried foods, and simple carbohydrates should be limited and eliminated, if possible. Avoidance of highly allergenic proteins, such as corn, wheat, and milk, can be beneficial in inflammatory conditions. The nightshade vegetables (i.e., green peppers, eggplant, tomatoes, white potatoes) should be avoided because they contain a toxin called solanine that irritates the joints, particularly in RA patients. The goal for RA patients is to reduce their toxic and allergenic load from all sources, including food, water, air, and household products. It has been wisely said that the less doctored the food you eat is, the less doctoring you will need.

Food allergies must be screened for in RA patients with laboratory testing such as enzyme-linked immunosorbent assay (ELISA) test. An even more comprehensive test that is sensitive to delayed food allergies is the Sage test (Sage Systems), which monitors white blood cell morphology changes after exposure to the challenge food proteins. (See Appendix B.)

REFERENCES

1. Balch JF, Balch PA: *Prescription for natural healing,* Wayne, NJ, 1990, Avery Publishing.
2. Barton-Wright EC, Elliott WA: The pantothenic acid metabolism of rheumatoid arthritis, *Lancet* 2:862-863, 1963.
3. Belch JJ, et al: Effects of altering dietary essential fatty acids on requirements for non-steroidal anti-inflammatory drugs in patients with rheumatoid arthritis: a double blind placebo controlled study, *Ann Rheum Dis* 47(2):96-104, 1986.
4. Bolton P, Bolton S: Is there a role for the chiropractor in the treatment and management of rheumatism? A clinical perspective, *J Austral Chiropr Assoc* 16(1), 1986.
5. Bougie J: Rheumatoid arthritis: early diagnosis and management, *Chiropr Techn* 5(4):140-145, 1993.
6. Brukner P: *Clinical sports medicine,* New York, 1993, McGraw-Hill.
7. Bucci LR: *Nutrition applied to injury rehabilitation and sports medicine,* Boca Raton, Fla, 1995, CRC Press.
8. Calcium pantothenate in arthritic conditions: a report from General Practitioner Research Group, *Practitioner* 224:208-211, 1980.
9. Cichoke AJ, Marty L: The use of proteolytic enzymes with soft-tissue athletic injuries, *Am Chiropr,* October 1981, p 32.

10. Clelend LG, et al: Clinical and biochemical effects of dietary fish oil supplements in rheumatoid arthritis, *J Rheumatol* 15(10):1471-1475, 1988.

11. Clemen M: Delivering effective force adjustments on patients with degenerative spinal conditions, *Int Rev Chiropr* 44:27-35, 1988.

12. Davidson A, et al: Red cell ferritin content: a re-evaluation of indices for iron deficiency anemia in the anemia of rheumatoid arthritis, *Br Med J* 289:648-650, 1984.

13. Fauci A, et al: *Harrison's principles of internal medicine,* ed 13, New York, 1994, McGraw-Hill.

14. Forbes CD, Jackson WF: *Color atlas and text of clinical medicine,* St Louis, 1993, Mosby.

15. Gatterman M: *Chiropractic management of spine related disorders,* Baltimore, 1990, Williams & Wilkins.

16. Grabowski RJ: *Current nutritional therapy,* San Antonio, Tex, 1993, Image Press.

17. Greidinger E, Hellmann DB: Arthritis: what to emphasize on the rheumatologic exam, *Consultant,* November 1995.

18. Grennan DM, et al: Serum copper and zinc in rheumatoid arthritis and osteoarthritis, *NZ Med J* 652:47-50, 1980.

19. Haldeman S: *Principles and practice of chiropractic,* ed 2, Norwalk, Conn, 1992, Appleton & Lange.

20. Hammer W: *Functional soft tissue examination and treatment by manual methods,* Gaithersburg, Md, 1991, Aspen Publishers.

21. Havsteen B: Flavonoids, a class of natural products of high pharmacological potency, *Biochem Pharmacol* 33(24):3933-3939, 1984.

22. Honkanen V, et al: Plasma zinc and copper concentrations in rheumatoid arthritis: influence of dietary factors and disease activity, *Am J Clin Nutr* 54:1082-1086, 1991.

23. Honkanen V, et al: Vitamins A and E, retinol binding protein and zinc in rheumatoid arthritis, *Clin Exp Rheumatol* 7:465-469, 1989.

24. Jamison J: The management of rheumatoid arthritis: considerations for chiropractic practice, *Chiropr J Austral* 24(3):83-90, 1994.

25. Janison J: Dietary intervention in rheumatoid arthritis, *J Can Chiropr Assoc* 31(3):141-146, 1987.

26. Kremer JM, et al: Dietary fish oil and olive oil supplementation in patients with rheumatoid arthritis, clinical and immunologic effects, *Arthritis Rheum* 33(6):810-820, 1990.

27. Liebenson C: *Rehabilitation of the spine,* Baltimore, 1996, Williams & Wilkins.

28. Litman K: A rational approach to the diagnosis of arthritis, *Am Fam Physician* 53(4):1295-1300, 1996.

29. *Manual of medical therapeutics (the Washington manual),* ed 27, Boston, 1992, Little, Brown.

30. *The Merck manual,* ed 16, Rahway, NJ, 1992, Merck Co.

31. Nelson W: Rheumatoid arthritis: a case report, *Chiropr Techn* 2(1):17-19, 1990.

32. Ng S: Rheumatoid arthritis—can diet be implicated? *J Austral Chiropr Assoc* 11(5):15-23, 1997.

33. Mullen A, Wilson CWM: The metabolism of ascorbic acid in rheumatoid arthritis, *Proc Nutr Sci* 35:8A-9A, 1976.

34. Niedermeier W, Griggs JH: Trace metal composition of synovial fluid and blood serum of patients with rheumatoid arthritis, *J Chronic Dis* 23:527-536, 1971.

35. Panush RS: Possible role of food sensitivity in arthritis, abstract of presentation at the VI International Food Allergy Symposium, Nov 13-14, 1987, *Immunol Allergy Pract* 10(3):124-125, 1988.

36. Panush RS, et al: Food-induced (allergic) arthritis, *Arthritis Rheum* 29(2):220-226, 1986.

37. Rakel RE: *Conn's current therapy,* Philadelphia, 1996, WB Saunders.

38. Rakel RE: *Textbook of family practice,* ed 5, Philadelphia, 1995, WB Saunders.

39. Resnick D: *Diagnosis of bone and joint disorders,* ed 2, Philadelphia, 1988, WB Saunders.

40. Rothwell RS, Davis P: Relationship between serum ferritin, anemia, and disease activity in acute and chronic rheumatoid arthritis, *Rheumatol Int* 1(2):65-67, 1981.

41. Scully RM, Barnes MR: *Physical therapy,* Philadelphia, 1989, JB Lippincott.

42. Seignalet J: Diet, fasting, and rheumatoid arthritis, *Lancet* 339:6809, 1992 (letter).

43. Svenson KL, et al: Reduced zinc in peripheral blood cells from patients with inflammatory connective tissue diseases, *Inflammation* 9(2):189-199, 1985.

44. Taraye JP, Lauressergues H: Advantages of combination of proteolytic enzymes, flavonoids and ascorbic acid in comparison with non-steroid inflammatory drugs, *Arzneimittelforschung* 27(1):1144-1149, 1977.

45. Tierney LM, McPhee SJ, Papadakis MA: *Current medical diagnosis and treatment,* ed 35, Norwalk, Conn, 1996, Appleton & Lange.

46. Watts DL: The nutritional relationships of copper, *J Orthomol Med* 4(2):99-108, 1989.

47. Werbach MR: *Nutritional influences on illness,* ed 2, Tarzana, Calif, 1996, Third Line Press.

48. Werbach MR, Murray MT: *Botanical influences on illness,* Tarzana, Calif, 1994, Third Line Press.

49. White AA, Panjabi MM: *Clinical biomechanics of the spine,* Philadelphia, 1990, JB Lippincott.

50. Yochum TR, Rowe LJ: *Essentials of skeletal radiology,* ed 2, Baltimore, 1995, Williams & Wilkins.

Degenerative Joint Disease (Osteoarthritis)

BRIAN BATENCHUK, LEW HUFF, AND DAVID M. BRADY

DEFINITION

A progressive, noninflammatory disease characterized by decreasing chondroitin sulfate with age that creates unsupported collagen fibrils followed by degeneration of the cartilage and its related structures. Osteoarthritis is the most common form of joint disease.

ETIOLOGY

Although the etiology remains unknown, it may be due to abnormal biomechanical stresses or genetic, endocrine, or metabolic causes.

Primary DJD

Unknown etiology, affecting people in their fifth to sixth decade, females 10:1, weight-bearing joints.

Secondary DJD

Known etiology (i.e., trauma), affecting people in their second to sixth decade, equal gender predilection, any joint affected.

Erosive Osteoarthritis

Inflammatory etiology, affecting people in their fourth to fifth decade, females 3:1, interphalangeal joints.

SIGNS AND SYMPTOMS

Location

Most common sites of involvement are the weight-bearing joints of the spine, hips, knees, AC joint, first metatarsophalangeal, first metacarpal-trapezium, and DIP joints of the hand. Any joint can be involved.

Pain Pattern

Joint pain and stiffness of involved segment. Stiffness and pain may follow inactivity. Most commonly the pain is a deep aching pain. DJD is characterized by brief morning stiffness and pain, which is relieved by rest.

Onset

Gradual onset, localized to a few joints at first.

Inspection

1. *Herberden's nodes:* Enlarged terminal interphalangeal joints are pathognomonic of the disease.
2. *Bouchard's nodes:* Swelling of the proximal interphalangeal (PIP) joints. Bony crepitus is the most common physical finding. Localized edema and erythema when acute.

Systemic Manifestations

Are absent.

LABORATORY TESTS/RESULTS

1. Laboratory studies are usually normal.
2. ESR and C-reactive protein may be slightly elevated.

IMAGING FINDINGS

1. Common radiographical signs include joint space narrowing, sclerosis/eburnation of subchondral bone in areas of stress, subchondral cyst formation (geodes), and osteophytes at articular margins or nonstressed areas.
2. Hand and foot signs include radial subluxation of the first

metacarpal base, Bouchard's nodes (osteophytes at PIP joint), and Herberden's nodes (osteophytes at DIP joint). Male-to-female ratio is 1:10.

3. Hip signs include superior migration of the femoral head (less frequently medial/axial); femoral and acetabular osteophytes, sclerosis, and cyst formation; and thickening/buttressing of the medial femoral cortex.

4. Knee signs include medial femorotibial compartment (usually first to be involved) and varus deformity.

5. Spinal signs include sclerosis and narrowing of the intervertebral zygapophyseal joints, and osteophytes usually associated with discogenic disease.

6. Erosive osteoarthritis is an inflammatory form of osteoarthritis. Postmenopausal females are predisposed to it. Common sites involved DIP and PIP joints of the hands; it is bilateral and symmetrical. Radiographical findings include "bird wing" ("sea-gull") joint configuration of central erosions; it may lead to bony ankylosis.

DIFFERENTIAL DIAGNOSIS

Differentially diagnose erosive osteoarthritis from rheumatoid arthritis, Wilson's disease, chronic liver disease, and hemochromatosis. (See Fig. 3.)

TREATMENT GOALS

1. Relieve pain.
2. Prevent progressive joint damage.
3. Maintain function and activities of daily living.
4. Nutritionally support cartilage.

MANAGEMENT PROTOCOL (OPTIONS)

- Chiropractic and physiotherapeutic treatment to maintain joint movement and strengthen weakened muscles.[12,15]
- Complications may include the following:
  1. **Spinal stenosis and lateral nerve entrapment syndromes**
  2. **Vertebral artery stenosis from compressive osteophytes, resulting in positional vertebrobasilar ischemia**

3. **Complete or incomplete osseous fusion across the joint and variable degrees in loss of function**

- Severe osteoarthrosis and spondylosis are indications for manual therapy. Mobilization without impulse, neuromuscular therapy, and muscular rehabilitation are beneficial.[15] *Rotary manipulation is contraindicated.*
- Pain-relieving modalities, such as ice packs, ultrasound, and weak electrical current stimulation (interferential therapy), are beneficial.[12]
- Instruct in the use of cane or assistive device and proper body mechanics.[13]
- Locally applied topical medications, such as methylsalicylate or capsaicin, may afford pain relief (decreases local levels of substance P).[13]
- Exercises:
  1. Quad-strengthening exercises are helpful with osteoarthritis of the knee.
  2. Isokinetic exercises moving the joint against resistance are beneficial.
  3. Aerobic exercises, such as walking or aquatic exercises, are beneficial and can decrease the number of clinically active joints, increase functional capacity, and reduce anxiety and depression.[12,13]
  4. Aquatic exercises decrease the joint-loading forces of the hip and knee.
  5. Gentle stretching and posture exercises can relieve symptoms and improve function.[12,13]
  6. Gentle ROM exercises increase ranges of pain-free motion.

NUTRITIONAL MANAGEMENT PROTOCOL (OPTIONS)

- Glucosamine sulfate (1500 mg per day in divided dosages). Supplies the needed nutrients for the production of healthy ground substance.
- Vitamin C (3000-6000 mg per day in divided dosages).
- Iron (glycinate) (8-12 mg per day in divided dosages).
- Alpha-ketoglutaric acid (15 mg per day in divided dosages).

The above three nutrients are required for the hydroxylation of L-proline to L-hydroxyproline, which is needed for the production of quality collagen.

- Calcium (400 mg tid)

- Vitamin E (200 IU per day)
- Zinc (glycinate) (12-18 mg per day divided dosages)
- Copper (glycinate) (600-900 µg per day in divided dosages)
- Manganese (glycinate) (4-6 mg per day in divided dosages)

The above provide antioxidant effects and serve as free radical scavengers to help remove cellular debris and promote healing. The zinc, copper, and manganese act as cofactors and catalysts for the potent antioxidant enzyme SOD and are therefore referred to as the *SOD induction complex.* Oral supplementation with SOD can be attempted; however, it has been reported that it is often destroyed in the stomach and intestinal tract before assimilation. SOD can be obtained in Cell Guard (Biotec Foods).

All of the above tissue-healing nutrients can be obtained in the formulary product Collagenics Intensive Care (Metagenics, Inc.). Other manufacturers make similar formulary products designed to aid in degenerative joint disease and usually contain glucosamine and/or chondroitin sulfate. Consult the catalog of the reputable vendors you use for alternate products.

HOME CARE PROTOCOL (OPTIONS)

1. Take warm soaks in tub at home.
2. Use cane, crutch, or walker if needed.
3. Modify home for easy access to tub, bathroom, and kitchen needs.
4. Use moist hot pack applications as instructed.
5. Establish a weight-loss program compatible with the patient's lifestyle.

REFERENCES

1. Balch JF, Balch PA: *Prescription for natural healing,* Wayne, NJ, 1990, Avery Publishing.
2. Bland JH, Cooper SM: Osteoarthritis: a review of the cell biology involved and evidence for reversibility, management rationally related to known genesis and pathophysiology, *Semin Arthritis Rheum* 14(2):106, 1984.
3. Bolton P, Bolton S: Is there a role for the chiropractor in the treatment and management of rheumatism? A clinical perspective, *J Austral Chiropr Assoc* 16(1), 1986.
4. Bucci LR: *Nutrition applied to injury rehabilitation and sports medicine,* Boca Raton, Fla, 1995, CRC Press.

5. Calcium pantothenate in arthritic conditions: a report from General Practitioner Research Group, *Practitioner* 224:208-211, 1980.

6. Clemen M: Delivering effective force adjustments on patients with degenerative spinal conditions, *Int Rev Chiropr* 44:27-35, 1988.

7. Dahnert W: *Radiology review manual,* Baltimore, 1991, Williams & Wilkins.

8. D'Ambrosio E, et al: Glucosamine sulfate: a controlled clinical investigation in arthrosis, *Pharmatherapeutica* 2(8):504-508, 1981.

9. Davis CD, Greger JL: Longitudinal changes of manganese-dependent superoxide dismutase and other indexes of manganese and iron status in women, *Am J Clin Nutr* 55:747, 1992.

10. Drovanti A, et al: Oral glucosamine sulfate in osteoarthritis: a placebo controlled double-blind investigation, *Clin Ther* 3(4):260-272, 1980.

11. Fauci A, et al: *Harrison's principles of internal medicine,* ed 13, New York, 1994, McGraw-Hill.

12. Gatterman M: *Chiropractic management of spine related disorders,* Baltimore, 1990, Williams & Wilkins.

13. Gowin KM, Schumacher HR: Osteoarthritis: practical steps to successful therapy, *Consultant,* September 1996.

14. Grabowski RJ: *Current nutritional therapy,* San Antonio, Tex, 1993, Image Press.

15. Haldeman S: *Principles and practice of chiropractic,* ed 2, Norwalk, Conn, 1992, Appleton & Lange.

16. Hammer W: *Functional soft tissue examination and treatment by manual methods,* Gaithersburg, Md, 1991, Aspen Publishers.

17. *Manual of medical therapeutics (the Washington manual),* ed 27, Boston, 1992, Little, Brown.

18. *The Merck manual,* ed 16, Rahway, NJ, 1992, Merck Co.

19. Niki E: Interaction of ascorbate and alpha-tocopherol, *Third Conference on Vitamin C* 498:187-189, 1987.

20. Rakel RE: *Conn's current therapy,* Philadelphia, 1996, WB Saunders.

21. Rakel RE: *Textbook of family practice,* ed 5, Philadelphia, 1995, WB Saunders.

22. Schwartz RI, et al: Ascorbate can act as an inducer of collagen pathway because most steps are tightly coupled, *Third Conference on Vitamin C* 498:172-184, 1987.

23. Taylor RB: *Manual of family practice,* Boston, 1996, Little, Brown.

24. Tierney LM, McPhee SJ, Papadakis MA: *Current medical diagnosis and treatment,* ed 35, Norwalk, Conn, 1996, Appleton & Lange.

25. Werbach MR: *Nutritional influences on illness,* ed 2, Tarzana, Calif, 1996, Third Line Press.

26. Werbach MR, Murray MT: *Botanical influences on illness,* Tarzana, Calif, 1994, Third Line Press.

27. White AA, Panjabi MM: *Clinical biomechanics of the spine,* Philadelphia, 1990, JB Lippincott.
28. Yochum TR, Rowe LJ: *Essentials of skeletal radiology,* ed 2, Baltimore, 1995, Williams & Wilkins.

Diabetes Mellitus

LEW HUFF, DAVID M. BRADY,
AND LIZA O. BANAAG-HUFF

DEFINITION

An inherited gene defect resulting in an abnormal insulin secretion and elevated blood glucose levels. There are two types: Type I, or insulin-dependent diabetes mellitus (IDDM), is the inherited juvenile type, which peaks at age 12. The juvenile type is insulin dependent and occurs 20 times more often in whites. Type II, or non-insulin-dependent diabetes mellitus (NIDDM), represents 80% of all diabetes. It is not insulin dependent and is also termed *adult-onset diabetes,* or *late-onset diabetes;* it increases in incidence after 40 years of age.

ETIOLOGY

May be due to direct damage of the islet cells, autoimmune destruction of the beta cells, viral infection, insulin insensitivity, or food allergy.

SIGNS AND SYMPTOMS

Classic Symptoms

Polyuria, polydipsia, polyphagia

Eye Signs

Recurrent blurred vision, diabetic retinopathy

Skin Signs

Boils, carbuncles, monilial vaginitis, pruritus

Other Signs

Weight loss despite a normal appetite, acetone breath, amenorrhea, asthenia

Neurological Signs

Decreased Achilles reflex, "stocking and glove" paresthesia, and foot paresthesia are late signs.

Diagnostic Criteria

Single glucose level in excess of 11 mmol/L (200 mg/dl) in the presence of classic symptoms, or three fasting glucose levels of greater than 140mg/dl (see Fig. 4).

DIFFERENTIAL DIAGNOSIS

Nephrogenic cause
Vascular disease
Neoplasms
Alcoholism

LABORATORY RESULTS

Glucosuria, ketonuria, proteinuria
Fasting glucose >140 mg/dl
Low immunoreactive insulin levels
Elevated glycosylated hemoglobin concentration
(300 to 1200 mg/100 ml)
Hyperlipidemia and hypercholesterolemia are common

TREATMENT GOALS

1. Reach a fasting glucose level within the reference range.[24]
2. Reach a 2-hour postprandial level of less than 150 mg/dl.[24]
3. Attempt to reach both of these goals without inducing wide glucose swings or hypoglycemia.[24]

These goals are usually more approachable for the NIDDM patient than for the IDDM patient.[24]

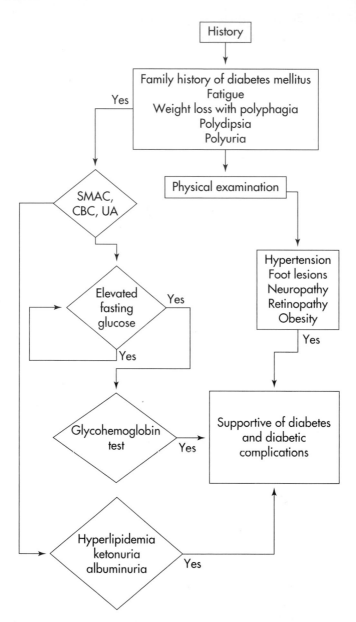

FIG. 4. Examination and diagnosis flow diagram for diabetes mellitus.

MANAGEMENT PROTOCOL (OPTIONS)

- Recommend weight-loss program for obese patients. Recommend diet modifications and modification of activity levels for all diabetic patients. Exercise, weight loss, and diet modification help decrease the amount of insulin needed.[24]
- Lifestyle modification:
  1. Avoid obesity and strive to achieve ideal body weight in Type II diabetes mellitus.
  2. Do moderate exercises regularly.
  3. Monitor blood glucose levels several times daily with home monitoring system. Alter diet to stay within normal glucose parameters.
- Dietary modifications:
  1. Eat small frequent meals instead of three large meals per day.
  2. Diet consisting of complex carbohydrates, protein (15% to 20% of calories), and fiber (30-40 g/day) is recommended.
  3. Eliminate or avoid simple sugars and refined carbohydrates, fried foods, alcohol, and tobacco.
  4. Avoid dairy products (Type I only).
  5. Some patients benefit more from a diet that is rich in fresh vegetables and fruits as the primary carbohydrate source, as opposed to pasta, potatoes, and grains. This diet is lower in complex carbohydrates and higher in lean protein and monounsaturated fats than the typical American Dietetic Association (ADA) diabetic diet. These concepts are fully explored in the book *The Zone,* by Barry Sears,[36] and tend to benefit patients with Type II diabetes and those with insulin insensitivity (syndrome X).
  6. Various studies are now linking modified food allergies, particularly cow's milk, as the trigger of the autoimmune response that may lead to IDDM in genetically susceptible children.[20,22]

NUTRITIONAL MANAGEMENT PROTOCOL (OPTIONS)

- Chromium picolinate (100 µg tid)
- Magnesium (200 mg tid)
- Vitamin C (1000 mg tid)

- Vanadyl sulfate (50 mg tid)
- Vitamin B_6 (pyridoxine) (50 mg tid)
- Vitamin B_{12} (cyanocobalamin) (100 µg tid)
- Vitamin B complex (50 mg tid)
- *Myo*-inositol (1.5 g tid)
- Omega-6 fatty acids (EPO) (750 mg tid)
- L-carnitine (100 mg tid)

Many of the above nutrients can be obtained in the formulary product Diabetic Nutrition (Progressive Research Labs, Houston) (see Appendix A).

Treat hypercholesterolemia and hypertriglyceridemia, when present, with the following nutrients (do not give omega-3 fatty acids to a patient with diabetes!).

Hypercholesterolemia:

- Niacin (500 mg daily in divided dosages: timed release on full stomach)
- Magnesium (aspartate) (1-3 g per day)
- Chromium with GTF (500-1000 µg per day)
- Bromelin (1-2 g per day)
- Vitamin E and selenium (400-800 IU and 50-400 µg daily, respectively, as antioxidants)
- Meta-Sitosterol (Metagenics, Inc.) (2 tablets tid provides 250 mg of mixed phytosterols, which bind dietary cholesterol in the gut.)
- Garlic capsules (2 capsules tid)
- Monitor chemistry, complete blood cell count (CBC), and UA every 8 weeks for complications of diabetes mellitus, including high glucose, elevated liver enzymes, hypercholesterolemia, hypertriglyceridemia, and sugar and ketones in urine, until well stabilized. Glycosylated hemoglobin (HbA1C) is the preferred test to monitor blood glucose.

HOME CARE PROTOCOL (OPTIONS)

- Adherence to diabetic diet, or "Zone" diet, is essential.
- Do home glucose monitoring.
- Perform moderate exercise daily.
- Get regular check-ups.

REFERENCES

1. Balch JF, Balch PA: *Prescription for natural healing,* Wayne, NJ, 1990, Avery Publishing.

2. Bedi T, et al: A study of serum B_{12} in various peripheral neuropathies, *J Assoc Physicians India* 21(6):473-479, 1969.

3. Bjorntorp P: Metabolic implications of body fat distribution, *Diabetes Care* 14:1132, 1991.

4. Cleary JP: Vitamin B_3 in the treatment of diabetes mellitus: case reports and review of the literature, *J Nutr Med* 1:217-225, 1975.

5. Clements RS Jr, et al: Dietary *myo*-inositol intake and peripheral nerve function in diabetic neuropathy, *Metabolism* 28:477, 1979.

6. *The clinical use of the trace element chromium (III) in the treatment of diabetes mellitus,* Harefuah, 1994 (in press).

7. Cunningham JJ: Altered vitamin C transport in diabetes mellitus, *Med Hypotheses* 26:263-265, 1983.

8. Davidson S: The use of vitamin B_{12} in the treatment of diabetic neuropathy, *J Fla Med Assoc* 15:717-720, 1954.

9. DCCT Research Group: The effects of intensive treatment of diabetes on the development and progression of long-term complications in insulin-dependent diabetes mellitus, *N Engl J Med* 329:977, 1993.

10. Elamin A, Tuvemo T: Magnesium and insulin-dependent diabetes mellitus, *Diabetes Res Clin Pract* 10:203-209, 1990.

11. Evans GW: Diabetes and aging: the chromium connection, *Today's Chiropractic* 23(2):40-42, 1994.

12. Fauci A, et al: *Harrison's principles of internal medicine,* ed 13, New York, 1994, McGraw-Hill.

13. Franz MJ, et al: Nutritional principles for the management of diabetes and related complications, *Diabetes Care* 17: 490, 1994.

14. Friday KE, et al: Omega-3 fatty acid supplementation has discordant effects on plasma glucose and lipoproteins in Type II diabetes, *Diabetes* 36(suppl 1):12A, 1987.

15. Ginter EM, Chorvathova V: Vitamin C and diabetes mellitus, *Nutr Health* 2:3-11, 1983.

16. Glauber H, et al: Adverse metabolic effect of omega-3 fatty acids in non-insulin dependent diabetes mellitus, *Ann Intern Med* 108(5):663-668, 1988.

17. Grabowski RJ: *Current nutritional therapy: a clinical reference,* San Antonio, Tex, 1993, Image Press.

18. Guyton AC, Hall JE: *Textbook of medical physiology,* ed 9, Philadelphia, 1996, WB Saunders.

19. Hotta N, et al: Effect of propionyl-L-carnitine on oscillatory potentials in electroretinogram in streptozotocin-diabetic Rats, *Eur J Pharmacol* 31(92-93):199-206, 1996.

20. Husby S, et al: Humoral immunity to dietary antigens in healthy adults: occurrence, isotype and IgG subclass distribution of serum antibodies to protein antigens, *Int Arch Allergy Appl Immunol* 77:416-422, 1985.

21. Jamal GA, et al: Treatment of diabetic neuropathy with gamma-linolenic acid (GLA) as evening primrose oil (Efamol), *J Am Coll Nutr* 6:86, 1987.

22. Karjalainen J, et al: A bovine albumin peptide as a possible trigger of insulin-dependent diabetes mellitus, *N Engl J Med* 327(5):302-307, 1992.

23. Khan MA, et al: Vitamin B_{12} deficiency and diabetic neuropathy, *Lancet* 2:768, 1969.

24. Lawrence D: *Fundamentals of chiropractic diagnosis and management,* Baltimore, 1991, Williams & Wilkins.

25. Levin ER, et al: The influence of pyridoxine in diabetic peripheral neuropathy, *Diabetes Care* 4:606, 1981.

26. *Manual of medical therapeutics (the Washington manual),* ed 27, Boston, 1992, Little, Brown.

27. Martin HE: Clinical magnesium deficiency, *Ann NY Acad Sci* 156:891-900, 1969.

28. McCann VJ, Davis RE: Serum pyridoxal concentrations in patients with diabetic neuropathy, *Aust NZ J Med* 8:259-261, 1978.

29. *The Merck Manual,* ed 16, Rahway NJ, 1992, Merck Co.

30. Mertz W: Effects and metabolism of glucose tolerance factor, *Nutr Rev* 33(5):129-135, 1975.

31. Nathan DM: Long-term complications of diabetes mellitus, *N Engl J Med* 328:1676, 1993.

32. Rakel RE: *Conn's current therapy,* Philadelphia, 1996, WB Saunders.

33. Rakel RE: *Textbook of family practice,* ed 5, Philadelphia, 1995, WB Saunders.

34. Reaven GM: Dietary therapy for non-insulin-dependent diabetes mellitus, *N Engl J Med* 319(13):862-864, 1988 (editorial).

35. Sakuria H, et al: Orally active and long-term acting insulin-mimetic Vanadyl complex, *Biochem Biophys Res Commun* 214(3):95-101, 1995.

36. Sears B, Lawren B: *The Zone,* New York, 1995, HarperCollins.

37. Steiner G: Editorial: from an excess of fat, diabetics die, *JAMA* 262(3):398-399, 1989.

38. Tierney LM, McPhee SJ, Papadakis MA: *Current medical diagnosis and treatment,* ed 35, Norwalk, Conn, 1996, Appleton & Lange.

39. Vandongen R, et al: Hypercholesterolaemic effect of fish oil in insulin-dependent diabetics, *Thromb Res* 43:643-655, 1986.

40. Venkatesan N, et al: Antidiabetic action of Vanadyl in rats independent of in vivo insulin-receptor kinase activity, *Diabetes* 40(4):492-498, 1991.

41. Vinik AI, et al: Diabetic neuropathies, *Diabetes Care* 15:1926, 1994.

42. Werbach MR: *Nutritional influences on illness,* ed 2, Tarzana, Calif, 1996, Third Line Press.

43. Werbach MR, Murray MT: *Botanical influences on illness,* Tarzana, Calif, 1994, Third Line Press.

44. Yale JF, et al: Hypoglycemic effects of peroxovanadium compounds in Sprague-Dawley and diabetic BB rats, *Diabetes* 44(11):1274-1279, 1995.

45. Zebrowski EJ, Bhatnagar PK: Urinary excretion pattern of ascorbic acid in streptozotocin diabetic and insulin treated rats, *Pharm Res Commun* 11(2):95-103, 1979.

Fibromyalgia

DAVID M. BRADY AND LEW HUFF

DEFINITION

A chronic disease characterized by widespread, chronic muscular pain, fatigue, and sleep disturbance. Also known as *fibrositis, fibromyositis, nonarticular rheumatism,* and *muscular rheumatism.* An estimated 3 to 6 million Americans are affected, with an increased incidence with women in the 35- to 60-year-old age-group. Female-to-male ratio is at least 5:1. Fibromyalgia is the second most common reason for a rheumatology referral.

ETIOLOGY

May be due to autoimmune response, decreased levels of serotonin, hypothyroidism, sleep disturbances, mitochondrial dysfunction, metabolic toxicity, or lack of physical fitness. Incidence often associated with industrial injuries, auto accidents, overuse, or repetitive stresses.

SIGNS AND SYMPTOMS

Palpation

Tender points over the vertebral border of the scapula, ischial tuberosity, L5, medial knee, medial epicondyle of elbow, trapezius bilaterally, base of skull, supraspinatus, second costosternal joint, gluteals, and greater trochanter. Tender points in muscle noted in upper and lower parts of body. Axial skeletal pain must be present in 11 of 18 anatomical points.

Timing

Pain waxes and wanes and is migratory.[9] Pain increases with weather changes and stress. Tender points persist during sleep.

Location

The body is divided into four quadrants: left, right, above the waist, and below the waist. The tender points are charted as to their locations in the quadrants. Tender points should be present in all four quadrants to support a diagnosis of fibromyalgia.

Comparison With Chronic Fatigue Syndrome

Chronic fatigue syndrome (CFS) has similar features: women in the 20- to 50-year-old age-group, absence of many objective findings, and absence of laboratory findings. Muscle pain predominates in fibromyalgia, whereas fatigue predominates in CFS.

Measurement

Sensitivity of tender points can be measured using a dolorimeter.

Other Manifestations

History of widespread pain above and below the waist, left and right sides, and midline. Widespread achiness, stiffness, fatigue, sleep disturbance, tension and migraine headaches, and restless leg syndrome.[7,37] Minimal exertion aggravates pain and increases fatigue. Objective signs of inflammation are absent.[35]

Systemic Manifestations

Fatigue, poor concentration, dizziness, poor memory, flushing, and paresthesias are reported. Headaches, premenstrual syndrome, pelvic pain, and irritable bowel syndrome are reported.[7,9]

Clinical Note

A number of controlled studies have shown that FMS is associated with irritable bowel syndrome, tension and migraine headaches, primary dysmenorrhea, chronic fatigue syndrome,

TMJ, myofascial pain syndromes, restless leg syndrome, and periodic limb movement disorders.[2]

DIFFERENTIAL DIAGNOSIS

Rheumatoid arthritis
Systemic lupus erythematosus
Chronic fatigue syndrome
Myofascial pain syndrome
Marked depression
Malingering

LABORATORY FINDINGS

Generally absent
Possible thyroid dysfunction
Low tryptophan levels[7]
Decreased serotonin[7]
Low IGF-1/somatomedin-C[7]
High substance P[7]

X-RAY FINDINGS

Absent

TREATMENT GOALS

1. Promote soft tissue healing.
2. Relieve pain and prevent recurrence.
3. Increase pain-free ranges of motion.
4. Restore preillness activities of daily living.

MANAGEMENT PROTOCOL (OPTIONS)

- *Manipulation:* Manipulate to correct any faulty spinal biomechanics. This may be marginally beneficial.
- *Physiotherapy:* May be of limited, palliative benefit. Hot moist packs may be of minor benefit. Physiotherapy does not provide any lasting improvements in the condition.
- *Rehabilitation:* Aerobic exercise is very important for patients with fibromyalgia; however, it is difficult because of the

fatigue and soreness. Mild activities, such as walking, should be started slowly and increased as tolerated. No anaerobic exercise should be performed, such as explosive high-demand activities of muscle groups (e.g., weightlifting, sprinting). Stretching exercises may be beneficial.[7] Exercise in short sessions, slowly increasing intensity and duration. Swimming and water-based therapy may be beneficial.[7]

- *Diet:* Eliminate coffee and alcohol.[7] Avoid or decrease consumption of refined sugars, sucrose, chocolate, and nicotine.[7]

NUTRITIONAL MANAGEMENT PROTOCOL (OPTIONS)

- Magnesium (glycinate) (600 to 1000 mg per day in divided dosages) Critical in the adenosine triphosphate (ATP) synthesis of mitochondrial respiration (cofactor in Krebs cycle). Competitive with aluminum (fibromyalgia patients show signs of aluminum toxicity).
- Malic acid (1200-2400 mg per day in divided dosages). Promotes aerobic metabolism as Krebs cycle intermediate. Causes excretion of aluminum from body (aluminum detoxifier).
- Manganese (20 mg per day in divided dosages). Promotes thyroid function as a cofactor in the hormonal cascades of the hypothalamic-pituitary-thyroid axis.
- Vitamins B_6 and B_1 (200 mg per day each in divided dosages). Promotes aerobic metabolism and ATP production as Krebs cycle cofactors. Supports neurological function and helps reduce stress.

All of the above nutrients may be obtained in the suggested ratios in Fibroplex (registered) (Metagenics, Inc.), a formulary product for fibromyalgia patients.

- *Codyceps sinensis* (Chinese caterpillar fungus) has also been used to promote ATP production because it is a rich source of adenosine. It can be obtained in the product Cordyphrine Pro (Metagenics, Inc.).

Clinical Notes

Any suggestion of hypothyroidism on laboratory analysis (i.e., low thyroid hormone fractions with an elevated TSH) should prompt supplementation with L-**tyrosine, thyroid glandular**

extract, and Atlantic Sea kelp (as a source of iodine). If nutritional support of the thyroid does not reduce the problem on follow-up laboratory assessment, the patient should be evaluated for hormone replacement therapy (HRT), preferably with natural thyroid hormone replacement, such as Armour Thyroid, which is made from desiccated pork thyroid.

Conditions that should be screened for in fibromyalgia patients include increased intestinal permeability (i.e., "leaky gut syndrome") and hepatic toxicity. Increased toxic load from a hyperpermeable gut, or an inability of the liver to adequately detoxify, can be the possible trigger of mitochondrial dysfunction, which possibly leads to fibromyalgia. Functional tests for these disorders are available through Great Smokies Diagnostic Labs. We prefer the use of Ultra Clear Sustain and Ultra Clear products (Health Comm, Inc.) for treating increased intestinal permeability and hepatic dysfunction, respectively. Refraining from using NSAID is essential to avoid increased intestinal permeability. A complete discussion of these techniques is beyond the scope of this book; however, research into the work of Jeffrey Bland will provide detailed techniques in handling these difficult problems.

A diet based on fresh (whole) foods is recommended. Foods of convenience, such as prepackaged, pre-prepared, "high-tech" foods, should be eliminated. Hydrogenated and partially hydrogenated oils and spreads should be avoided. (Yes, use butter instead of margarine!) The goal for fibromyalgia patients is to reduce their toxic load from all sources, including food, water, air, and household products. It has been wisely said that "The less doctored the food you eat, the less doctoring you will need."

Food allergies must be screened for in patients resistive or refractive to the above therapies with laboratory testing such as ELISA or radioallergosorbent test (RAST). An even more comprehensive test that is sensitive to delayed food allergies is the SAGE test, which monitors white blood cell morphology changes after exposure to the challenge food proteins (see Appendix B).

REMEMBER: Fibromyalgia is a metabolic disorder and not merely a musculoskeletal disorder. Standard physical medicine techniques are not generally curative and may in fact worsen the patient's symptoms. For example, do not treat the tender points (Tes) of FM like trigger points (TrPs) found in myofascial pain syndromes by applying ischemic compression. You will needlessly cause the patients pain and possibly make them worse. It must be managed from a biochemical perspective as described above.

HOME CARE PROTOCOL (OPTIONS)

- Aerobic exercises, fast walking, dancing, yoga, and meditation techniques may be beneficial.
- Go to bed at the same time each night and set room temperature at or below 70° F.

REFERENCES

1. Abraham GE, et al: Management of fibromyalgia: rationale for the use of magnesium and malic acid, *J Nutr Med* 3:49-50, 1992.
2. American College of Rheumatology, Wolfe F, et al: Criteria for classification of fibromyalgia, Multicenter Criteria Committee, *Arthritis Rheum* 33(2):160-172, 1990.
3. Bensky D, Gamble A: *Chinese herbal medicine: materia medica,* Seattle, 1986, Eastland Press.
4. Brostoff J, Scadding GK: *Complexes in food induced arthralgia.* Paper presented at the XII International Congress of Allergy and Clinical Immunology, October 1985, Washington, DC.
5. Brozell D: Fibromyalgia: clinical concepts, *CCA J* 21(8):40-41, 1996.
6. Cartette S, Lefrancois L: Fibrositis and primary hypothyroidism, *J Rheumatol* 15:1418-1421, 1988.
7. Chan Ho A: Fibromyalgia syndrome, *Resident Reporter* 1(1), 1996.
8. Chen QT, et al: *Paecilomyces sinensis* sp. nov. and its connection with *Cordyceps sinensis, Acta Mycologica Sinica* 3:24-28, 1988.
9. Clauw DJ: Fibromyalgia: more than just a musculoskeletal disease, *Am Fam Physician* 52(3):843-851, 1995.
10. Denmeen AM, et al: Joint complaints and food allergic disorders, *Ann Allergy* 51:260-263, 1983.
11. Domingo JL, et al: Citric, malic and succinic acids as possible alternatives to deferoxamine in aluminum toxicity, *Clin Toxicol* 26(1,2):67-79, 1988.
12. Eisinger J, Ayavou T: Transketolase stimulation in fibromyalgia, *J Am Coll Nutr* 9(1):56-57, 1990.

13. Eisinger J, et al: Donnees actuelles sur les fibromyalgies: magnesium et transaminases, *Lyon Mediterranee Med* 24:11585-11586, 1988.

14. Fauci A, et al: *Harrison's principles of internal medicine,* ed 13, New York, 1994, McGraw-Hill.

15. Ghayoumi A: Multidisciplinary approach to fibromyalgia, *J Chiropr* 31(11):83-86, 1993.

16. Golding DN: Is there an allergic synovitis? *J Roy Soc Med* 83(5):312-314, 1990.

17. Lawrence D: *Fundamentals of chiropractic diagnosis and management,* Baltimore, 1991, Williams & Wilkins.

18. Liu B: *Chinese medicinal fungi,* ed 3, Taiyuang, China, 1984, Shanxi People's Press.

19. Liu XJ, et al: Isolation and identification of the anamorphic state of *Cordyceps sinensis, Acta Mycologica Sinica* 8:34-40, 1994.

20. Lowe JC: Results of an open trial of T3 therapy with 77 euthyroid female fibromyalgia patients, *Clinical Bulletin of Myofascial Pain* 2(1):35-37, 1997.

21. Lowe JC: T3-induced recovery from fibromyalgia by a hypothyroid patient resistant to T4 and desiccated thyroid, *Journal of Myofascial Therapy* 1(4):26-31, 1995.

22. Lowe JC: Thyroid status of 38 fibromyalgia patients: implications for the etiology of fibromyalgia, *Clinical Bulletin of Myofascial Therapy* 2(1):47-64, 1997.

23. *Manual of medical therapeutics (the Washington manual),* ed 27, Boston, 1992, Little, Brown.

24. Martin J: Understanding fibromyalgia, *J Am Chiropr Assoc* 33(12), 1996.

25. *The Merck manual,* ed 16, Rahway, NJ, 1992, Merck Co.

26. Millan SB: Fibromyalgia: when the patient hurts all over: *Fam Pract Recert* 18(6), 1996.

27. Neeck G, Riedel W: Thyroid function in patients with fibromyalgia syndrome, *J Rheumatol* 19:1120-1122, 1992.

28. Rakel RE: *Conn's current therapy,* Philadelphia, 1996, WB Saunders.

29. Rakel RE: *Textbook of family practice,* ed 5, Philadelphia, 1995, WB Saunders.

30. Reiffenberger D: Fibromyalgia syndrome: a review, *Am Fam Physician* 53(5):1698-1712, 1996.

31. Rowe AH: Allergic fatigue and toxicemia, *Ann Allergy* 17:9-18, 1959.

32. Schneider MJ: Tender points/fibromyalgia vs. trigger points/myofascial pain syndrome: a need for clarity in terminology and differential diagnosis, *J Manipulative Physiol Ther* 18:398-406, 1996.

33. Scully RM, Barnes MR: *Physical therapy,* Philadelphia, 1989, JB Lippincott.

34. Taylor RB: *Manual of family practice,* Boston, 1996, Little, Brown.

35. Tierney LM, McPhee SJ, Papadakis MA: *Current medical diagnosis and treatment,* ed 35, Norwalk, Conn, 1996, Appleton & Lange.
36. Werbach MR: *Nutritional influences on illness,* ed 2, Tarzana, Calif, 1996, Third Line Press.
37. Yunus MB: Fibromyalgia syndrome: blueprint for a reliable diagnosis, *Consultant,* June 1996.

Hypertension

LEW HUFF, LIZA O. BANAAG-HUFF,
AND DAVID M. BRADY

DEFINITION

A condition of high blood pressure often referred to as *the silent disease* because there may be no symptoms until late in the disease process. Blood pressure may vary throughout the day. Hypertension has been defined as a persistent systolic blood pressure of at least 140 mm Hg or diastolic blood pressure of at least 90 mm Hg.[6]

Mild hypertension: Diastolic 90-104
Moderate hypertension: Diastolic 105-114
Severe hypertension: Diastolic >115
Upper limits of normal may be 160/95 mm Hg

ETIOLOGY

Primary hypertension is idiopathic, whereas secondary can be due to kidney disease, tumor, and other causes. Secondary hypertension collectively accounts for about 5% of the hypertensive population. Blacks are affected more often than whites and males more often than females. Hypertension is linked to heredity, smoking, obesity, and excessive salt intake. Hypertension affects 50% of people over 65 years of age.

SIGNS AND SYMPTOMS

Diagnostic Criteria

High blood pressure may be diagnosed with three readings averaging greater than 140 mm Hg systolic or greater than 90 diastolic at least 1 week apart in a resting patient. A patient whose blood pressure goes down after periods of rest has labile hypertension; one half of such patients go on to develop sustained hypertension. Studies show that an elevated systolic pressure has as great or greater importance than the diastolic pressure in estimating cardiovascular risk.[14]

Other Findings

Early-morning suboccipital headaches, light-headedness, fatigue, or tinnitus is possible. Paroxysmal nocturnal dyspnea is possible.

Eye Signs

Retinal hemorrhage, A-V nicking, and cotton-wool patches may be noted.

DIFFERENTIAL DIAGNOSIS

Renal disease
Hypothyroidism
Adrenal disease
Cushing's disease

ESSENTIAL TESTS

CBC, SMAC, UA, blood urea nitrogen (BUN)
Sodium, chloride, CO1
Cortisol, T4, hematocrit
Cholesterol, triglycerides
Chest x-ray, electrocardiogram (ECG)

COMMON FINDINGS

Low specific gravity of urine, increased BUN and creatinine, anemia, proteinuria, and granular casts in urine may be noted.

X-RAY FINDINGS

Rib notching or cardiac enlargement may be noted.

Clinical Note

Specific-contact short-lever arm spinal adjustments may cause a hypotensive effect in a medicated hypertensive patient that may lead to complications (e.g., hypotension). Because a medicated hypertensive patient's blood pressure may fall below normal while he or she is undergoing chiropractic care, it is advised that the blood pressure be closely monitored and medications adjusted, if necessary, by the patient's medical physician.[17]

MANAGEMENT PROTOCOL (OPTIONS)

- Patients with increased diastolic blood pressure (115 mm Hg and above) should be referred for evaluation and medical treatment.[1]
- Mild hypertension with no additional coronary risk factors or target organ damage may be treated with nonpharmacological methods.
- After a trial period of nonpharmacological treatment (6 to 12 months) with little or no reduction of blood pressure, referral for medical evaluation is needed. A trial of 1 to 2 months is reasonable for a patient with mild hypertension accompanied by some evidence of target organ damage or those with several risk factors.[1]
- The first steps in nonpharmacological treatment of mild hypertension:
  1. Weight reduction
  2. Restriction of alcohol intake
  3. Restriction of sodium intake
  4. Discontinuation of smoking
  5. Moderate aerobic exercises[1,3,16]
  6. Supplemental nutrition program
- A patient should not be started on antihypertensives until it is established that his or her blood pressure elevation is sustained.
- *Exercise Therapy:* A daily exercise program will lower blood pressure.[1,3,15]
- *Diet Considerations:*
  1. Restrict sodium intake.

2. Increase potassium intake in the form of bananas, apricots, oranges, melons, dates, asparagus, broccoli, and raisins.
3. Increase calcium intake (1000-2000 mg daily).
4. Adhere to a caloric restriction diet.
5. Decrease alcohol intake.[1,3,15]
6. Decrease phosphorus intake (e.g., soda).

NUTRITIONAL MANAGEMENT PROTOCOL (OPTIONS)

- Calcium (1500 mg daily)
- Magnesium (1000 mg daily)
- Selenium (200 µg daily)
- Garlic (500 mg tid)
- Coenzyme Q10 (100 mg daily)
- Taurine (3 g daily)
- Vitamin C (3000 mg daily)
- Potassium may need to be supplemented if patient is on hypertensive medications; monitor blood work to make final decision

HOME CARE PROTOCOL (OPTIONS)

- Start a moderate exercise program under physician's advise.
- Start a weight-reduction program.
- Cease smoking.

REFERENCES

1. Amidon TM: Hypertension: a four-article symposium, *Postgrad Med* 100(4), 1996.
2. Balch JF, Balch PA: *Prescription for natural healing,* Wayne, NJ, 1990, Avery Publishing.
3. Black HR, et al: The emerging role of chronotherapeutics in managing hypertension, *Am J Hypertens* 9(4):34S-39S, 1996.
4. Fauci A, et al: *Harrison's principles of internal medicine,* ed 13, New York, 1994, McGraw-Hill.
5. Grabowski RJ: *Current nutritional therapy,* San Antonio, Tex, 1993, Image Press.
6. Grimm RH, et al: Long-term effects on plasma lipids of diet and drugs to treat hypertension, *JAMA* 275(20):1549-1556, 1996.

7. Kamimura M: Anti-inflammatory activity of vitamin E, *J Vitaminol* 18(4):204-209, 1972.

8. Lawrence D: *Fundamentals of chiropractic diagnosis and management,* Baltimore, 1991, Williams & Wilkins.

9. Levy D, et al: The progression from hypertension to congestive heart failure, *JAMA* 275(20):1557-1562, 1996.

10. MacMahon S, et al: Blood pressure, stroke, and coronary heart disease, *Lancet* 335(8692):765-774, 1990.

11. *Manual of medical therapeutics (the Washington manual),* ed 27, Boston, 1992, Little, Brown.

12. McKnight M, Deboer K: Preliminary study of blood pressure changes in normotensive subjects undergoing chiropractic care, *J Manipulative Physiol Ther* 11:261-266, 1998.

13. *The Merck manual,* ed 16, Rahway, NJ, 1992, Merck Co.

14. Mootz R: Conservative management of patients with mild hypertension, *Top Clin Chiropr* 2(1):37-44, 1995.

15. Moser M: Management of hypertension, Part I, *Am Fam Physician* 53(7):2295-2302, 1996.

16. Plaugher G, Bachman T: Chiropractic management of a hypertensive patient, *J Manipulative Physiol Ther* 16(8):544-549, 1993.

17. Plaugher G, Bachman T: Chiropractic management of hypertension: a case study, *Transactions of the Consortium for Chiropractic Research,* June 1992.

18. Plaugher G, et al: Randomized clinical trial of chiropractic adjustments and brief massage treatment for essential hypertension: a pilot study, *Proceedings of the Chiropractic Centennial Foundation,* July 1995.

19. Rakel RE: *Conn's current therapy,* Philadelphia, 1996, WB Saunders.

20. Rakel RE: *Textbook of family practice,* ed 5, Philadelphia, 1995, WB Saunders.

21. Reynolds E, Baron RB: Hypertension in women and the elderly, *Postgrad Med* 100(4):58-63, 1996.

22. Scully RM, Barnes MR: *Physical therapy,* Philadelphia, 1989, JB Lippincott.

23. Tierney LM, McPhee SJ, Papadakis MA: *Current medical diagnosis and treatment,* ed 35, Norwalk, Conn, 1996, Appleton & Lange.

24. Weaver K: Magnesium and its role in vascular reactivity and coagulation, *Contemp Nutr* 12(3), 1987.

25. Werbach MR: *Nutritional influences on illness,* ed 2, Tarzana, Calif, 1996, Third Line Press.

26. Werbach MR, Murray MT: *Botanical influences on illness,* Tarzana, Calif, 1994, Third Line Press.

27. Zellner C, Sudhir K: Lifestyle modifications for hypertension: the many benefits are worth the effort, *Postgrad Med* 100(4):75-79, 1996.

Osteoporosis

LEW HUFF AND DAVID M. BRADY

DEFINITION

A condition of low bone mass resulting from excessive bone resorption surpassing bone formation. Also known as *brittle bones,* osteoporosis is the most common systemic disorder of the 50-year-old and over age-group. There is an increase incidence with postmenopausal females after a hysterectomy. It is technically defined as a decrease in bone mass in the absence of a mineralization defect. The clinical sequelae result from fractures of the vertebrae, hip, humerus, wrist, or tibia.

Type 1 occurs primarily in postmenopausal females and is characterized by a decrease in trabecular bone mass and fractures. *Type 2* is characterized by a loss of both cortical and trabecular mass and usually occurs in both males and females 70 years old and older. This is commonly associated with a fracture of the femur neck, proximal fibula, or tibia and the proximal humerus.

ETIOLOGY

May be due to immobilization, fracture, disk prolapse, hormonal disorder, lack of physical activity, lack of estrogen, chronic low intake of calcium, or malabsorption syndrome. Risk factors are postmenopausal women with a low skeletal mass, poor musculature, sedentary lifestyle, smoking, excessive alcohol intake, and certain medications, particularly corticosteroids.

SIGNS AND SYMPTOMS

Pain Pattern

Ranges from asymptomatic to severe back pain. Sharp, nagging, deep, and dull pain. Acute pain may radiate around the flank into the abdomen. Episodes of pain usually subside within several days to a week.

LOCATION

Spontaneous fractures and vertebral collapse, usually of thoracic and lumbar spine

Inspection

Rounded shoulders, increased thoracic kyphosis, loss of height reported.

DIFFERENTIAL DIAGNOSIS

Malnutrition
Hyperparathyroidism
Osteomalacia
Steroid use
Calcium deficiency

X-RAY FINDINGS

Loss of trabeculae
Fractures of vertebrae
Demineralization
Erylenmeyer flask deformities
Celery stalking appearance
Penciling of vertebrae
NOTE: Patient must have 30% bone loss to be detected by conventional x-rays.

SPECIALIZED TESTS

Most precise diagnostic tool is dual energy x-ray absorptiometry.[3]

Bone protein assay: Measures osteocalcin, bone-specific alkaline phosphatase, and metabolites of collagen 1. Measured in 2-hour timed samples of urine.[3]

LABORATORY RESULTS

Serum calcium and alkaline phosphatase are normal. Parathyroid hormone may be abnormal.

LABORATORY ASSESSMENT OF CHOICE

Osteoporosis risk evaluation. Pyridinium and deoxypyridinium metabolites of bone reabsorption in urine (Great Smokies Diagnostic Labs) is one of the most sensitive, lowest-cost, side-effect-free screening tools available (see Appendix B).

TREATMENT GOALS

1. Relieve musculoskeletal pain.
2. Restore normal strength and stability to bones and joint structures.
3. Restore preillness activities of daily living.

MANAGEMENT PROTOCOL (OPTIONS)

- *Prevention:*
    1. Prevention is directed at achieving and maintaining optimal bone mass through diet, exercise, and avoidance of medications and smoking.
    2. Women should ingest at least 800 mg of calcium daily throughout life.
    3. Good dietary sources of calcium:
        a. Green leafy vegetables
        b. Non-fat or low fat milk products
        c. Calcium-fortified orange juice
        d. Canned sardines or salmon
        e. Corn tortillas
        f. Citrus fruits
        g. Sunflower seeds, almonds, Brazil nuts, and hazelnuts
- Hydroculator packs, bed rest, and low-force manipulation and soft tissue techniques to relieve musculoskeletal pain.[11]
- *Exercise:*
    1. Weight-bearing exercise 3 times per week (walking, jogging, weight training)
    2. Extension and isometric exercises minimize vertebral compression

- *Lifestyle Factors:*
  1. Do not smoke.
  2. Limit alcohol and caffeine intake.
  3. Obtain counseling about appropriate shoes, gait training, and proper lighting of house and areas of activity.
- Refer for hormone replacement therapy if severe.

NUTRITIONAL MANAGEMENT PROTOCOL (OPTIONS)

Calcium:
- Young adults: 800 mg calcium per day
- Pregnant or lactating women: 1200 mg calcium per day
- Postmenopausal women: 1 g elemental calcium per day

Supplemental calcium: Microcrystaline Hydroxy Apatite form preferred (500-1000 mg per day).

Vitamin D:
- Adults: 400 IU per day
- Seniors: 800 IU per day

REFERENCES

1. Balch JF, Balch PA: *Prescription for natural healing,* Wayne, NJ, 1990, Avery Publishing.
2. Bellantoni M: Osteoporosis prevention and treatment, *Am Fam Physician* 54(3):986-992, 1996.
3. Clemen M: Delivering effective force adjustments on patients with degenerative spinal conditions, *Int Rev Chiropr* 44:27-35, 1988.
4. Fauci A, et al: *Harrison's principles of internal medicine,* ed 13, New York, 1994, McGraw-Hill.
5. Grabowski RJ: *Current nutritional therapy,* San Antonio, Tex, 1993, Image Press.
6. Lawrence D: *Fundamentals of chiropractic diagnosis and management,* Baltimore, 1991, Williams & Wilkins.
7. Lindsay R: Osteoporosis update: strategies to counteract bone loss, prevent fracture, *Consultant* 36(7), 1996.
8. *Manual of medical therapeutics (the Washington manual),* ed 27, Boston, 1992, Little, Brown.
9. *The Merck manual,* ed 16, Rahway, NJ, 1992, Merck Co.
10. Murtagh J: *General practice,* New York, 1994, McGraw-Hill.
11. Raisz L: Osteoporosis: 13 questions physicians often ask, *Consultant* 35(7), 1995.
12. Rakel RE: *Conn's current therapy,* Philadelphia, 1996, WB Saunders.

13. Rakel RE: *Textbook of family practice,* ed 5, Philadelphia, 1995, WB Saunders.
14. Tierney LM, McPhee SJ, Papadakis MA: *Current medical diagnosis and treatment,* ed 35, Norwalk, Conn, 1996, Appleton & Lange.
15. Werbach MR: *Nutritional influences on illness,* ed 2, Tarzana, Calif, 1996, Third Line Press.
16. Werbach MR, Murray MT: *Botanical influences on illness,* Tarzana, Calif, 1994, Third Line Press.

Appendix A

Nutritional Product Manufacturers

The following vendor contacts are being provided for products and services, which were mentioned in the text.

1. **Allergy Research Group:** 1-510-639-4572
2. **Bio-Tech:** 1-800-345-1199

Manufacturer of Lithate, a lithium aspartate supplement that, in selected patients, may substitute for the prescription drug lithium carbonate.

3. **Biotec Foods:** 1-800-331-5888

Manufacturer of Cell-Guard (superoxide dismutase [SOD]).

4. **HealthComm, Inc.:** 1-800-228-1911

Call HealthComm, Inc. for technical and seminar information concerning the "functional medicine" techniques of Jeffrey Bland, PhD, for the management of chronic health conditions, such as chronic fatigue syndrome, fibromyalgia, gastrointestinal disorders, and toxicity. To order HealthComm products, such as UltraClear Plus (detoxification), UltraClear Sustain (gastrointestinal disorders), and UltraInflamX (chronic inflammatory disorders), call Metagenics, Inc. (see below).

5. **Metagenics, Inc.:** 1-800-692-9400

In addition to the Metagenics product line mentioned in the text, Metagenics, Inc. is also the distributor of all HealthComm, Inc. products. These include UltraClear Plus and UltraClear Sustain for hepatic detoxification and the treatment of intestinal permeability disorders.

6. **Murdock Madaus Schwabe/Natures Way:** 1-800-489-1500

7. **Nutri-West:** 1-800-443-3333
8. **Professional Health Products:** 1-800-929-4133
9. **Progressive Research Labs:** 1-713-365-9336
10. **Thorne Research:** 1-800-228-1966

Appendix B

Specialty Clinical Laboratories

1. **Great Smokies Diagnostic Laboratory:** 1-800-522-4762
This laboratory provides clinical data relating to hepatic dexotification and functional gastrointestinal problems via their Liver Detoxification Profiles, Intestinal Permeability Test, and Complete Digestive Stool Analysis (CDSA). They also offer food allergy testing via the ELISA method, hair analysis, *H. pylori* antibodies, urinary pyridinium and deoxypyridinium excretion for osteoporosis screening, and an array of other useful and unique tests. This laboratory is very helpful when treating chronic fatigue syndrome, fibromyalgia, and chronic digestive and toxicity problems.

The labs below provide food allergy testing and other selected specialty tests.

2. **Meridian Valley Clinical Labs:** 1-206-859-8700
3. **MetaMetrix Labs:** 1-800-221-4640
4. **Immuno Labs:** 1-800-231-9197
5. **Diagnos-Techs:** 1-800-878-3787
6. **Sage Systems:** 1-800-491-9511
This laboratory provides unique food allergy testing that does not depend on the normal ELISA method of testing predominantly IgG allergy pathways. The Sage System uses changes in white blood cell morphology after exposure to various food proteins. This method tends to pick up latent and delayed allergies missed on ELISA.

7. **SpectraCell:** 1-713-621-3101

This laboratory provides a metabolic nutrient analysis that measures the antioxidant function of a patient and intracellular nutrient status, using various challenges to cultures of the patient's living white blood cells.

Appendix C

Outcome Assessment Questionnaires

Oswestry Low Back Pain Disability Questionnaire

Patient Name _____   Date _____

Please Read:
This questionnaire has been designed to give the doctor information as to how your back pain has affected your ability to manage in everyday life. Please answer every section, and mark in each section only the one box that applies to you. We realize that you may consider that two of the statements in any one section may relate to you, but please just mark the one box that most closely describes your problem.

SECTION 1   PAIN INTENSITY

( ) I can tolerate the pain I have without having to use painkillers.
( ) The pain is bad, but I can manage without taking painkillers.
( ) Painkillers give me complete relief from pain.
( ) Painkillers give me moderate relief from pain.
( ) Painkillers give me very little relief from pain.
( ) Painkillers have no effect on the pain, and I do not use them.

SECTION 2   PERSONAL CARE (WASHING, DRESSING, ETC.)

( ) I can look after myself normally without causing extra pain.
( ) I can look after myself normally, but it causes extra pain.
( ) It is painful to look after myself, and I am slow and careful.
( ) I need some help but manage most of my personal care.
( ) I need help every day in most aspects of my self-care.
( ) I do not get dressed, wash with difficulty, and stay in bed.

SECTION 3 LIFTING

( ) I can lift heavy weights without extra pain.
( ) I can lift heavy weights, but it causes extra pain.
( ) Pain prevents me from lifting heavy objects, but I can lift them if they are conveniently placed (e.g., on a table).
( ) I can lift only very light weight.
( ) I cannot lift or carry anything at all.

SECTION 4 WALKING

( ) Pain does not prevent me from walking any distance.
( ) Pain prevents me from walking more than 1 mile.
( ) Pain prevents me from walking more than ½ mile.
( ) Pain prevents me from walking more than ¼ mile.
( ) I can only walk using a cane or crutch.
( ) I am in bed most of the time; I have to crawl to the toilet.

SECTION 5 SITTING

( ) I can sit in any chair as long as I like.
( ) I can only sit in my favorite chair as long as I like.
( ) Pain prevents me from sitting for more than 1 hour.
( ) Pain prevents me from sitting for more than ½ hour.
( ) Pain prevents me from sitting more than 10 minutes.
( ) Pain prevents me from sitting at all.

SECTION 6 STANDING

( ) I can stand as long as I want without extra pain.
( ) I can stand as long as I want, but it gives extra pain.
( ) Pain prevents me from standing for more than 1 hour.
( ) Pain prevents me from standing for more than 30 minutes.
( ) Pain prevents me from standing for more than 10 minutes.
( ) Pain prevents me from standing at all.

SECTION 7 SLEEPING

( ) Pain does not prevent me from sleeping well.
( ) I can sleep well only by using tablets.
( ) Even when I take pills, I have less than 6 hours sleep.
( ) Even when I take pills, I have less than 4 hours sleep.

( ) Even when I take pills, I have less than 2 hours sleep.
( ) Pain prevents me from sleeping at all.

SECTION 8   SEX LIFE

( ) My sex life is normal and causes no extra pain.
( ) My sex life is normal but causes some extra pain.
( ) My sex life is nearly normal but is very painful.
( ) My sex life is severely restricted because of pain.
( ) My sex life if nearly absent because of pain.
( ) Pain prevents any sex life at all.

SECTION 9   SOCIAL LIFE

( ) My social life is normal and gives me no extra pain.
( ) My social life is normal but increases pain.
( ) Pain has no significant effect on my social life apart from limiting energetic interests (e.g., dancing).
( ) Pain has restricted my social life; I do not go out much.
( ) Pain has restricted my social life to my home.
( ) I have no social life because of pain.

SECTION 10   TRAVELING

( ) I can travel anywhere without extra pain.
( ) I can travel anywhere, but it gives me extra pain.
( ) Pain is bad but, I manage journeys over 2 hours.
( ) Pain restricts me to journeys less than 1 hour.
( ) Pain restricts me to journeys less than 30 minutes.
( ) Pain prevents me from traveling except to the doctor or hospital.

Roland/Morris Disability Questionnaire

Name _____ Date _____ Time _____

When your back hurts, you may find it difficult to do some things that you normally do. This list contains some sentences that people have used to describe themselves when they have back pain. When you read them, you may find some that stand out because they describe you today. As you read the list, think of yourself today, and put a check beside the number of the sentence. If the sentence does not describe you, then leave the space blank and go on to the next one. Remember, only check the sentence if you are sure that it describes you today.

___ 1. I stay at home most of the time because of my back.

___ 2. I change position frequently to try to get my back comfortable.

___ 3. I walk more slowly than usual because of my back.

___ 4. Because of my back, I am not doing any of the jobs that I usually do around the house.

___ 5. Because of my back, I use a handrail to get upstairs.

___ 6. Because of my back, I lie down to rest more often.

___ 7. Because of my back, I have to hold onto something to get out of an easy chair.

___ 8. Because of my back, I try to get other people to do things for me.

___ 9. I get dressed more slowly than before because of my back.

___ 10. I only stand up for short periods of time because of my back.

___ 11. Because of my back, I try not to bend or kneel down.

___ 12. I find it difficult to get out of a chair because of my back.

___ 13. My back is painful most of the time.

___ 14. I find it difficult to turn over in bed because of my back.

___ 15. My appetite is not very good because of my back.

___ 16. I have trouble putting on my socks (or stockings) because of the pain in my back.

___ 17. I only walk short distances because of my back pain.

___ 18. I sleep less well than usual because of my back.

___ 19. Because of my back pain, I get dressed with help form someone else.

___ 20. I sit down for most of the day because of my back pain.

___ 21. I avoid heavy jobs around the house because of my back.

___ 22. Because of my back pain, I am more irritable and bad tempered with people than usual.

___ 23. Because of my back pain, I go upstairs more slowly than usual.

___ 24. I stay in bed most of the time because of my back.

Pain Disability Index

Name _____   Date _____

The rating scales below measure the impact of chronic pain in your everyday life. We want to know how much your pain is preventing you from doing your normal activities. For each of the 7 categories of life activity listed, circle the one number that best reflects the level of disability you typically experience. A score of 0 means no disability at all. A score of 10 means that all the activities that you would normally do have been disrupted or prevented by your pain. Your rating should reflect the overall impact of pain in your life and not just when the pain is at its worst. Make a rating for every category. If you think that a category does not apply to you, circle 0.

FAMILY/HOME RESPONSIBILITIES

This category refers to activities related to the home and family. It includes chores and duties performed around the house (e.g., yard work) and errands or favors for other family members (e.g., driving the children to school).

0	1	2	3	4	5	6	7	8	9	10
No Disability		Mild		Moderate		Severe		Total Disability		

RECREATION

This category includes hobbies, sports, and other leisure-time activities.

0	1	2	3	4	5	6	7	8	9	10
No Disability		Mild		Moderate		Severe		Total Disability		

SOCIAL ACTIVITY

This category includes parties, theater, concerts, dining out, and other social activities that are attended with family and friends.

0	1	2	3	4	5	6	7	8	9	10
No Disability		Mild		Moderate		Severe		Total Disability		

OCCUPATION

This category refers to activities that are directly related to one's job. This includes nonpaying jobs as well, such as that of a homemaker or volunteer worker.

0	1	2	3	4	5	6	7	8	9	10
No Disability		Mild		Moderate		Severe		Total Disability		

SEXUAL BEHAVIOR

This category refers to the frequency and quality of one's sex life.

0	1	2	3	4	5	6	7	8	9	10
No Disability		Mild		Moderate		Severe		Total Disability		

SELF-CARE

This category includes personal maintenance and independent daily living activities (e.g., taking a shower, driving, getting dressed).

0	1	2	3	4	5	6	7	8	9	10
No Disability		Mild		Moderate		Severe		Total Disability		

LIFE-SUPPORT ACTIVITY

This category refers to basic life-supporting behaviors, such as eating, sleeping, and breathing.

0	1	2	3	4	5	6	7	8	9	10
No Disability		Mild		Moderate		Severe		Total Disability		

INDEX